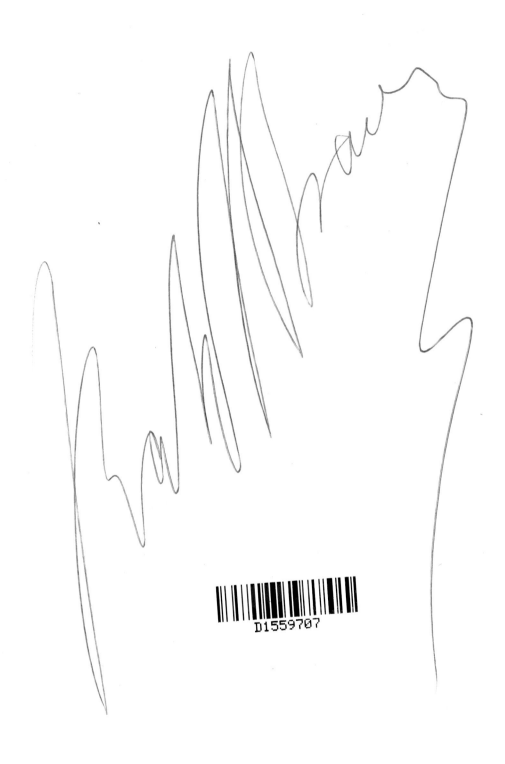

Hyperthermia
and Cancer

Hyperthermia and Cancer

George M. Hahn

Stanford University School of Medicine
Stanford California

PLENUM PRESS ● *NEW YORK AND LONDON*

Library of Congress Cataloging in Publication Data

Hahn, George M., 1926—
  Hyperthermia and cancer.

Includes bibliographical references and index.
  1. Cancer—Treatment. 2. Thermotherapy. 3. Heat—Physiological effect. I. Title.
[DNLM: 1. Fever therapy. 2. Neoplasms—Therapy. QZ 266 H148h]
RC271.T5H33 1982   616.99'40632   82-12368
ISBN 0-306-40958-5

© 1982 Plenum Press, New York
A Division of Plenum Publishing Corporation
233 Spring Street, New York, N.Y. 10013

Printed in the United States of America

Dedicated to the memory of
DAVID HAHN: 1950−1962

Preface

Hyperthermia as a tool for the treatment of malignant disease is rapidly becoming a clinical reality. In this book I am attempting to summarize the known biological and physical underpinnings that have led to this development. I also present a compilation of existing clinical results, limited as these are. My aim is to provide oncologists and other physicians with up-to-date information on this modality, which is both new and old, as well as to make available to biologists, physicists and engineers summaries of currently available information on specific areas of hyperthermic research.

Many people have helped me with this book. Specifically, thanks are due to Drs. William Dewey, Jean Dutreix, Peter Fessenden, Gloria Li, and Jane Marmor. Their suggestions have been invaluable. I hope that not too many errors and omissions have crept into the volume, but in any case, for these I have only myself to blame. I also wish to express my appreciation to David Betten and Marie Graham for their help.

Most of this material was written while I was on sabbatical leave on the shores of Lake Atitlan in Guatemala. There I enjoyed the hospitality of a gracious, friendly, and proud people who deserve better than fate seems to have in store for them.

George M. Hahn

Contents

1

Introduction
Historical and General Comments

Hundreds of years ago, the Greek physician Parmenides said that given the means to induce fevers he would be able to cure all illnesses. Presumably he meant to include cancer, since malignancies were described in early Greek literature. The effects of elevated temperatures on human physiological functions and, in particular, on the healing process have fascinated clinicians and researchers for many years. Hippocrates described in detail many febrile diseases and commented extensively on the beneficial role of fever. A Roman, Celsus, catalogued the clinical symptoms of inflammation and noticed their association with fevers.

Today, the induction of elevated temperatures (hyperthermia), either locally or over the whole body, has become quite feasible. Whether or not this is a realization of Parmenides's wish is somewhat questionable. Fever is a unique form of hyperthermia in that it is not associated with the failure of a thermal regulatory system but rather with a change in the "set point," i.e., the temperature about which regulation is exerted. This is true not only in humans but also in a wide range of animals. The point is perhaps most graphically illustrated in a fascinating set of experiments involving a poikilotherm, the desert iguana, *Disposaurus dorsalis* (Kluger *et al.*, 1973). These animals were placed in a box in which a thermal gradient had been established by heating one end of the container and cooling the opposite end. The "normal" iguanas consistently settled in one temperature zone. This very primitive regulation, their own motion, established the set point for normal lizards. The reptiles were then injected with a known reptilian pathogen (e.g., *Pasteurella hemolytica*). They promptly moved to a warmer zone, thus inducing a "fever." After further injection with appropriate doses of sodium salicylate, which is a well-known antipyretic agent, the iguanas returned to the cooler location. In these experiments, the movement of the animal was a direct, visual demonstration of the change in "set point" of their thermal regulatory system.

1

Other forms of hyperthermia, such as heat stroke, the clinical syndrome called malignant hyperthermia, or pharmacologically induced hyperthermias, seem to involve the failure of one or more regulatory systems (Stitt, 1979).

There is one important point that I have not discussed so far. When talking about hyperthermia, what range of temperatures is meant? Before answering this question it is necessary to look at the range of core body temperatures of various animals, as measured under nonpathogenic situations. For humans, the "normal" body temperature has been reported to vary from 35.1 to 37.7°C, while camels seem to show the widest variation in temperature, 34 to 40°C. All other mammals fall somewhere in this range. Obviously, during fevers temperatures may rise to higher values; the maximum in man seems to be about 41.5 to 42°C before severe central nervous system symptoms are encountered. Birds tend to be at higher temperatures; their normal range starts at 37°C, with the highest temperature, a surprising 43.3°C, reported for the abert towhee (Swan, 1974). By hyperthermia I mean temperatures above those encountered under either pathogenic or normal situations. For mammalian cells, temperatures of 42°C or higher may then be regarded as hyperthermic. Obviously a different range needs to be established for avian cells, with hyperthermic temperatures beginning at about 43.5°C. Unicellular organisms can withstand or adapt to much higher temperatures. The eukaryotes capable of withstanding the highest temperatures are the thermophilic fungi. For these there may be an absolute temperature limit slightly above 60°C (Tansey and Brock, 1972). Prokaryotes can exist right up to the boiling point of water. For example, members of the genus *Sulfolobus* have been found in springs whose normal temperature is 97°C, where these organisms reproduce, apparently happily, in water whose pH is 2.4! Brock (1978) has presented an interesting argument for the inability of eukaryotes to evolve members capable of growing at temperatures above about 60°C. Functionally, the thermophilic fungi are quite similar to those prokaryotic heterotrophs that are able to grow at high temperatures. Both are aerobes and can grow on media containing single compounds. Enzymes and other macromolecules of both types of organisms are equally heat stable. Cellular functions such as active transport (and presumably the establishment of pH gradients) occur in both types of organisms at high temperatures; hence, the plasma membrane for both prokaryotes and eukaryotes must be heat stable. The critical difference between prokaryotes and eukaryotes that allows the former to grow at higher temperatures, Brock argues, is therefore neither at the plasma membrane level nor at the macromolecular level but at an intermediate level of organization. All eukaryotes have membranous intracellular organelles (e.g., nuclei and mitochondria). It is argued, and it seems to me to be a reasonable argument, that the inability of eukaryotes to grow at high temperatures resides in their inability to retain the integrity of these intracellular membranes. These membranes differ from plasma membranes in that the former must allow for the passage, by diffusion, of large macromolecules. To be able to do this, they must of necessity be relatively leaky and hence not heat labile. Thus, the argument goes, it would be impossible for eukaryotes to construct intracellular membranes that are both thermally stable and functional. I have given considerable space to this argument because of the possible role of membranes in determining the heat death of mammalian cells.

In this book I will deal only peripherally with the effect of fevers on cancer, because I plan to concentrate on the application of externally induced hyperthermias against tumors. That is not to say that fever may not have beneficial effects for some cancer patients. One need only to read the literature of Busch (1866), Fehleisen (1883), and others, particularly Coley (1893), to convince oneself that tumor regression and extension of life span may well be associated with the deliberate or accidental exposure of patients to fever-inducing illnesses or with the injection of pyrogenic bacterial toxins to induce fevers. Much of this literature has been reviewed by Selawry et al. (1957; 1958). Pertinent to assessing the role of fever may also be the frequently quoted observation that the rate of cancer incidence is lower in countries whose population is affected by endemic malaria (Dietzel, 1975). However, there are obvious limitations to the role pyrogen-induced fevers can play. The maximum temperature inducible in humans without incurring risks of severe toxic effects is about 42°C. However, as I will show in subsequent chapters, the optimum temperature for treatment of tumors may be much higher. Fevers of necessity raise the temperature in all parts of the body. Yet differential heating of specific malignant tissue is almost surely desirable in those patients suffering from localized or partially localized disease. Finally, after an induction of a fever, cooling is not accomplished very quickly or reproducibly. As a result, it is difficult to speak with any precision of the temperature–time profile resulting from the administration of the pyrogen. Reproducible temperature–time profiles may be of great importance if hyperthermia treatments are to be standardized.

The current expectation that heat should have a useful role in the clinical management of cancer is based not just on the historical anecdotes discussed but on results from recent biological experiments, on the development of equipment designed and capable of heating arbitrary volumes of human tissue, and on preliminary clinical trials. My plan in this monograph is to describe first the existing experimental evidence that indicates that tumor cells *in situ* should be more sensitive to hyperthermia than normal tissue. This evidence includes the possibility that at least some neoplastic cells are inherently more sensitive to heat than their normal counterparts, although the data supporting this optimistic view are opposed by almost as many negative results. Much more conclusive evidence exists that indicates that the milieu of at least a large fraction of cells in solid tumors makes these particularly heat sensitive. Cells in a poor nutritional environment and cells at low pH appear to be easily inactivated by exposures to temperatures that do not impair the proliferative ability of the cells in a more favorable environment. Many tumors have low blood flow rates; cells away from capillaries may therefore be in precisely the states identified with increased heat sensitivity. I will then proceed to discuss the potential of hyperthermia in conjunction with radiation therapy and chemotherapy. In the case of the interaction of hyperthermia and X irradiation, the evidence is incontrovertible: cells become much more radiation sensitive if exposed to elevated temperatures either shortly before, during, or immediately after irradiation. At present, the question of whether normal tissue is equally sensitized remains unanswered. The interactions of drugs and hyperthermia in cell inactivation present a complicated picture; either appreciable sensitization or protection by hyperthermia can be seen, depending upon the drug and the time sequence of exposure. Unfortunately, only a very limited body of data is available. This field, which deserves much more attention than it has been receiving, offers considerable potential for improving the treatment of patients. In my opinion, most of the benefit to be derived from hyperthermia depends critically on the ability to induce and measure locally elevated temperatures. The physiology of tumors, particularly the inability of many neoplasms to exchange blood rapidly with their normal surroundings, makes it highly desirable to accomplish heating *via* the local deposition of energy. For this reason I shall devote considerable space to describing the means of doing so, either by ultrasound or by electromagnetic techniques. The final chapter will be devoted to a summary of the somewhat limited clinical experience available today.

The literature that I have cited in these chapters is largely limited to works dealing with mammalian systems. I have attempted to quote most of the pertinent results, but the number of papers published that deal with hyperthermia is enormous, and they appear in journals covering many disciplines. Therefore I have undoubtedly omitted many potential references. I apologize to the investigators involved and assure them that no slight is intended.

When it comes to experiments not dealing with mammalian systems, I have selected only those results specifically relevant to points not covered sufficiently by mammalian data. This by no means implies that work on other organisms has not been done or is less interesting. In fact, two books have appeared within the last few years that deal with areas not covered here. A volume by Alexandrov (1977) primarily describes work on plants and plant cells and makes available to Western readers the vast Soviet literature on the effects of both heat and cold. While the book is not exactly easy to read, I cite it here because it points out clearly how dangerous specialization and parochialism can be. Had mammalian cell biologists been aware of the data described by Alexandrov, many of the recent experimental results obtained with mamalian cells could have been anticipated. Heat-induced heat resistance (thermotolerance) and the effects of ethanol and deuterium oxide on heat sensitivity, to cite only a few examples, were all known to the plant physiologists. The second book is that of Brock (1978); I have already quoted extensively from that work. This delightfully written volume presents a wealth of material on the ways unicellular organisms have evolved to deal with high-temperature environments. Very likely some of the material presented there is also relevant to more complicated biological structures such as mammalian cells.

While the orientation of my book is clinical, I have attempted to include in it much of the currently available information on heat effects as they relate to mammalian cellular and tumor biology. My aim is to attract not only clinicians, but also radiobiologists, tumor biologists, and cell biologists in general. The study of hyperthermia is one of the most fascinating areas of cellular biology active today. It involves many disciplines, from membrane biophysics to histology and morphology. Much of the work that I will discuss originated in my laboratory. This has its advantages and disadvantages. The advantages, e.g., close familiarity with the work and acute awareness of experimental limitations, are obvious. The disadvantages are perhaps less visible. It is impossible to work in a field for many years and not form specific prejudices. I am sure some of these will appear throughout the exposition, and I make no apologies for them. Of course, I do try to present a balanced view, even on subjects where my own inclinations lead me to adopt a particular point of view. For example, I think that damage to membraneous structures is the most likely lesion leading to heat-induced cell death. At the same time I point out in the text that this is far from being a closed subject, and that other "targets," such as chromosomes, may well have equal or greater importance. It must be remembered that only within the last ten years have effects of hyperthermia on cells and tissues been investigated in a systematic way. Very likely, as new knowledge is accumulated, new prejudices will replace the old.

2

Mammalian Cell Survival Responses after Exposure to Elevated Temperatures

2.1. INTRODUCTION

Current concepts of cancer treatment focus on the killing of neoplastic cells. In the case of surgery this is accomplished by excision and physical removal of the cancerous tissue. Radiation and drug treatments require the inactivation *in situ* of the vast majority of individual malignant cells. This must be done without damaging normal tissue to the point where its function is permanently compromised. For many normal tissues such as bone marrow, skin, and the lining of the gastrointestinal tract, functional level is largely determined by the number of stem cells that have maintained reproductive integrity at the end of the radiation or drug treatment. For all of these reasons, the survival kinetics of malignant and normal cells exposed to heat are of considerable importance. Experiments are much easier to perform on cultured cells than on cells *in vivo*, although of course the contribution to cancer research of such investigations depends on their ability to predict behavior of cell populations *in vivo*. Historically, in research on heat effects the tissue culture studies enjoy a rather unique position. It is largely the results of such studies that have fanned the current clinical interest, not the reverse, as tended to be the case with radiotherapy and chemotherapy.

Most of the data that I present in this chapter come from experiments directed toward answering the following critical question: Are malignant cells in tumors frequently or perhaps even invariably more heat sensitive than are cells of surrounding normal tissue? There are at least two possibilities whose realization could lead to an affirmative answer. It is conceivable that the process of malignant transformation itself could involve a step that would cause cells to become more heat sensitive. Many tem-

7

perature-sensitive (ts) mutants have been isolated. These are cells that, when compared to the wild genotype, have a more restricted temperature range for their complete activity. At so-called "nonpermissive" temperatures one or more of the mutants' functions is inhibited. It is not inconceivable that malignant cells frequently or even invariably might also be functional mutants. In that case, the particular function affected at the nonpermissive temperature would be maintenance of reproductive integrity. The other possibility to be considered is that *in vivo* the physicochemical environment of tumor cells is such as to make these unusually heat sensitive. An investigation of this eventuality requires the specification of such a milieu and the examination of how each individual parameter associated with tumor environment affects survival kinetics.

While I have dwelled at length on the use of tissue culture data for clinical purposes, these do not constitute the only reasons for studying the effects of heat on cells. There are also basic aspects of cellular thermal biology that are well worth examining. For example, mammalian cells are capable of accommodating themselves within a temperature range that, to be sure, is limited to about $37 \pm 5°C$. Both short- and long-term adaptive strategies seem to be involved. These fascinating phenomena appear to be examples of the abilities of cells to deal with a variety of stresses, and their study should therefore have evolutionary and ecological implications.

2.2. HEAT SENSITIVITY OF MAMMALIAN CELLS: DEFINITION

When performing an experiment in which the effect of heat on the proliferative capacity of cells is determined, what is really being measured? The glib answer, "the cells' thermostability," requires a definition of the term thermostability. Alexandrov (1977) distinguishes between primary and general thermostability. The former he defines in terms of the response of organisms in the absence of all of the following: repair, adaptation during heat exposure, or a possibly deleterious postexposure environment. General thermostability is the response under the environmental conditions of the particular experiment and includes the effects of the assay procedure.

In experiments involving mammalian cells it is not at all clear that the concept of primary thermostability as proposed by Alexandrov is either very meaningful or even measurable. As will amply be demonstrated later in this chapter, apparently minor variations in the microenvironment of the cells can effect major changes in their ability to withstand the stresses caused by heat. Our knowledge about possible intracellular repair mechanisms of heat-induced damage is essentially nonexistent. How then are we to know which external influence modifies repair and which does not?

This leaves the nonspecific term of general thermostability. But any measurement that includes effects of environmental and assay conditions can provide only relative, not absolute, data on heat responses. It is, for example, reasonable to ask: What is the relative survival of specific normal and transformed cells treated under identical conditions? But it is neither meaningful nor useful to ask: What is the thermostability of, say, HeLa cells? The experiments to be described in this chapter will compare either heat responses of one cell line under different environmental conditions or heat responses of two or more different cell lines (or strains) with experimental conditions kept as constant as possible.

Finally, thermostability is perhaps too specific a term to describe various heat responses. It has too much the connotation of molecular stability. While indeed heat death of cells may be a result of the excessive lability of specific macromolecules, no definitive proof supporting such a hypothesis exists. Furthermore, "cellular heat sensitivity" is a term that has become accepted in the Western literature, and I will continue to use it; but it must be kept in mind that it is meaningful only as a quantity of comparison.

2.3. ASSAYS

How is the heat sensitivity of cells to be measured and quantified? To avoid possible misinterpretation of survival data, it should be recognized that as the temperature changes many parameters in the cells' surroundings may also change. Tissue culture cells are always maintained in aqueous media. Hence, the effect of temperature on the properties of water may be of some concern. Brock (1978) lists several changes in the physical and chemical characteristics of liquids as temperature increases. These include density, viscosity, heat capacity, pH, ionization, and solubility of oxygen and other gases. These changes become quite important when temperature differences are large. Then a change observed in some cellular response might be attributed to heat, while actually it may have resulted from a heat-induced modification of the cells' surroundings. However, the temperature changes under discussion in this chapter are less than 10°, from 37 to a maximum of 47°C. For such small differences, the absolute temperature increases only from 310 to 320° Kelvin, a change of about 3%. Except in media where phase changes may be occurring in that temperature range, the properties of the cells' surroundings may be considered constant.

For cancer studies, the one cellular parameter of supreme importance is the cells' capacity for unlimited proliferation. To attempt to measure it either directly or indirectly, a variety of techniques have been employed. Among these are: cataloguing the morphology of individual cells (Schrek, 1966); measuring cell migration (Friedgood, 1928); measuring the growth or death of entire cultures (Pincus and Fischer, 1931); utilizing dye exclusion—trypan blue (Strom *et al.*, 1977), erythrosin B (Moressi, 1964), or lisamine green (Overgaard, 1975); injecting tumor cells treated *in vitro* into syngeneic hosts (Giovanella *et al.*, 1970); inhibiting respiration (Cavaliere, *et al.*, 1967; Dickson and Suzanger, 1976); using microphotography (Landry and Marceau, 1979); incorporating tritiated thymidine (Euler *et al.*, 1974; Landry and Marceau, 1979); counting the number of cells per colony (Landry and Marceau, 1979); analyzing cell multiplication without correction for growth delay and the presence of heat-sterilized cells (Giovanella *et al.*, 1973; 1976; Goss and Parsons, 1977); analyzing cell multiplications with corrections for dead cells and division delay (Kase and Hahn, 1976); and evaluating colony forming ability (Westra and Dewey, 1971; Palzer and Heidelberger, 1973; Hahn, 1974; Gerner and Schneider, 1976; Kase and Hahn, 1976). This list is surely not exhaustive, and the references listed are certainly not complete. Not all the techniques used yield unequivocal survival data. Harris (1966) has shown conclusively that survival experiments using dye exclusion can lead to very misleading results when this technique is applied to hyperthermia experiments. Testing for the cells' ability to give rise to colonies, and perhaps the injection of graded numbers of treated tumor cells into syngeneic hosts to test for the cells' ability to induce tumors, can lead to an unambiguous definition of survival. Even the latter technique may yield spurious results if, as has been suggested by Mondovi *et al.* (1972), heating changes the hosts' immune response against the injected cells. Cell multiplication, particularly the change of cell number with time, very likely can be translated into survival only if corrections for treatment-induced changes in kinetic parameters are made. These include growth delay, the number of heat-sterilized cells that may be capable of multiplying one or more times before heat-death is expressed, and the rate at which dead cells are removed from the population. This has been discussed recently by Hahn (1980). Quantifying the inhibition of respiration (Dickson and Suzanger, 1976) would be an attractive and rapid assay; but until experiments have been performed that demonstrate correlations between survival curves obtained with this assay and those based on colony-forming ability, the validity of equating the inhibition of respiration with cell killing is difficult to judge. The other assays described earlier either measure quantities not strictly related to cellular survival, or can best be described as pseudo-quantitative.

Two criticisms have been leveled recently against the use of colony formation as an assay for survival of heated cells. First, Lin *et al.* (1977) demonstrated that many heat-treated cells rapidly lose their ability to attach to growth surfaces. They point out that these cells may escape the assay procedure. Secondly, Bass *et al.* (1978) indicate that because the plasma membrane is very likely involved in hyperthermic cell death, damage from trypsinization, a procedure usually required for plating of single cells but that also affects the plasma membrane, may interact with damage from hyperthermia. Therefore, death attributed to heat may have been caused, at least partically, by the proteolytic enzyme.

Because the great majority of hyperthermia studies that I am going to quote do use colony formation as the assay of choice for cell survival experiments, these criticisms deserve some consideration before I proceed. I will discuss the experiments of Lin *et al.* (1977). These investigators exposed monolayers of heated or unheated Chinese hamster cells to trypsin (0.125% + 0.2 g/liter EDTA; 2–4 min at 37°C) and then showed that only a fraction of the heated cells were able to attach to the growth surface, while essentially all unheated control cells were able to do so. The fraction of unattached cells correlated with the time the cells had spent at the elevated temperature (43°C). In another set of experiments, the workers first trypsinized cells, then heated them while these were suspended in medium, and finally plated the cells for colony formation. Again, only a fraction of the heated cells were able to attach and then form colonies.

Based on these results, the authors conclude that their work ". . . demonstrates a flaw in experiments using inhibition of colony formation to measure the impact of hyperthermia alone, or together with other variables, on the reproductive viability of cells: cells that do not attach, cannot form colonies and other experimentation is required to evaluate their reproductive viability." There are, however, several difficulties with the study and with the conclusions drawn. First of all, the authors are in error when they state that the experimental procedures followed by them are representative of techniques employed by earlier investigators. For example, Westra and Dewey (1971), one of the groups whose work is mentioned specifically as possibly being flawed, used a procedure of trypsinizing cells, plating them at the appropriate cell densities, and only several hours later exposing them to heat. Most other investigators followed a similar sequence. Attachment of cells to the petri dishes occurred well before heating. For these experiments, the demonstration that some heated cells may not be able to attach to growth surfaces appears to be irrelevant. Secondly, even in those studies where the sequence of operations performed was similar to that of Lin *et al.* (1977), the concentration of trypsin employed was usually much lower, and EDTA was avoided completely. For example, Hahn (1974) used 0.5% trypsin without any additional EDTA, for 1–4 min at 37°C; Gerner *et al.* (1976) also used 0.5% trypsin without EDTA, and exposed cells to the enzyme at room temperature, rather than at 37°C. Use of the potent trypsin–EDTA mixture might, at least in part, account for the findings of Lin and his associates. Furthermore, even if some heated cells are unable to attach, it needs to be shown by some other technique that these cells had retained their ability to proliferate before concluding that the colony formation technique is inappropriate. In one study such data were sought. Kase and Hahn (1976) present survival data based on two different assays: colony formation, and cellular growth corrected for division delay and for the presence of heat-sterilized cells. While the colony formation assays involved plating of heated, trypsinized cells, the latter experiments did not. Yet both assays gave more or less similar survival results. Similarly, Power and Harris (1977) exposed cells to heat before and after trypsinization and attachment and found that both procedures yielded similar survival data.

Thus, the contention that trypsinization may seriously modify heat responses does not seem to be in line with experimental results. In any case, studies can readily be performed to give quantitative answers to the objections listed by Lin *et al.* and Bass *et al.* It is somewhat surprising that neither of these research teams performed the appropriate control experiments before impugning such a large body of experimental data. Most other laboratories involved in cellular studies carefully examined possible trypsin effects and used procedures that minimized or bypassed them. In the absence of specific results to the contrary, it is reasonable to accept as valid the available heat survival data from experiments using the colony formation assay. Nevertheless, it is useful to keep in mind the possibilities of experimental artifacts whenever trypsinization of heated cells is part of the exposure protocol.

2.4. SURVIVAL OF CELLS EXPOSED TO SINGLE HEAT TREATMENTS

Survival curves obtained from cells exposed to elevated temperatures for various lengths of time can be grouped into three classes according to the shape of the survival patterns. One class is exemplified by curves generated from HeLa cells heated at temperatures between 41 and 45°C for periods of up to 5 hr. Survival was exponential over the entire time range, as shown in Figure 2.1. A different type of survival curve is obtained with Chinese hamster ovary (CHO) cells (Westra and Dewey, 1971). For the results shown in Figure 2.2, cells were heated to temperatures ranging from 43.5 to 46.5°C. Cells from most other lines yield survival curves somewhat like those of Figure 2.2. These are characterized by a shoulder; only for longer exposure times does the shape become log-linear. Survival values of Figure 2.1 can be represented by an equation of the type:

$$S = S_0 e^{kt}$$

where S is the survival at any time, S_0 is the survival at the time of heat initiation, k is the inactivation rate at the particular temperature, and t the duration of exposure.

A similar formulation can be used for the data of Figure 2.2, provided that it is only applied to the log-linear portion of the survival curve, i.e., for $t \gg 1/k$. Following the example of radiobiology, it has become customary in studies measuring cellular inactivation by heat to replace k by

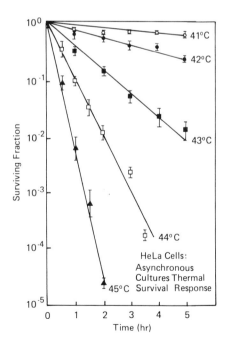

Figure 2.1. Exponential survival curves. HeLa cells were exposed to the indicated temperatures for various durations. Survival was assayed by colony formation. Note the complete absence of a shoulder, implying an inability to sustain sublethal damage. Data from Gerner *et al.* (1975) with permission.

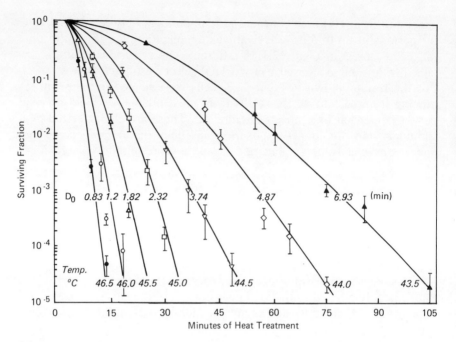

Figure 2.2. Sigmoidal survival curves. CHO cells were exposed to the indicated temperatures for various lengths of time. Temperature control was to ±0.1°. Exposure was several hours after trypsinization. Survival was assayed by colony formation. Both slopes and shoulder widths are a function of temperature. The shoulder does not result from artifacts of warm-up periods and therefore suggests an ability to sustain sublethal damage. Data from Westra and Dewey (1971) with permission.

a quantity $1/D_0$. Here D_0 is the time required (at the temperature of interest) to reduce cell survival on the exponential part of the curve to $1/e$ times its initial value. For the two cell lines of Figure 2.1 and 2.2, a graph of the values of $1/D_0$ vs. temperatures above 43°C produces an interesting result. Although the absolute values of the inactivation rates are very different for each cell line, in all cases an increase of one degree in temperature has associated with it a halving of D_0 (or a doubling of the rate constant, k).

A third type of survival curve is seen in Chinese hamster cells heated at temperatures below 43°C (Figure 2.3). The initial portion of the survival curves looks very much like that of the graphs of Figure 2.2; however, at longer exposures, the survival curve becomes concave upward until by about 4 hr it reaches a new, much shallower slope. The final inactivation rate is much smaller than that seen at the initiation of treatment. Because

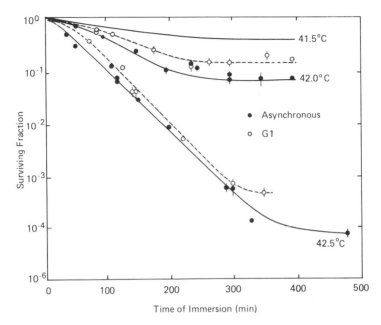

Figure 2.3. Survival curves showing resistant "tails". Asynchronous (solid lines) or synchronous G1 (broken lines) CHO cells were treated as described in Figure 2.2. The G1 cell survival closely mimics that of the asynchronous population. At temperatures below 43° the survival curves appear to be changing continuously until the resistant tails are reached. Data from Sapareto *et al.* (1978) with permission.

of the continuous bending of the curve, it is difficult to define one specific inactivation rate except for the terminal portion of the curve. Elsewhere the inactivation rate is continuously changing.

Survival curves having shapes more or less like those of Figure 2.3 are not unknown in radiobiology. They are usually associated with radiation inactivation of a heterogeneous population of cells, some radiation sensitive, some resistant. Small doses of irradiation inactivate primarily the sensitive subpopulation, so that the initial portion of the curve is steep. At larger doses it is the resistant cells that define the shape of the survival curve. There are also other circumstances that can give rise to such curves. Some of the cells may be in an environment where they are partially protected, either physically or chemically, from the effects of irradiation. Finally, in asynchronous populations, a fraction of the cells could occupy a portion of the cell cycle in which the cells are resistant to killing. This last possibility is of particular importance when cell killing by chemotherapeutic agents is concerned.

Can any of these possibilities explain the shape of the curves of Figure 2.3? To test for the possibility of the existence of one or more resistant subpopulations, enrichment experiments have been performed by several investigators. These have consisted typically of killing off the "sensitive" cells in a one-, two-, or three-step procedure and then testing cell populations derived from survivors for resistance to hyperthermia. Results of such studies were almost uniformly negative. With only very few exceptions, cell populations genetically resistant to heat have not been found. Yet survival curves such as those of Figure 2.3 have been observed for almost all cell lines. Careful control of environmental conditions in most experimental protocols insures that all the cells find themselves in a more or less homogeneous milieu. Thus it is very unlikely that external conditions, either physical or chemical, protect a small fraction of the cells. Finally, plateau phase cells, i.e., cells that have largely stopped proliferating because of density inhibition, also show survival curves of this type (Li and Hahn, 1980a). Cells in the plateau phase of growth are almost entirely in the Gl, or at least in a Gl-like, part of the cell cycle. Hence the third possibility, namely that cell cycle events are responsible for the development of the resistant "tail" of the survival curve, can be ruled out. A final possibility exists that might serve as an explanation for the concavity of the survival curves of Figure 2.3. Several inducible repair systems have recently been shown to operate in bacteria (e.g., Hanawalt *et al.*, 1979). It is not inconceivable that a similar mechanism or one involving biophysical adaptation operates during hyperthermic exposure. This could explain the "thermotolerant" state that is observed after cells have been exposed continuously for 4–5 hr at temperatures in the range of about 39 to 42°C. This subject matter will be discussed further in a later section devoted to thermotolerance (2.6.2.).

2.4.1. Stable Heat-Resistant Variants

As has just been said, the finding of stable, heat-resistant mutants of mammalian cells is rare. This is not because investigators have not tried. For example, Giovanella *et al.* (1979) carried out a careful search for heat-resistant sublines. He reports a negative result. Similarly, several attempts in my laboratory were unsuccessful. There are only about five reports (Selawry *et al.*, 1957; Harris, 1967; 1969; 1980; Reeves, 1972) in the literature that demonstrate the existence of such variants, and three of these deal with the same cell subline (Harris, 1967; 1969; Reeves, 1972). The first report that suggests the isolation of heat-resistant cell populations is that of Selawry *et al.* (1957). These authors exposed three types of human cells to elevated temperatures. The cells were HeLa cells, those derived from a biopsy specimen from a carcinoma of the larynx, and cells obtained from the peripheral blood of a patient affected with monocytic leukemia. These were exposed at 42°C to multiple treatments that lasted for up to 168 hr. Measurements were made of the "latent period" (defined as the time interval between the end of the heat application and the appearance of the first new mitoses) and of the LD_{100}s (the minimum heat–time profiles required to completely inhibit the growth of cultures for one month or longer). The findings for HeLa cells were as follows: in wild-type populations, a 1-hr exposure resulted in a latent period of 26 days, while the LD_{100} at 42°C was about 12 hr. HeLa cells derived from survivors of three exposures at 42°C of 168 hr each had a latent period of only 6 hr, while the LD_{100} had increased to several days. Somewhat similar observations were made for the other two cell lines.

Heat resistance was maintained for up to 3 months in spite of intervening growth of the cells at 36°C, or of "maintenance" for 3 months at 24 to 26°C. A long period of growth delay may well occur after such a long storage at this low temperature; furthermore, because of the lack of experimental detail presented by the investigators about the growth conditions, it could be that these cells simply had not re-adapted to the lower temperatures (Li and Hahn, 1980b). Thus, there is some uncertainty about the genetic stability of the heat resistance. Nevertheless, it appears likely that Selawry *et al.* (1957) did encounter true resistant variants.

No doubts exist in the case of a heat-resistant line described by Harris and associates (Harris, 1967; 1969; Reeves, 1972). These authors harvested a number of clonal isolates from populations of previously heated pig kidney cells. Some of these were obtained by alternate exposures of populations of cells to 47°C followed by subculture at 37°C. Several of the kidney cell strains obtained from cells surviving the repeated heat exposures proved to be heat resistant. In addition, heat-stable strains were isolated from cells that survived heat exposure that reduced the initial population by a factor of 10^{-5}. The heat-resistant variants did not differ from wild-type cells with respect to cell morphology, growth rate, or chromosomal pattern. The demonstration that heat-resistant sublines could be isolated from clonal populations directly, that is, without extensive preheating, demonstrated that the variant did not arise by adaptation. Heat-resistant cells must have been present in the original population. Reeves (1972) compared some biochemical properties of normal and heat-resistant pig kidney cell lines. He concluded that the development of heat resistance was associated with changes in membrane permeability. Specifically, the heat-resistant cells showed a decreased loss of uridine or uridine-containing materials under heat stress. Another difference found was that macromolecular synthesis, interrupted by heating, recovered more rapidly in the resistant lines than in the wild type. Whether the recovery of synthesis simply reflected higher survival in the resistant strain, or if the resumption of synthesis was responsible for the higher survival, is not known.

Recently Harris (1980) has also reported on the isolation of heat-resistant sublines of Chinese hamster cells. The isolation of the stable, heat-resistant cells required thermal exposures that reduced viability by a factor of 10^{-5}, just as was the case for the pig kidney cells. This was achieved by heating logarithmically growing Chinese hamster cells at 44.5°C for 60 to 75 min. Harris then set up three-phase procedures to enrich cultures with stable, resistant variants by cyclic exposure of the cells to 44.5°C with intervening recovery periods at 37°C. Figure 2.4 shows survival curves obtained from two stock lines (129-5 and B150), as well as survival curves from three variant populations isolated at the first, second, and third phases of the cyclic experiment. The latter lines were designated 296, 418B, and 456-1, respectively. While the D_0 value of stock cultures exposed to 44.5°C varied between 4.6 and 5 min, the D_0 for the most resistant line (456-1) was increased to 26.3 min. These differences in D_0's can give rise to tremendous variation in survival. For example, 75 min of heating at 44.5°C resulted in a million-fold survival difference between the resistant and sensitive cells. Contrary to the behavior of the pig kidney

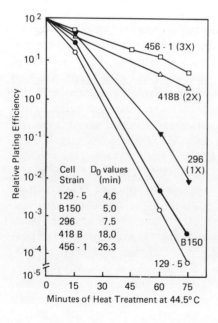

Figure 2.4. Selection of stable, heat-resistant cell populations. V–79 Chinese hamster cells were exposed to various heating regimens and heat-resistant survivors were isolated. This procedure was repeated up to three times. Both resistant and stock cultures were exposed to 44.5° for the times indicated on the abscissa. The survival responses of the parent line (129–5) and of the resistant strains are strikingly different. Data from Harris (1980) with permission.

cell variants, the Chinese hamster cells showed a distinctive pattern of growth and clonal morphology. Colonies formed by the heat-resistant 456-1 cells were much smaller, because of reduced growth rates, and the cells tended to grow in parallel and palisading arrays. This gave the colonies a jagged and angular appearance, in contrast to the round and well-defined colony shape of the heat-sensitive parent lines. Harris suggested that the difference between the parent line and the sublines might lie in differences in membrane components, and that different lipids might give rise to different membrane fluidities. Stiffness of the membranes would then provide both a rationale for increased heat resistance as well as an explanation for the morphological alterations.

2.4.2. Stable Heat-Sensitive Variants

The search for variants of mammalian cells that are unusually temperature sensitive presents quite a different picture. A wide range of so-called "ts" mutants have been isolated. The subject is of considerable current interest, and there are several recent reviews (e.g., Simchen, 1978). It must be recognized at the outset that a ts mutant, as the term is used by geneticists, is not necessarily temperature sensitive in the same sense as the variants of the last paragraph are temperature resistant. A ts mutation, by definition, results in a phenotype that in the wild type, but not in the mutation, is capable of multiplication and/or function at the "nonpermissive" temperatures. In other words, the ts mutant has a more restricted "permissive" temperature range than does the wild type. For most ts mutatations the permissive temperature of the mutants is in the lower part of the wild type's normal temperature range. There are, however, also so-called "cold-sensitive" mutants; these have permissive temperatures in the upper part of the wild type range. I emphasize again that a ts mutation does not necessarily imply inability of the mutated cell to survive at higher temperature, but only refers to its ability to multiply or fulfill the specific ts function. In fact, most selection procedures depend upon the ability of the ts mutant cell to remain in a quiescent state at the nonpermissive temperature while still maintaining reproductive integrity. Such mutant cells, upon being returned to the permissive temperature, resume growth.

A wide array of ts mutants have been isolated. Some of these have temperature-sensitive steps in DNA synthesis, some in RNA synthesis, and some in cell cycle progression or protein synthesis. While the biochemical defects are relatively easy to demonstrate, a temperature-sensitive gene product has been specified only in a few situations. Surprisingly, no data exist that compare survival at hyperthermic temperatures of ts mutants to that of appropriate wild-type controls. Data in this direction would be of considerable interest. Di Mayorca *et al.* (1973) have demonstrated that about half of chemically transformed BHK cells also show a temperature-sensitive mutation. If, as suggested by Wallach (1977), the temperature-sensitive function is membrane associated, perhaps because of defective membrane proteins or lipids or reduced amounts of sterols, then it may very well be that ts mutants are less able to survive at higher temperatures. A membrane-altered temperature-sensitive mammalian cell mutant has been described by Ceri and Wright (1977), consistent with Wallach's suggestion.

2.4.3. Sensitivities of Normal and Malignant Cells

There have been many reports, some of which go back at least 100 years, claiming that malignant cells are more heat sensitive than their normal counterparts. The subject has been reviewed several times in the last few years (Cavaliere *et al.*, 1967; Suit and Shwayder, 1974; Strom *et al.*, 1977). Currently, many investigators accept the "selective thermosensitivity of cancer cells" as established experimental fact. Unfortunately, an examination of the existing evidence does not lead to quite such an optimistic evaluation. The older literature contains data obtained from experiments in which the assay procedures that were used are no longer considered reliable, such as dye exclusion or morphological criteria. The results from these investigations not surprisingly are far from uniform. To compare numbers, six or seven reports claim enhanced thermal sensitivity of neoplastic cells, two reports find no difference, and three reports show that the opposite may be true; i.e., that malignant cells may be more heat resistant. When such diverse findings are coupled with the very likely situation that negative reports are frequently either not submitted for publication or not accepted by the scientific journals, it is somewhat difficult to see how a recent book based on these data could justifiably be termed "Selective Heat Sensitivity of Cancer Cells."

Things don't get any better when one looks at the more recent data. If I restrict myself to investigations in which the assay to test cell survival was the ability to form colonies, then only four studies have been reported in which the sensitivity *in vitro* of normal and neoplastic cells was compared. Chen and Heidelberger (1969) clearly showed that mouse prostate cells, upon being transformed by carcinogenic hydrocarbons *in vitro*, in parallel acquired a pronounced heat sensitivity. On the other side of the fence, Harisiadis *et al.* (1975) compared survival of "normal" liver cells with those obtained from a closely associated hepatoma. The hepatoma cells were found to be slightly more resistant to heat than the normal liver cells. Kase and Hahn (1975) compared the colony-forming abilities of heat-treated WI38 cells, a human fibroblast strain, to those of similarly treated SV-40 transformed WI38s. The latter were shown to be malignant by their ability to grow as tumors in nude, (i.e., immune deficient) mice. It was found that during exponential growth, the normal cells were somewhat more resistant than their transformed counterparts. However, when the same experiment was repeated, but with the cells at very high cell density (approximately $1-3 \times 10^7$ cells/dish) the difference in heat sensitivities disappeared (Kase and Hahn, 1976).

There are two other recent works (Giovanella *et al.*, 1973; 1978) that strongly indicate that malignant cells in general tend to be more sensitive than their normal counterparts. Unfortunately, perhaps because of the difficulty in cloning human cells, and particularly normal human cells, these studies used cell number as the criterion for survival. Equal numbers of cells were seeded into individual compartments on "microwell plates." These are plastic dishes, subdivided into several growth areas. The individual areas are separated from one another by partitions and so have the appearance of individual wells. Dishes with equal numbers of cells in each microwell were heated and then returned to incubators at 37°C. At several time points, cells in each well were counted. Survival was expressed as the ratio of cell number in a heated well to that in an unheated control. The "survival" values so obtained invariably were lower for malignant cell populations than were those for cells obtained from normal tissue of comparable histology.

Some questions need to be raised about the assay employed. The problem with using cell number as a measure of reproductive capacity is that there are several factors other than survival that can influence the number of countable cells in a microwell. These include: the presence in the population of doomed, reproductively dead cells; differential rates of detachment of heat-inactivated cells; and differentiated effects of heating on division delay and on subsequent proliferation rates. These must all be measured individually before cell number can be used to determine survival. In one study that compared the survival of human WI38 cells and their virally transformed counterparts, it was shown that without appropriate measurements of each one of these parameters the use of cell number can lead to highly misleading estimates of survival parameters (Kase and Hahn, 1976).

Recently developed techniques have make it possible to test rigorously if any correlation exists between malignancy and heat sensitivity. A strain of mouse embryo fibroblasts, designated 10T1/2, has been developed by Heidelberger and his associates (Reznikoff *et al.*, 1973). Cells from this strain show a low spontaneous transformation rate but can be transformed *in vitro* by a variety of agents, both physical and chemical. Transformed cells can be isolated, and their offspring then give rise to substrains. It is possible to measure the heat sensitivities of the "normal" as well as the transformed strains. The heat responses of cells from three X-ray- and one methylcholanthrene-transformed substrains were compared to that of 10T1/2 cells (Hahn, 1980). These cells from the various strains were also tested for their ability to form tumors in syngeneic hosts, some of which had been rendered immune deficient by X irradiation. It was found that the transformed cells varied greatly in their ability to induce tumors. Those from one of the X-ray-transformed strains appeared to be nonmalignant; even 10^6 cells injected into the hosts did not produce any tumors. This paralleled the behavior of the untransformed cells. Another similarly transformed strain required an average of 10^5 cells to induce tumors in 50% of the injected sites, while another X-ray transformant required only 10^3 cells. Finally, the methylcholanthrene-transformed strain proved to be the most malignant of all: less than 10 cells were required, on the average, to initiate tumors. When the heat sensitivities of the transformed strains and the parent line were compared, it was found that during exponential growth at least, the "normal" 10T1/2 cells were slightly more resistant. But this difference was very minor. It manifested itself as an increase of 10 to 20% in the width of the shoulder of the survival curve. However, as the plateau phase and high cell density were reached, this difference disappeared. In these density-inhibited cells, no differences could be demonstrated between the heat response of "normal" cells or of any of the transformed strains. Indeed, the most malignant cell strain, that transformed by methylcholanthrene, had survival kinetics almost identical to those of the normal cells.

The conclusions that can be drawn from these diverse results appear to be as follows. Although studies demonstrating increased heat sensitivity of malignant cells clearly exist, there are enough contradictory reports to strongly suggest that this sensitivity is not a general characteristic of all malignant cells. From the clinical treatment viewpoint, this may not be too important. The requirement that all malignant transformations entail a thermosensitive step is unnecessarily restrictive. Even if only 20 or 30% of malignancies were sufficiently thermosensitive so that treatment with whole body hyperthermia could destroy enough malignant cells to induce remissions, this would warrant extensive clinical applications. Probably even this is optimistic, for as Giovanella and Mondovi (1977) have pointed out, "Unfortunately, the size of the difference in thermal sensitivity between normal and neoplastic cells is not great." Based on the data presented here, I might add, if indeed this difference exists at all.

2.4.4. Influence of Ploidy, Cell Density, and Cell Cycle on Heat Sensitivity

Lücke-Huhle (1978) examined the relative sensitivities to 42°C of diploid and tetraploid sublines obtained from V-79 Chinese hamster cells. She found that exponentially growing tetraploid cells were somewhat more resistant to heat than were the diploid cells (D_0 ratio of about 1.4 : 1), while plateau phase cells showed no differences in heat response. Exponentially growing cell populations were composed of about 50% S phase cells and 40% G1 cells, as determined by cytofluorometry. After 4 hr at 42°C, essentially all G1 cells had proceeded into S phase, again as demonstrated by cytofluorometric studies. Because plateau phase cells have a DNA complement similar to those of G1 cells, this suggests that any difference in heat sensitivities between the diploid and tetraploid cells may be measurable only in the S phase. An additional and interesting finding was that there was no difference between the heat responses of diploid and of tetraploid cells when these were grown as spheroids. There is only one additional work that suggests ploidy as a determinant of heat sensitivity of cells. In another eukaryotic system, Wood (1956) found that tetraploid yeast cells were substantialy more resistant to heat than their diploid cousins.

The study by Lücke-Huhle just cited also demonstrated that plateau phase V-79 cells were consistently more heat resistant than exponentially growing cells when sensitivity was measured under matched growth conditions (monolayers or spheroids). Human WI38 cells, as well as the SV–40-transformed counterparts, also showed increased resistance when growing at high densities (Kase and Hahn, 1975; 1976), while V-79 cells were found to be more resistant when exponentially growing (Schulman and Hall, 1974). This latter finding seemed to confirm an earlier study with HA-1 Chinese hamster cells (Hahn, 1974). Furthermore, EMT6/Az cells were also found to be more sensitive in plateau phase (Gerner et al., 1979), as were ENJ ascites tumor cells (Bichel and J. Overgaard, 1977). It seems very likely that these conflicting results relate to the lack of standardized environmental factors, particularly nutrition, pH, and cell densities per se, rather than to true differences in the thermal response of cells in different growth stages.

An aspect that influences the heat sensitivity of most cells is that of their position in the reproductive cycle. Cells from most lines seem to follow the general pattern demonstrated by Westra and Dewey (1971) for CHO cells. These authors synchronized cells utilizing the mitotic "shake-off" technique originally developed by Terasima and Tolmach (1963a,b).

In this method, advantage is taken of the reduced ability of the rounded, mitotic cells to adhere to their growth surface. Vigorous shaking of medium-covered monolayers preferentially dislodges mitotic cells. In order to obtain a sufficiently large number of cells, harvested mitotic cells are plated at 4°C; at that temperature their forward passage in the cell cycle is arrested, apparently without major trauma associated with the cold shock. Cells from several harvests can then be pooled. Upon being returned to 37°C, the cells initiate progression into the cycle as a closely synchronized cohort. At specified times after transfer to 37°C, Westra

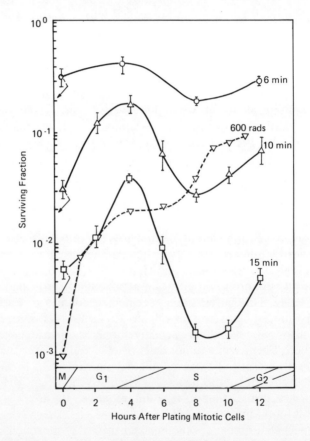

Figure 2.5. Age response patterns of heated cells. CHO cells were synchronized using the mitotic shakeoff procedure, and then exposed to 45° for the indicated durations at various times after harvest. The age response pattern of cells exposed to 600 rad of X irradiation is shown for comparison. The arrows indicate the magnitude of uncertainty introduced by cell division during the experiment ("multiplicity correction"). Data from Westra and Dewey (1971) with permission.

and Dewey exposed cells to 45.5°C for durations of 6, 10, or 15 min. The "age responses" so obtained are shown in Figure 2.5. Most sensitive were mitotic and late S phase cells. The most heat-resistant cells appeared to be these in early G1, although cells in G2 may have been equally resistant. In experiments involving cells synchronized by the shakeoff technique, accurate determination of the response of G2 cells is particularly difficult because of the considerable amount of desynchronization that occurs between the time of harvest and entry into G2.

The results of Westra and Dewey and those of other workers agree quite well, but there are two exceptions. Reeves (1972) compared the age responses of pig kidney cells and those of the heat-resistant variant described in Section 2.4.2. He induced synchrony *via* the double thymidine block described by Bootsma (1965). The presence in the medium of concentrations of thymidine in excess of 10^{-3}M slows DNA synthesis to the point that cells accumulate at the G1/S interface. Replacement of the thymidine-containing medium with fresh nutrients allows the passage of a partially synchronized cell population. Survival curves of M, G1, S, and G2 cells were obtained. Reeves saw no differences in responses with respect to position in the cell cycle in cells from either strain and hence concluded that cells in all portions of the cell cycle responded similarly to heat. Palzer and Heidelberger (1973) combined the thymidine block and mitotic shakeoff techniques to obtain a sufficient number of synchronized HeLa cells without having to resort to cold storage. The variations of survival within the cell cycle measured after exposure of the HeLa cells from 6 to 120 min at 42°C were not very pronounced. It is conceivable that in the experiments of Reeves and those of Palzer and Heidelberger the use of thymidine somehow reduced the variation in heat sensitivities. Alternatively, Palzer and Heidelberger suggested that the low temperature exposure associated with most mitotic shakeoff procedures increased the differences in heat responses. However, unpublished control experiments performed by Kapp and Hahn did not show any such effect resulting from short term (approximately 2 hr) storage at 4°C.

On balance, it seems reasonable to conclude that those cells that are most sensitive to heat exposure are mitotic cells and late S phase cells. This latter result is particularly intriguing because late S phase cells are unusually resistant to X irradiation, and this finding therefore suggests one rationale for the combination, in the clinic, of these two modalities.

2.5. MODIFICATIONS OF HEAT RESPONSES

In this section I am going to discuss how the environment of cells modifies their heat response. In particular, I am going to spend some time on the available evidence that indicates that cells in a tumorlike milieu may be more sensitive than cells in an environment similar to that found in normal tissue. The existence of hypoxic cells in human tumors has long been suspected and is frequently quoted as a reason for some failures of radiation therapy. It is however worthwhile to point out that the occurrence of such cells has unequivocally been demonstrated only in murine tumors. There they arise either because in actively metabolizing tissue the diffusion distance of oxygen is limited to about 100μm, or because of the possible temporary blockage of some tumor blood vessels (Brown, 1979).

Less well known, though perhaps not surprising in view of the hypoxic state of many cells in solid tumors, is the acidity of most neoplasms. A compilation of published data is shown in Table 2.1 (Gerweck, 1978). While there is considerable variation in the absolute value of the pH measured even in normal tissues, each individual result indicates a lower pH in the intracellular fluid of tumors when compared to that of normal tissue.

Finally, cells in tumors are very likely nutritionally deprived, although data on this aspect are hard to come by. Glucose consumption increases in hypoxic regions, hence it is very likely that microregions of solid tumors

TABLE 2.1
TISSUE FLUID pH OF NORMAL AND MALIGNANT TISSUES[a]

Investigator	Tumor types	Tissue fluid pH		Assay conditions
		Normal	Tumor	
Gullino et al.[b]	Rat, n = 5	7.33 ± 0.00	7.05 ± 0.09	In vivo
Eden et al.[c]	Rat, n = 8	7.39 ± 0.12	7.03 ± 0.12	In vivo
Ashby[d]	Human, melanomas	7.43 ± 0.08	6.78 ± 0.09	In vivo
Naeslund and Swenson[e]	Human, gynecological, n = 5	7.57 ± 0.25	6.89 ± 0.28	In vivo
Meyer et al.[f]	Human, various, n = 14	6.60 ± 0.38	6.21 ± 0.29	Surgical specimens

[a]L.E. Gerweck, 1978, with permission.
[b]Guillino et al., 1965.
[c]Eden et al., 1955.
[d]Ashby, 1966.
[e]Naeslund and Swenson, 1953.
[f]Meyer et al., 1948.

are in a state of hypoglycemia. Similarly, serum proteins may be in short supply, since their diffusion distance is also limited.

For these reasons, comparisons of the survival of cells heated under experimental protocols involving modifications of extracellular pH and manipulations of oxygen, glucose, and serum concentrations in the cells' medium are of clinical importance. I am also going to describe experiments in which the heat response of cells is measured in media whose water has been replaced by deuterium oxide, and the effects on heat sensitivity of increasing the hydrostatic pressure during the thermal exposure. While these latter two factors have little relevance to cancer treatment, the experiments are of interest for the discussion, in Chapter 4, of the possible mechanisms responsible for heat-induced cell death.

2.5.1. Modification by Changes in pH

Investigation of the effect of pH on the heat sensitivity of mammalian cells has largely been the work of three groups, those of Von Ardenne, Gerweck, and Overgaard. Von Ardenne (Von Ardenne and Reitnauer, 1970; Von Ardenne, 1971) has examined the relationship between cell glycolysis, pH, and heat damage. His group has also made rather strong claims regarding the role of glucose in acidifying the intracellular milieu. However, most of the quantitative investigations *in vitro* were carried out by Gerweck and his associates and by Overgaard's group. Typical results of survival responses at different pH values are those shown in Figure 2.6, taken from Gerweck's work (Gerweck, 1977). In these experiments, cells were cultured in McCoy's medium containing 10% calf and 5% fetal calf sera. The pH was adjusted by varying the sodium bicarbonate or hydrochloric acid concentrations. Changes in pH, particularly below 7.0, affected survival at all the temperatures tested. The biggest effect was seen at 42°C, where lower pH sharply increased the cytotoxic efficacy of the heat exposures. The major effect appeared to be the inhibition of the development of thermotolerance. This is clearly shown by comparing the results obtained at 42°C with those obtained at the higher temperature, since above 43° thermotolerance does not develop in these cells during heating (section 2.6.2.).

At the higher temperatures, the differences between survival at pH 7.4 and 6.7 were much reduced, although in absolute terms they were still appreciable. For example, at 43°C, 90 min of incubation at pH 7.4 yielded survival of about 10^{-1}, while this was reduced to 10^{-3} at 6.7.

Gerweck also investigated the question of whether pH changes in the medium either before or after exposure were as effective in modifying survival as pH changes during the time the cells were heated. His results

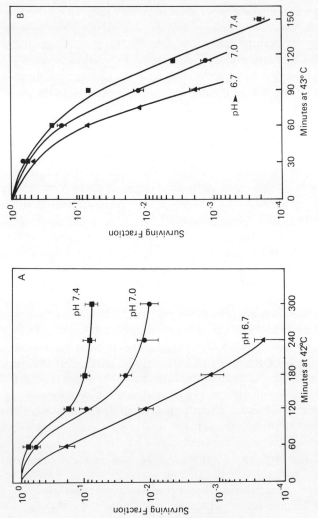

Figure 2.6. Influence of pH during heating on survival. CHO cells were exposed to 42 (A) or 43°C (B) for various lengths of time. The pH was adjusted to the indicated values. Survival was measured by colony formation. At the lower temperature, the major role of pH appeared to be the modulation of the time of appearance of the resistant "tail" of the survival curve, while at the higher temperature the slopes of the survival curves were primarily affected. Data from Gerweck (1977) with permission.

showed that preincubation in slightly acidic medium somewhat sensitized cells, while incubation at pH 6.7 after heating had no effect on survival, provided heating and earlier incubation had been carried out at pH 7.4. Similar results were also found by Freeman *et al.* (1977), who showed that at 45.5°C there was a continuous increase in heat sensitivity as the pH was varied from 7.35 down to pH 6.65, although the major change occurred below a pH of 7.0. Overgaard (Overgaard and Overgaard, 1975; Overgaard, 1976) worked with L182 ascites tumor cells. They were heated in suspension in Eagle's medium (no serum) and the pH was varied from 7.2 to 6.4. The temperature was 42.5°C and exposure time 60 min. Two assays to determine viability were employed: cells were stained with lissamine green, or 10^6 treated cells were injected into mice to test for the cells' ability to form tumors. The survival of cells removed from the heat suspensions immediately after the incubation period showed a strong dependence on pH during heating. Cells that had been heated at pH 7.2 were able to form tumors in 100% of the hosts. Those cells heated at pH 6.4 were incapable of initiating tumors. The major change occurred between pH values of 7.2 and 7.0. In that narrow pH interval, the reduction in observed tumor "takes" was from 100% to 33%. This diminution in ability to form tumors may have occurred over an even smaller range of pH values: a graph of percent tumor "takes" v. pH indicates that 100% tumor takes would occur somewhere in the neighborhood of pH 7.1 to 7.15.

In this study the effect of low pH in the postincubation medium was also investigated. Unfortunately, here all the survival measurements were done with dye exclusion, and it has been established many times that this is an unsatisfactory assay, particularly after hyperthermia. Overgaard (1975) also performed ultrastructural examination, indicating however that if acidic conditions (pH 6.4) were maintained after a heat exposure at low pH, cell lysis was accentuated. The number of cells having lesions in their plasma membranes as well as those showing increased lysosomal activity increased. It should be kept in mind that incubation was not only at acid pH, but also in medium in the absence of serum. It has since been demonstrated that posttreatment incubation of heated cells in buffer, in the absence of serum, accentuates heat killing, but that under such conditions cytotoxicity is not affected directly by pH changes between 6.7 and 7.4 (Li *et al.*, 1980a).

In another work Nielsen and Overgaard (1979) investigated the role of extracellular pH on the survival of the same L182 cells used in the previous study. In the new investigation, heat exposure was performed in a Krebs–Ringer phosphate buffer that was, however, supplemented with 10% fetal calf serum. Heating under these conditions resulted in very different survival responses. Now, using inhibition of colony formation as the assay, it was found that survival curves changed only in a minor way as the pH was varied between 7.2 and 6.5; only below 6.5 was there an appreciable pH effect. The temperature of exposure in these experiments was 42°C, as compared to 42.5°C in the earlier study. It is difficult to see that half a degree of temperature difference would cause such a marked change in the ability of pH to modify heat response. This is particularly true in view of the results of Gerweck, discussed earlier, who showed that as the temperature is increased above 42°C, effects of pH changes on survival are reduced. Two explanations come to mind that could resolve these discrepancies. The ability of cells to form tumors in animals depends not only on viability, but also on the immune response the animal is able to mount against foreign cells. It may be that the data from the earlier Overgaard study reflect not only cell killing but also modification of host responses. The other explanation, which I find more plausible, is that during one study serum was present during heating, while it was missing in the other work. Serum, as will be discussed in the next section, provides some protection to cells during heating and may also modify the influence of pH.

2.5.2. Nutrients

2.5.2.1. Serum

The role of nutrients in modifying cell sensitivity seems to be closely associated with that of pH. There are three reports citing experiments indicating that under certain conditions pH changes in the range of 6.4 to 7.2 do not affect cell survival (Euler *et al.*, 1974; Dickson and Oswald, 1976; Li and Hahn, 1980a). These three studies have one feature in common, namely that heating was performed in media containing no serum. In the three investigations, incubation medium in each case consisted of a buffer, supplemented with glucose. The converse also appears to be true: each study in which heating was carried out in medium containing serum reported the pH modification of survival kinetics. Serum, even at pH 7.4, has been shown to be a protective agent if present during heating (Hahn, 1974). This is shown in Figure 2.7.

The importance of nutrient modulation on heat sensitivity, particularly in densely growing cells, is frequently overlooked. The reason I am emphasizing densely growing cells is that these can rapidly deplete medium of one or more component and therefore may modify their nutrient environment during the course of an experiment. This is illustrated in Figure 2.8, in which survival of EMT6/ST cells during plateau phase is

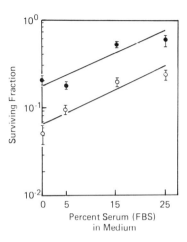

Figure 2.7. The effect of nutrient environment on cell survival. HA–1 cells in the plateau phase of growth were heated in media supplemented with the indicated percentage of fetal bovine serum. Closed circles: 43°, 2 hr; open circles: 43°, 3 hr. The correlation between survival and serum concentrations reflects changes in the environment during heating. Data from Hahn (1974), with permission.

shown. In these experiments, the medium was renewed at zero time. The cells were then either exposed to heat immediately or returned to 37°C incubation for various lengths of time and then exposed to the elevated temperature. Heating was for 120 min at 43°C. Thus the only variable in this experiment was the elapsed time between medium renewal and the application of the 120-min heat pulse. Reduction in survival value by

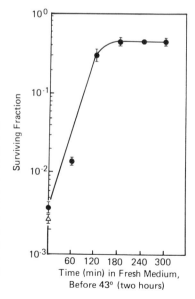

Figure 2.8. The effect of nutrient environment on cell survival. EMT6/ST cells were grown to confluence without medium exchange. At 0 time the medium was renewed. Cells were exposed to 43°C (2 hr) at various times thereafter. Survival was assayed by colony formation. The open triangle represents survival from controls, which were heated before the medium renewal. The increase in survival was not associated with an influx of cells into the most resistant S phase and therefore reflects exclusively the change in nutrient environment before heating. Unpublished data from Sanchez and Hahn.

almost two orders of magnitude occurred as this interval increased from 0 to 8 hr. These results make it very clear that the heat sensitivity of densely growing cells (and perhaps of other populations) is strongly dependent on specific details of the protocol employed, including the precise timing of medium exchanges. It may very well be that the different results I have discussed earlier with respect to the survival kinetics of such cultures result from differences in "feeding schedules", pH variations, and perhaps availability of oxygen.

2.5.2.2. Oxygen

As mentioned earlier, the presence of hypoxic cells in tumors is frequently thought to be one of the factors responsible for radiotherapeutic failures. Inactivation of acutely hypoxic cells requires two to three times the X-ray dose needed for the killing of oxygenated cells. For that reason the role hypoxia plays in modifying the heat sensitivity of cells is of considerable interest. Again the data are conflicting. In what appears to be the earliest study of this subject, the response of exponentially growing Chinese hamster cells to 43°C was found to be independent of the presence or absence of oxygen during heating (Hahn, 1974). Later studies more or less consistent with this finding were those of Power and Harris (1977), Bass et al. (1978), and Gerweck et al. (1979). Bass et al. found a slight protective effect of hypoxia against the killing of HeLa cells exposed to 43°C. In all these experiments, hypoxia was induced by displacing oxygen dissolved in the growth medium with nitrogen or with nitrogen–CO_2 mixtures.

Several other reports suggest that oxygen acts to protect cells against hyperthermic death. In all of these (Hahn, 1974; Schulman and Hall, 1974; Harisiadis et al., 1975; Kim et al., 1975b), experimental design depended on the cells' respiration to induce hypoxia. Hahn (1974) used plateau phase cells overlaid with 9 ml of medium. Such cells, at a density of about 10^7 cells/cm^2, become hypoxic because oxygen cannot diffuse rapidly enough through the 9 ml of medium to balance the amount consumed. The cells were truly hypoxic, as was verified by direct measurement and also by determining the cells' radiation response. These density-inhibited cultures were found to be slightly more sensitive to exposure at 43°C than similar cultures overlaid with only 2 ml of medium. The reduced depth of the medium overlay permits the diffusion of adequate amounts of oxygen. In a similar vein, Kim et al. (1975b) induced hypoxia by utilizing the oxygen depletion capability of a large number of heavily irradiated, but actively metabolizing, "feeder" cells. These were added to the cells whose proliferative ability was to be assayed. In one experiment, a suspension of live HeLa cells at a concentration of 10^5 cells/ml was supplemented with 30–60 times this number of heavily irradiated "feeder" cells. Small amounts of this cell mixture (0.6 ml) were then sealed in 1-ml plastic pipettes. These were incubated at 37°C for 8 hr before heating commenced. During that time the respiratory activity of the feeder layer depleted essentially all available oxygen. A somewhat similar technique was utilized by Hall and associates (Schulman and Hall, 1974; Harisiadis, *et al.*, 1975) to obtain hypoxic cells. When cells made hypoxic in this manner were tested for heat sensitivity, it was found that they were appreciably more readily inactivated than their well-oxygenated counterparts. The roles of pH and nutritional factors were not appreciated at the time these experiments were done; however, today it must be assumed that the response of the cells was not simply a result of their hypoxia, but a combination of chronic hypoxia, low pH, and nutrient deficiency. As has been suggested earlier, precisely these conditions obtain in many solid tumors. Therefore, although the results of these experiments may not describe effects of hypoxia *per se,* they very likely do have clinical relevance.

2.5.2.3. Glucose

Closely connected with the roles played by pH, oxygen, and serum in determining cellular heat sensitivity is that of glucose. I am not now discussing the various suggestions by Von Ardenne and Reitnauer (1976) that glucose infusions can lead to hyperacidifications of tumors. This subject will be discussed later. What is of interest here is the fact that low glucose concentrations, and particularly the absence of glucose, can cause cells to exhibit greatly enhanced heat responses. An attempt to assess the importance of glucose in determining the heat sensitivity of cells, particularly of densely growing cells, presents some serious experimental problems. Glucose is used by cells at a rapid rate; yet glucose is required to maintain viability of heated cells (Hahn, 1974). For hyperthermia experiments, which may take several hours to complete, it is therefore difficult to maintain low glucose concentrations at constant levels over the durations of the experiment. For this reason most experimenters instead of working at low external glucose levels have used glucose analogues that competitively inhibit glucose transport to reduce intracellular glucose concentrations. At low analogue concentrations the cells are able to utilize glucose normally, and hence depletion proceeds rapidly. At analogue concentrations that greatly exceed those of the amount of glucose present, inhibition of glycolysis becomes appreciable. Then relatively constant intracellular concentrations of glucose can be maintained at arbitrary levels and for long durations.

One study in which the glucose analogue 2-deoxy-D-glucose was utilized showed that increased heat sensitivity could be demonstrated at analogue concentrations below 10^{-1} mg/ml, while at a concentration of 10 mg/ml maintained for 24 hr heat sensitivity was similar to that of cells in full medium and essentially independent of glucose concentrations (Hahn, 1974). This very limited study, which examined only a very restricted range of glucose concentrations, therefore concluded that the role of glucose as a protective agent, while clearly existing, did not rival the importance of other factors such as pH and serum in determining heat sensitivity. As long as any glucose was available, the cells maintained their heat resistance.

Quite different results were seen by Song *et al.* (1977), who used 5-thio-D-glucose as an inhibitor of glycolysis. Even at 37°C, the presence in the medium of this analogue was shown to be selectively toxic to hypoxic cells. Because of the dependence of hypoxic cells on glycolytic pathways for energy metabolism, this result emphasizes the interrelationship between the availability of oxygen and other nutrients. Starting with this result, Kim *et al.* (1978) then showed that this selective effect of the glucose analogue on hypoxic cells was greatly magnified at elevated temperatures. Typical results are shown in Figure 2.9. Of particular interest was the finding that even at relatively low temperatures, and at analogue concentrations that have no effect whatsoever at 37°C, 5-thio-D-glucose efficiently killed hypoxic HeLa cells. For example a 4-hr exposure of such cells to 41°C killed about 30% of the cells when no glucose

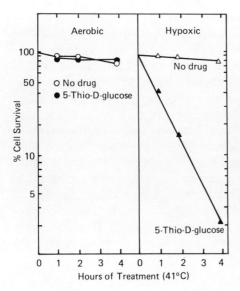

Figure 2.9. The role of glucose in determining the heat response of hypoxic cells. HeLa cells were heated to 41°C for the indicated time under either aerobic or hypoxic conditions, and in the presence of the glucose analogue 5-thio-D-glucose. This agent competitively inhibits glucose transport. The increased killing of hypoxic cells at the elevated temperature in the presence of the inhibitor illustrates the cells' need for glucose to maintain viability during heating. Data from S. H. Kim *et al.* (1978), with permission.

analogue was added to the medium; however, in the presence of 5 mM 5-thio-D-glucose, killing was increased to the point where only 2% of the cells survived. In these studies no data are presented on the pH of the medium during heating, but the method used to induce hypoxia, as well as the description of the culture conditions, makes it reasonable to assume that the pH in which the cells found themselves was maintained in the region of 7.0 and 7.5. Hence, sensitization in the presence of the analogue probably reflects its inhibition of glucose utilization. Glucose starvation before heat exposure can result in greatly increased heat sensitivity, as shown in two other studies (Haveman and Hahn, 1981; Nagle *et al.*, 1981).

2.5.2.4. Conclusion—Nutrients and pH

Data presented in the last sections indicate that there is a close connection between the pH, the presence or absence of nutrients, and the degree of availability of oxygen in determining the heat sensitivity of mammalian cells. This implies that specification during an experiment of one of these factors, say pH, is not sufficient to define the heat response. Similarly, it is very likely that the question of whether or not mammalian cells require the presence of oxygen for survival during heat exposure cannot be answered without specifying data on the pH of their surroundings, as well as on nutrient factors. The results on increased heat sensitivity of cells at low glucose concentrations also point clearly to the necessity of using caution about accepting the proposition that reducing the pH by increasing the glucose concentrations either *in vitro* or *in vivo* will necessarily increase the heat sensitivity of cells. It may very well be that increasing the glucose concentrations might decrease the pH, but any benefits so achieved would be negated by increased resistance owing to the richer nutrient environment created.

2.5.3. Protective Agents

I can hardly envision that deuterium oxide D_2O or increased hydrostatic pressure will play a role in the clinical use of hyperthermia. Nevertheless, the action of these two agents is described here because their role in modifying the cytotoxicity of hyperthermia has biological implications, which are discussed in more detail in Chapter 4.

2.5.3.1. Deuterium Oxide

Protection of mammalian cells against hyperthermic damage by D_2O was first described by Wenzel and Stohr (1970), and Maurer and Wenzel (1977). Though plant cell biologists had made a similar observation even earlier (reviewed by Alexandrov, 1977), the work was not exploited any further. The protective ability of D_2O was "rediscovered" in my laboratory in the last few years (G.M. Hahn *et al.*, 1978b). Figure 2.10. demonstrates some unpublished work of Fisher *et al.* In the experiments shown, graded amounts of D_2O were substituted for H_2O, and the D_2O-substituted media was used to overlay the cells during heating. At least over the range of 0 to 70% substitution, there was a dose-dependent protection by D_2O against the cytotoxicity of the 43°C exposure. Why 100% D_2O substitution resulted in less protection than that seen with 70% is not understood, but may reflect a lethal effect of D_2O not related to its protective function. Curiously, the latter phenomenon was observable only at 43°C; at 45°C the presence of D_2O also protected cells, and 100% D_2O protected more than 70%. Other unpublished experiments showed that the D_2O needed to be present during heating. D_2O administered either immediately or for several hours before or after heating had no protective effect, provided that during heating the medium contained D_2O. The results could be interpreted to show that 100% D_2O shifted the heat response of these cells by 2°. In other words, the same level of cytotoxicity seen in H_2O medium at 43°C was seen at 45°C in medium with 100% D_2O. In this sense, D_2O acts as a true temperature-modifying agent.

2.5.3.2. Hydrostatic Pressure

Increased hydrostatic pressure can also protect against heat-induced damage. This is shown in Figure 2.11. In this experiment cells were exposed to 45°C for 1 hr inside a pressure vessel. It can be seen that pressure is very effective in protecting cell survival. Because of equipment limitations, the experiment was not extended above 3000 p.s.i., but in the range of 0 to 3000 p.s.i. there was a more or less linear increase in the logarithm of the surviving fraction as pressure was increased.

2.6. SURVIVAL OF CELLS EXPOSED TO MULTIPLE HEAT TREATMENTS

When cells are exposed to heat more than once, their responses to doses other than the first depend on several factors. Those of major importance are: (1) recovery from sublethal or potentially lethal injuries, and the possible interactions of remnant lesions with those newly inflicted; (2) redistribution of cells in the cell cycle and the resulting change in heat sensitivity of the cell population; (3) thermotolerance, i.e., heat-induced resistance in part or all of the cell population. I will now examine each

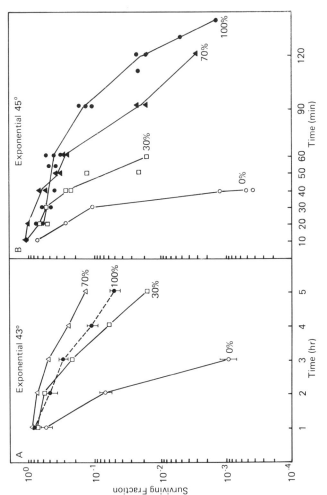

Figure 2.10. Protection against heat-induced cytotoxicity by deuterium oxide. Exponentially growing HA–1 cells were exposed to 43 (A) or 45°C (B) in media in which the H_2O had been replaced by D_2O to the indicated percentage. In all cases the percent replacement refers to the medium (without serum) only; 15% serum, which had not been dialyzed against D_2O, was added to all cultures. Protection is seen at all D_2O replacement levels. The somewhat reduced protection at 100% replacement in panel A is anomalous, and indicates that the D_2O action is complex. Data from Fisher *et al.* (1982).

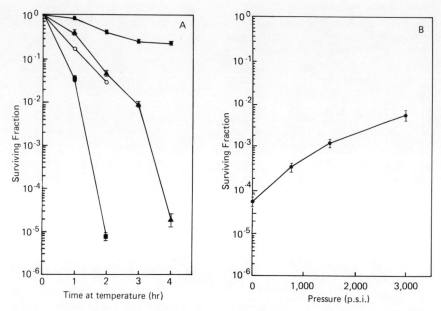

Figure 2.11. Protection against heat-induced cytotoxicity by increased hydrostatic pressure. Panel A: HA–1 cells were heated for the time indicated on the abscissa, either unpressurized or pressurized. ▲: 42.9°, unpressurized; ●: 42.9°, 2500 p.s.i.; ■: 43.7°, unpressurized; ○: 43.7°, 3000 p.s.i. Panel B: HA–1 cells were exposed to 44.0°C for 90 min at pressures ranging up to 3000 p.s.i. In both panels, the increased survival at elevated pressures is a measure of the protection afforded against heat-induced damage. Data from Minton *et al.* (1980), with permission.

of these factors individually, although as I will demonstrate, separation of recovery effects from the development of thermotolerance is not easy.

2.6.1. Recovery Phenomena

Most survival curves obtained from cells exposed at constant elevated temperatures for different durations of time show an initial shoulder. While the shoulder may in part result from artifacts, particularly the time required for a culture to reach the equilibrium temperature, it is very likely that for most experimental conditions the shoulders on the survival curves imply an ability of the cells to sustain a level of damage. Since this damage does not lead to cell lethality, it is called sublethal. Recovery from sublethal damage after exposure of cells to, for example, ionizing radiation, has been studied in great detail (Elkind *et al.*, 1967). In general, irradiated cells recover between adjacent doses. This is shown by a reduced cytotoxicity of the "split" dose as compared to a single irradiation. The differences in observed survivals are related to the width of the shoulder of the survival curve. When attempts were made to do similar split-dose experiments, after heat exposure it was found that not only did cells recover, but they "overrecovered," that is the cells appeared to be much more resistant to the second dose than they were to the first. This overrecovery has been termed "thermotolerance" (Section 2.6.2.). Because of the occurrence of thermotolerance during the time that recovery from sublethal damage might be expected to happen, the question of whether or not the cells recover from sublethal damage or if thermotolerance is a totally unrelated phenomenon is difficult to answer. There appears to be only one system in which the two phenomena (thermotolerance and recovery from sublethal damage) could be separated. Nielsen and Overgaard (1979) performed two-fraction experiments on L182 ascites cells. They exposed these cells to two 42°C exposures, each one of 1.5-hr duration, with a variable interval at 37°C between treatments. While they also showed the overrecovery phenomenon, in their hands maximum expression of thermotolerance did not occur until the fractionation interval was 10 hr. During the first 4 hr of separation of the two doses, the shape of the survival curve indicated that the measured increase in survival resulted almost exclusively from restoration of the shoulder. Thermotolerance did not seem to become appreciable until about 6 hr. Thus, in these cells there appeared to be recovery from heat-induced sublethal damage.

Multiple-fraction experiments were also performed by Palzer and Heidelberger (1973). They found that fractionating the dose was less efficient in cell killing than giving the dose without fractionation. On the basis of these results they concluded that recovery from sublethal damage did occur. However, their results very likely were also influenced by the development of thermotolerance, so that their conclusion may not have been warranted.

Another type of recovery of X-irradiated cells has been termed "repair of potentially lethal damage." This recovery is defined operationally by changes in survival induced by modification of the cells' environment after treatment (Phillips and Tolmach, 1966). Recovery is said to occur if increases in survival are seen over that obtained by a specified, standard treatment. Again Palzer and Heidelberger were the first to turn their attention to quantifying possible repair of potentially lethal, heat-induced damage. They exposed HeLa cells to 43°C for 3 hr and then added inhibitors of DNA synthesis (2 mM thymidine) or protein synthesis (cycloheximide, 1 ug/ml). In the presence of either drug survival increased

by 100 to 200% over controls. Survival increased with increasing duration
of application of the inhibitors. Thus they concluded that heated HeLa
cells could recover from potentially lethal damage.

Plateau phase cells were used by Li *et al.* (1980a) to measure recovery
from potentially lethal damage. Cells were heated (43°C) in the density-
inhibited state. The survival of some of the treated cells was assayed
immediately by trypsinization followed by replating at much lower cell
densities. Other cells were maintained in the density-inhibited state for
various lengths of time so that recovery could take place, and survival
was assayed at preselected time points. The methods used by Palzer and
Heidelberger (1973) and by Li *et al.* have one thing in common: proliferation following exposure is inhibited for various lengths of time, either
by the presence of a metabolic inhibitor, or by the maintenance of density
inhibition. In plateau phase cells recovery also occurred but only under
very restricted conditions. First of all, the survival level in cells explanted
immediately after heating had to exceed about 10^{-3}. If cell killing exceeded that level no recovery was observed, as shown in Figure 2.12. In
the experiment whose results are depicted in that figure, survival was
measured immediately after heating and 24 hr later. Maximum recovery
was seen after an exposure of about 120 min. After 24 hr the survival

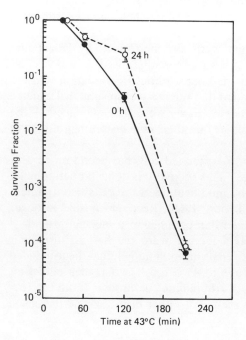

Figure 2.12. Recovery from heat-induced potentially lethal damage. Plateau phase HA–1 cells were heated in
medium supplemented with 15% fetal
calf serum. Temperature and time were
as indicated. Cells were either explanted immediately after the heat exposure (closed symbols) or 24 hr later
(open symbols). Recovery was observed only if the survival level was
in the range of 10^0 to 10^{-3}. Heating
in media without serum or in a buff-
ered balanced salt solution, prevented any subsequent recovery. Data
from Li *et al.* (1980a), with permission.

increased from about 2×10^{-2} to about 2×10^{-1}, i.e., a factor of 10. On the other hand, when heating was carried out for 210 min, survival was 10^{-4}, both in the cells explanted immediately and in those maintained in the density-inhibited state for 24 hr. At the lower survival level, no recovery from potentially lethal damage was seen. Whether or not recovery occurred also depended on both the nutrient conditions during the initial treatment and the milieu in which recovery was allowed to proceed. Cells heated in Hanks' Balanced Salt Solution showed little or no recovery. After heating in medium, cells maintained at a pH of 7.5 showed greater recovery than those maintained at a pH of 7.0. In these aspects, recovery from potentially lethal heat damage is very different from recovery from damage inflicted by X irradiation. There maximum recovery is seen if cells are irradiated and then maintained in the balanced salt solution. Furthermore, pH effects are minimal and the amount of recovery observed after X irradiation is dose-dependent—the more damage, the more recovery.

2.6.2. Thermotolerance

Perhaps one of the most intriguing aspects of thermal biology is the finding that one nonlethal heat treatment of mammalian cells can modify, and at times drastically so, their subsequent response to elevated temperatures. This phenomenon has already been alluded to several times.

2.6.2.1. Nomenclature

The change in heat response induced by the initial heat treatment has been variously called *induced thermal resistance*, *thermal tolerance*, or *thermotolerance*. The term induced thermal resistance is perhaps the most precise; however, Gerner (personal communication) points out that it may have a possibly unwarranted, mechanistic connotation. Resistance induced in prokaryotes by ionizing or by UV radiation is associated with *de novo* synthesis of a specific enzyme or enzyme system. No evidence exists that such a process is involved in the development of resistance to heat. Hence, Gerner suggests it might therefore be desirable to use a term not implying such a specific mechanism. On the other hand, tolerance dose has a specific connotation to radiotherapists. In clinical terminology it defines the maximum dose that can be given to normal tissue without running excessive risks of causing either acute or chronic damage to normal tissue. Therefore the term thermal tolerance may also involve a misleading connotation. Furthermore, heat does induce the synthesis of new proteins (so-called heat shock proteins). Although no evidence exists definitely linking them to heat resistance, such an association cannot be ruled out. The term resistance is more descriptive than is tolerance, and for this reason my own personal preference would be to continue using induced thermal resistance. However, by now thermotolerance has become accepted in the literature and I will continue to use this term.

2.6.2.2. Definition of Thermotolerance

Not only nomenclature, but also the operational definition of thermotolerance involves some difficulty. Henle and Dethlefsen (1978) define thermotolerance exclusively in terms of the change in slope of the heat survival curve. This might be useful from the viewpoint of molecular biology, but it is an excessively restricted definition for practical considerations. Neither the patient nor the therapist is too concerned whether a tumor becomes heat resistant because of changes in the slope or in the width of the shoulder of the survival curve obtained from the cells that make up the tumor. For this reason and others to be discussed in Chapter 4, I will define thermotolerance as any heat-induced increase in heat resistance, whether the shoulder or the terminal slope of the survival curve is affected. Thermotolerance must be transient; the genetically transmitted heat resistance as described by Harris (1980) is specifically excluded. Again, there are both practical and theoretical reasons for doing so. Heat resistance permanently affects a cell line or a tumor. No amount of clever timing can bypass such resistance. On the other hand, thermotolerance decays sufficiently rapidly so that its effects can be circumvented by appropriate fractionation. It is also possible that entirely different molecular events govern thermotolerance than govern genetically determined resistance.

Operationally, there are at least two ways by which heating can induce thermotolerance. It can be done *via* continuous heating at relatively low temperatures (42.5°C or less for most cell lines) or by heat-dose fractionation at temperatures from 39 to 47°C or higher. Obviously, this latter method works over a much wider temperature range than the former. The two- (or more) fraction regimen must be interrupted by culture of the cells at or near physiological temperatures.

2.6.2.3. Experimental Demonstration of Thermotolerance

Probably the first indication of induction of thermolerance by continuous heating of mammalian cells comes from the work of Palzer and Heidelberger (1973). These authors heated cells at 42°C, and demonstrated the development of the resistant "tail" of the survival curve. They clearly

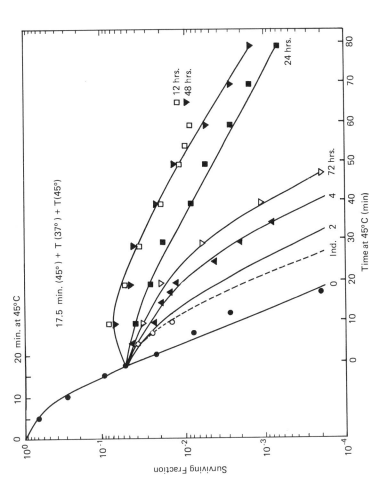

Figure 2.13. Induction of thermotolerance. CHO cells were heated to 45°C for 17.5 min and then returned to 37°C incubation. At the times shown in the graphs, they were then exposed to a second 45° dose for the time indicated on the abscissa. Survival expected if complete recovery from sublethal damage had taken place is shown by the dotted line. Actual survival greatly exceeded the expected values. Cells showing heat-induced resistance to heat are said to be thermotolerant. Data from Henle and Leeper (1976), with permission.

identified the transient nature of the phenomenon, by pointing to "numerous unsuccessful attempts to produce an enrichment of cells resistant to hyperthermic killing in mixed populations that had survived prolonged exposure to 42°C." As the most likely explanation for their findings, they postulated a selection of phenotypically resistant cells, possibly occupants of a particularly heat-resistant part of the cell cycle. Thus, while they demonstrated the existence of the phenomenon, they erred in interpreting it.

The first two-fraction experiment that rather clearly showed the induction of thermotolerance was also not interpreted as such (Westra, 1971). Similarly, Gerweck and Dewey (1975) interpreted what appeared to be "overrepair" as a combination of repair from sublethal damage plus progression of cells into a heat-resistant part of the cell cycle.

It remained for Henle and Leeper (1976) and Gerner and Schneider (1976) to show conclusively that the resistance induced in the cells by one heat exposure exceeded any result to be expected either from recovery from sublethal damage or from progression of cells into a resistant part of the cell cycle or from a combination of these. Results from Henle and Leeper are shown in Figure 2.14. Cells were given an initial exposure of 45°C for 17.5 min and then incubated at 37°C for graded intervals. At the end of that time, the cells were given another exposure to 45°C that varied between 0 and 80 min. On the graph are also shown the expected survival values if complete recovery of sublethal damage occurred. What is very clear is that not only has recovery from sublethal damage possibly occurred, but that survival has increased dramatically over and beyond that expected from full recovery. After 30 min of exposure, complete recovery would have resulted in survival of the two heat treatments of somewhere in the neighborhood of 10^{-4}. However, if between 12 and 48 hr intervened between the two exposures, survival was well above 10^{-2}. In other words, the initial 17.5 min exposure at 45°C resulted in reduced cell killing twelve hr later by a factor of better than 100. By 72 hr, there was still a remnant of resistance noticeable, but the survival curve much more resembles that of the initial cell population. Henle and Leeper (1976) were also able to show that if the incubation temperature between the two doses was a temperature other than 37°C, very different survival kinetics were obtained. For example, if the incubation temperature was 40°C, a reduction rather than an increase in survival was observed. This observation has led to the definition of a new term, "step-down" heating (no new field of science seems to be happy without its specialized jargon), i.e., heating for short times at high temperatures followed by longer exposures at temperatures below 42.5°C. Incubation at 0°C completely blocked the development of thermotolerance, but did not reduce survival.

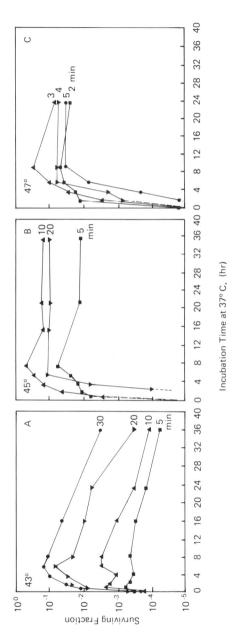

Figure 2.14. Kinetics of induction of thermotolerance. Plateau phase cultures of HA-1 cells were exposed to temperatures of 43° to 47°C for the times indicated in each graph. The cells were then returned to 37° incubation for the times indicated on the abscissas, and at that time given a uniform second treatment (45°; 45 min). Survival variations therefore reflect the induction of thermotolerance after the conditioning dose. There is no indication of any development of tolerance during the initial heating period. Data from Li *et al.* (1982b), with permission.

Both the duration and the temperatures required for the induction of this resistance to heat have been investigated. Of major interest are the kinetics of induction of thermotolerance, the temperature dependence of the rate at which the phenomenon can be induced, the time and temperature required for its initiation, and finally the rate of disappearance of tolerance. These factors appear to be interrelated. For example, in CHO cells, Henle *et al.* (1978) have shown that the D_0 of cells initially exposed for 5 min to 45°C rose to a maximum of about 11 min (versus about 3 min for controls) 2 hr after the conditioning doses. However, if the treatment was 10 min at 45°C, the development of thermotolerance appeared to be both somewhat delayed in time and more effective. The peak of resistance occurred now at 8 hr, with a D_0 of 15 min (i.e., 5 times that of the control value). These investigators also looked at the behavior of the extrapolation number of survival curves from preheated cell populations. A 10-min exposure to 45°C raised the extrapolation number from about 3 to about 14 within 2 hr. It then dropped back to the control value by approximately 5 hr. This interchange, the rapid increase in extrapolation number in the early period followed by a large increase in apparent D_0 raises the possibility that the "D_0" in these experiments really only related to the initial portion of the survival curve and that the terminal portion (which would give the "true" D_0) was never reached.

As far as the minimum temperature required for the induction of thermal tolerance is concerned, Henle *et al.* and Joshi and Jung (1979) were able to show that some resistance could be induced even by temperatures as low as 38°C.

Rather remarkable changes in survival parameters owing to the induction of thermotolerance were demonstrated by Li and Hahn (1980a) and Li *et al.* (1982b). Chinese hamster cells (HA-1) were grown to plateau phase. In this density-inhibited state there is very little proliferation (Hahn and Little, 1972); hence, cell cycle effects are minimized. Almost 90% of the cells have the 2C DNA content of G1 cells. Plateau phase cultures were given conditioning treatments at temperatures ranging from 43 to 47°C and for periods that varied between 2 and 30 min. Some of the cells were then challenged immediately by a second treatment at 45°C (45 min). The others were returned to 37°C for 2 to 30 hr and then given a similar exposure. Survival of the 45°C (45 min) treatment in the absence of preheat, was about 6×10^{-5}. At the completion of the conditioning dose, no evidence of thermotolerance was seen. But, as can be seen from Figure 2.15, survival of this same dose changed to almost 100% in cells that had been exposed 4 hr earlier to a conditioning dose of 45° (20 min). It is difficult to think to another biological event where an apparently minor treatment can cause such a tremendous modification of survival kinetics!

Another interesting feature of Figure 2.14 is the interrelationship between the duration and the temperature of the conditioning dose required to achieve a given level of thermotolerance. Typically, a reduction of one degree requires a doubling of the duration to achieve a similar effect. This is very reminiscent of the cell killing results, where a similar time-duration relationship was observed.

Below 43°C the induction of thermotolerance behaves very differently. Li *et al.* (1982b) performed experiments exactly like those discussed in the previous paragraph, except that the temperature of the initial treatment was reduced to 41 and 42°C, and the duration of the exposure was increased up to 240 min. Data are shown in Figure 2.15. Obviously, both the kinetics of induction, as well as the times required for this induction, were very different at these lower temperatures. Thermotolerance had developed almost completely during the conditioning dose. It is noteworthy that the time–temperature relationship observed for conditioning doses given above 43°C also holds for those at lower temperatures. However, between 42 and 43°C, a major change in response occurs, so that between those specific temperatures that relationship between time and temperature fails to hold.

If the conditioning dose was at temperatures below 43°, quite different results are seen. As was shown in Figure 2.15 immediately upon com-

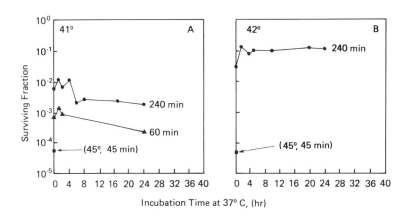

Figure 2.15. Kinetics of the induction of thermal tolerance. Plateau phase cultures of HA–1 cells were treated as described in Figure 2.14, except that the temperature of the initial treatment was reduced to either 41 or 42°C. Note that for each curve, survival was essentially at its maximum at 0 time, showing that thermotolerance had developed during heating. Note also the long durations of the initial treatments (60–240 min). Data from Li *et al.* (1982b), with permission.

pletion of an initial incubation at 41°C, cells show what is essentially maximum thermal tolerance. These results can be modified somewhat by varying environmental conditions. This subject is currently under considerable study. For example, Gerweck (1977) has shown that development of thermal tolerance *via* continuous heating can be delayed at pH below 7.4; while Nielsen and Overgaard (1979) have indicated that pH can also affect induction and expression of split-dose tolerance. Similarly, Li and Hahn (1980a) have shown that nutrient effects can somewhat modulate the expression of thermal tolerance. However, the general characteristics of induction and development of thermotolerance proceeds over a wide range of external conditions.

2.6.2.4. Step-Down Heating

If, after an initial conditioning exposure at 43°C (or higher), cells are immediately tested for their heat responses at various temperatures, results of the type shown in Figure 2.16 are observed. When the second treatment is at 42.5° or lower, this type of experiment is referred to as "step-down" heating (Henle *et al.*, 1978). In panel B the conditioning exposure was at 45°C for 10 min, while panel A shows control curves of HA-1 cells not exposed to any preheating. The survival curves shown in panel B are exponential, i.e., without shoulders. The slopes of the curves obtained at temperatures of 43°C or higher is similar to that of unheated controls (A). What is interesting is that at temperatures below 43°C, the curves are also exponential, do not show the characteristic, resistant "tail" seen in many experiments done with previously unheated cells, and are much steeper. The ability of a high-temperature pulse to sensitize cells to a later exposure at lower temperatures is obvious when the results are compared to survival curves of cells not previously heated (A). However, this "step-down" heating has no effect on cells previously made thermotolerant; specifically, a high temperature pulse does not abolish the thermotolerance developed earlier. This is shown in Figure 2.17.

2.6.2.5. Decay of Tolerance

A subject that has not been discussed at all is the rate of decay of tolerance. This topic is obviously of considerable concern, because the effects of fractionated heat treatments clearly depend, in part, upon the kinetics of the disappearance of tolerance. Initially, experiments by Gerner *et al.* (1979) indicated that thermal tolerance was only associated with that gen-

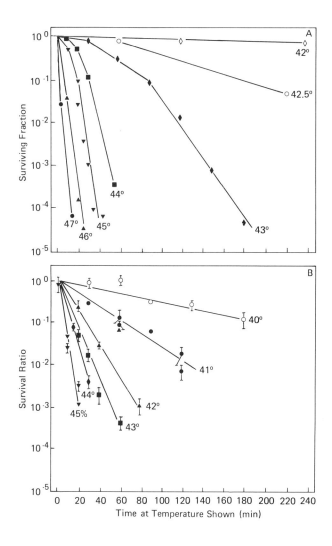

Figure 2.16. Step-down heating: survival of cells following a 45°C exposure. Plateau phase HA–1 cells were heated to 45°C for either 0 (A) or 20 min (B). The cells were then immediately exposed to the indicated temperatures for the times shown on the abscissas of each panel. The differences between the curves in panels A and B are twofold: no shoulders are seen in survival curves from the preheated cells, and the slopes of curves obtained from preheated cells subsequently exposed to temperatures below 43°C are markedly steeper than those from control cells. Unpublished data from Li and Hahn.

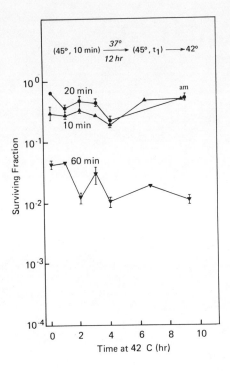

Figure 2.17. Survival kinetics of thermotolerant cells following a 45°C exposure. Plateau phase HA–1 cells were made thermotolerant by exposing them to 45°C (10 min) and returning them to the incubator for 12 hr. They were then subjected to a "step-down" procedure as in Figure 2.16. However, the high-temperature (45°C) pulse did not abolish thermotolerance, as shown by the resistance to 42°C heating, thus showing that thermotolerant cells are not subject to stepdown sensitization. Unpublished data from Li and Hahn.

eration of cells in which it had been induced. In HeLa cells, division immediately abolished the thermotolerant state. In other cells this has not been found to be the case. For example, Chinese hamster cells (HA-1) as well as EMT6 mouse sarcoma cells were able to pass thermotolerance on to daughter cells, although the level of tolerance in daughter cells appeared to be reduced (Sanchez and Hahn, unpublished). Division was not required for the loss of thermotolerance, since in plateau phase cells there was also a gradual disappearance of the tolerant state (Gerner *et al.*, 1979; Li and Hahn, 1980a). Obviously in such density-inhibited cultures, which show very little mitotic activity, loss of resistance could not have been associated with cell division. One way of attempting to assess the importance of proliferation in affecting the rate of decay of tolerance is to compare directly tolerance kinetics in actively growing and in density-inhibited cultures. Results of such an experiment with EMT6 cells are shown in Figure 2.18. Clearly, induction of tolerance was very similar in the two cultures. Decay was somewhat slower in the density-inhibited state. Since decay of tolerance is not affected by pH or by nutritional environments, the more rapid decay rate in actively proliferating cultures very likely reflects the influence of cell division.

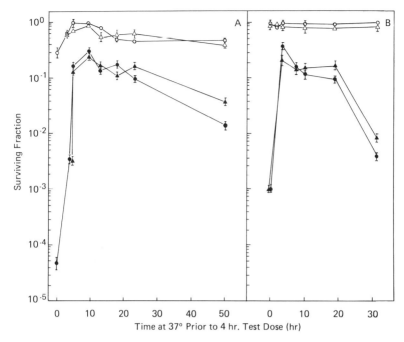

Figure 2.18. Decay of thermotolerance in proliferating or in nonproliferating cells. EMT6 cells, either in the plateau (A) or the exponential growing (B) phase were exposed to a conditioning dose of 43°C (2 hr). The cells were returned for incubation at 37° at either pH 7.4 (circles) or pH 7.0 (triangles) for the times indicated on the abscissa. At the indicated time, cells were then either explanted to assay survival (open symbols) or given a 4-hr dose of 43°C (closed symbols). The closed symbols therefore indicate the kinetics of induction and decay of tolerance. pH is seen to have little if any effect on the kinetics; the rate of induction of tolerance seems also to be independent of proliferative state. However, decay of tolerance appears to proceed more rapidly in proliferating cultures. Unpublished data from Sanchez and Hahn.

The data presented in Figure 2.18 show that both cultures retain a level of thermotolerance for at least 30 hr and probably somewhat longer. The reduced rate of disappearance of resistance in plateau phase cultures if found to apply to other cell lines may have useful clinical consequences, since it my indicate that some normal, slowly proliferating tissue retain tolerance to a greater degree than the more rapidly proliferating tumor cells.

2.6.2.6. A Model

Li and Hahn (1980a) have proposed an operational model for the dissection of what appears to be a complicated body of phenomena currently lumped under the thermotolerance label. They suggest that there are three individual and separate effects involved. The first is the induction of thermal tolerance ("trigger"). This is followed by the expression (development) and finally the decay of tolerance. The trigger of tolerance can occur at any temperature above the normal growth temperature of the cells and indeed may be occurring there also, since obviously "tolerance" is a relative term. However, its expression occurs only in the limited range of temperatures, namely between 37 and 41°C. (The numbers used here are for Chinese hamster HA-1 cells normally grown at 37°C; it is quite possible, indeed probable, that other temperatures are appropriate for other cell lines, as is indicated, for example, by the results of Nielsen and Overgaard (1979), who suggest that L182 cells do not develop thermotolerance at 42°C.) Some decay of thermal tolerance occurs immediately upon the initiation of development. Induction (or triggering), development (or expression), and decay may all have their unique temperature, pH, and nutrient dependence. Under certain circumstances, the phenomena can be examined individually. For example, in medium in which D_2O replaces H_2O, triggering occurs but the expression of thermotolerance is suppressed (Li, Fisher, and Hahn, unpublished).

This model has some practical and theoretical implications. From a practical point of view, it would explain the otherwise difficult to understand experiment involving fractionated hyperthermic treatments at 38°C followed by 45°C ("step-up") or the reverse order ("step-down"), such as those reported by Henle et al. (1978) and by Joshi and Jung (1979). The latter authors found that an exposure of cells to 38°C protected against an immediate subsequent exposure to 45°C; on the other hand, pre-exposure to 45°C sensitized cells to subsequent exposures to 41°C. The interpretation of these results in terms of the model presented by Li and Hahn (1980a) would be that during the 38°C exposure there was both an induction and an expression of thermal tolerance; therefore, at the time of exposure to 45°C, the cells were already thermotolerant and protected. On the other hand, an earlier exposure of 45°C, while inducing a trigger, postponed the subsequent development of thermal tolerance. Hence, the cells then exposed to 41°C were considerably more sensitive. The theoretical implications are discussed in Chapter 4. I point out here that both Joshi and Jung, as well as Henle et al., interpreted their results in terms of the interaction either of different types of damage or of potentially lethal lesions, while the emphasis is placed by Li and Hahn on the role of tolerance.

I have already pointed out several times that in addition to the very intriguing biological aspects of thermal tolerance, the phenomenon may have considerable clinical importance. Hyperthermia of tumors invariably involves attempts to manipulate treatment parameters in such a way as to maximize damage to the tumor while not exceeding the tolerance level of critical normal tissue. Obviously, any treatment that can modify cell survival by many orders of magnitude must be taken into account in considering attempts at hyperthermic eradication of solid malignancies. On the one hand, if normal tissue and tumor are affected equally, the only aspect of treatment that really needs to be considered is the modification of heat dose. This would still be important because temperature and duration of individual treatments would have to be adjusted to compensate for the development of tolerance. On the other hand, if either the development or the decay of tolerance were different in normal tissue than in tumors, advantage could be taken of such differences by timing fractions to coincide with periods where the tumor is relatively less protected than the normal tissue. Also, if the development of thermotolerance could be shown to be a feature associated with all normal tissue, it would not seem difficult to elevate the temperature of particularly critical organs to, say 41°C without raising the tumor temperature. This could be accomplished by appropriate geometric isolation of the deposition of energy. After a period that would permit the development of thermotolerance in the heated tissue, tumor treatment would be carried out with the tumor at normal sensitivity to hyperthermia and the normal tissue protected by the previous heat exposure. Obviously, the reverse condition could lead to treatment disaster. This two-edged aspect of thermotolerance will surely be investigated in considerable detail in the near future.

2.7. SUMMATION

Most mammalian cells are rapidly inactivated at temperatures above 41 to 42°C. The shape of the survival curve depends upon the temperature: survival curves from cells exposed to temperatures below 42°C have a resistant "tail", whereas from cells exposed to temperatures greater than 43°C, they do not. Values of D_0s for inactivation at 44.5° and at pH 7.4 range from about 4 to 25 min, the high values being associated with the few stable, heat-resistant variants isolated to date. Many temperature-sensitive mutants have been found whose heat response places them at the lower limit of the quoted sensitivities.

The attractive hypothesis that malignant cells are frequently or even invariably more heat sensitive than their normal counterparts is not borne out by existing data. While, to be sure, several reports indicate that malignancy and heat sensitivity are correlated, an equal number of investigations dispute this. Furthermore, among malignant strains derived from a common source, no correlation has been found between degree of malignancy and heat sensitivity.

When looking for other determinants of heat sensitivity, the data on ploidy and on growth stage are contradictory; hence it is unlikely that these are the primary factors that determine heat sensitivity. Experiments on synchronized cells have shown that cells in early or mid G1 are the most heat resistant, while mitotic cells and those in late S are particularly sensitive.

The heat senstitivity of cells can be modulated by relatively minor changes in their surroundings. Low pH, reduced serum, and chronic oxygen or glucose deprivation all act to make cells highly heat sensitive. These factors are by no means independent. For example, cells in medium without serum are much less affected by pH changes; on the other hand, oxygen-deprived cells are much more sensitive to changes in glucose availability. Thus it is very likely that one metabolic pathway is affected by all these factors, and that this pathway somehow modulates heat sensitivity. Both D_2O and elevated pressures during heat are capable of reversing a limited amount of heat effects.

Multiple exposures of cells to heat involve recovery phenomena as well as the induction of thermotolerance. These factors are difficult to test individually. Thermotolerance manifests itself immediately upon the completion of heating below 43°C; above that temperature a sojurn at or near 37°C is required. Both the shoulder and the slope of the survival curve may reflect the development of the resistant state. Decay of tolerance takes up to 72 hr or longer; induction is much more rapid, requiring at most about 8 hr. Recovery from sublethal damage (restoration of the shoulder) very likely occurs also, though its unequivocal demonstration is not easy. Recovery from potentially lethal damage is observed only in the presence of adequate nutrients and then only if the survival level does not go below about 10^{-3}.

3

Thermal Enhancement of the Actions of Anticancer Agents

3.1. INTRODUCTION

It is hardly surprising that heat increases the rate at which some drugs inactivate cells. For example, one would readily predict that any cytotoxic reaction not governed by enzymatic or permeability limitations would follow an Arrhenius type law, i.e., the rate constant governing the reaction would increase more or less exponentially with temperature. Indeed, the killing of cells by several agents behaves in this manner (e.g., the nitrosoureas). Furthermore, it is not unreasonable to suspect that drugs whose entry into the cell is limited by membrane permeabilities might find it easier to enter the cell at higher temperature, since permeabilities to most substances are increased with temperature. The temperature dependence of the action of such agents would not necessarily follow Arrhenius kinetics. Again, examples of such behavior can be found (e.g., adriamycin).

On the other hand, there is no reason *a priori* to suspect that the direct actions of other modalities, X irradiation for example, are necessarily modified by mild heat. The ultimate survival of cells is, however, determined not only by the damage done during exposure, but also by subsequent enzymatic repair. Hence, heat damage to specific proteins might be reflected as reduced survival. Evidence, though indirect, bears out this expectation. Additionally, some effects of heat on drug action have been found that could not be predicted from known effects of drug action. Because of the variety of the interactions between heat and anticancer agents, this field is very intriguing, not only because of the potentials for clinical application, but also because of the wide range of biological phenomena involved. Curiously, except for the interaction of X rays and heat, the subject has received little attention from either cell biologists or cancer chemotherapists.

3.2. THERMAL ENHANCEMENT OF RADIATION SENSITIVITY

Since X irradiation is currently the second most important means of cancer treatment (next to surgery), it is not surprising that in the last few years investigators have quite carefully examined the interaction of ionizing irradiations with hyperthermia. It has now been demonstrated amply that the cytotoxic effects of low LET (linear energy transfer) radiations are magnified if irradiation is carried out at elevated temperatures. Two early studies (Belli and Bonte, 1963; Smith and McKinley, 1967), although primarily concerned with the temperature range of 0 to 37°C, did indicate that at higher temperatures synergistic effects might be expected. For example, Smith and McKinley (1967) investigated the ability of irradiated and heated bone marrow cells to take up ^{59}Fe after these cells were injected into unirradiated hosts. This ability was blocked completely if cells irradiated with 100 rad had previously been kept at 40°C for 6 hr. Irradiation alone had much less of an effect, while heat alone was completely ineffective.

Since these studies, a large number of investigations have greatly extended these rather tentative observations (Westra and Dewey, 1971; Ben-Hur *et al.*, 1972; 1974; Robinson and Wizenberg, 1974; Harisiadis *et al.*, 1975, 1978; Joshi *et al.*, 1977). The findings more or less agree. Typical features found are illustrated in Figure 3.1, from the work of Robinson and Wizenberg (1974). Heating shortly before, during, or immediately after X irradiation modifies both the extrapolation number and the D_0 of

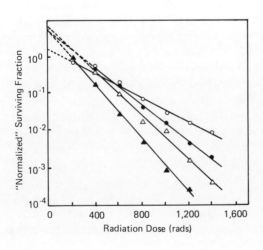

Figure 3.1. Radiation survival curves for Chinese hamster cells subjected to thermal treatment (2 hr before, during, and after irradiation). Irradiation was timed so as to be during the middle of the heating period. The curves are normalized to a surviving fraction of 1.0 at zero radiation dose. Note that heating before, during, and immediately after X irradiation modifies both the extrapolation number and the D_0 of the X-ray survival curves. ○: 40°C; ●: 42.0°C; △: 42.5°C; ▲: 43.0°C. Data from Robinson and Wizenberg (1974) with permission.

the X-ray survival curve. Both of these are reduced, even when cell killing data are corrected for the cytotoxicity of heat in the absence of irradiation. There seems to be little question that heating during rather than before or after irradiation maximizes cell killing (Sapareto *et al.*, 1979). Whether heating is more effective before or after irradiation depends upon the cell line examined. This is illustrated by Figure 3.2, taken from the work of Li and Kal (1977). Two cell lines, a Chinese hamster line (HA-1) and a tissue-culture-adapted mouse sarcoma line (EMT6), were heated to 43°C and irradiated with graded doses of X rays. For the HA-1 cells, irradiation after heating was most cytotoxic; for EMT6 the reverse order resulted in least cell survival. In these experiments conditions were standardized, so that the only variables were the cell line and the order of treatments; obviously no generalizations can be made.

3.2.1. Upper Limit of Heat Sensitization

Several of the studies cited have shown that in general, increased exposure at any one temperature or increased temperature at a fixed duration of thermal exposure increases the magnitude of the interaction of X rays and heat. What has not been completely answered is whether or not there is an upper limit to the effect of heat on radiosensitivity (saturation). Three sets of data are pertinent to this point (Loshek *et al.*, 1977a, b; Sapareto *et al.*, 1979; unpublished data of Li and Hahn). I will start with the results of Loshek *et al.* These investigators define as the interaction coefficient the ratio of the slopes of the survival curves with and without heat. This quantity is more frequently called *thermal enhancement ratio* (TER) by other investigators. The slopes were measured in the log-linear portion of survival curves of CHO cells. A plot of the interaction coefficient *vs.* the duration of exposure at 42 and 43°C is shown in Figure 3.3. The authors interpret their results as showing no saturation. To quote them: "The value of the TER is dependent on the magnitude of the hyperthermia dose." In accordance with this interpretation, they draw a straight line to indicate a linear relationship in Figure 3.3. Their data only partially justify this; indeed, the TER increases linearly between 0 and 75 min. But longer exposures appear not to lead to concomitant increases in TER; thus, saturation seems indicated. This latter result is consistent with the data of Li and Hahn, Figure 3.4, obtained at 43°C. At that temperature, after 30 min of heating, the slope of the survival curves of X-irradiated HA-1 cells seem to reach a maximum value; beyond that, any additional killing is attributable to the increased exposure at 43°C.

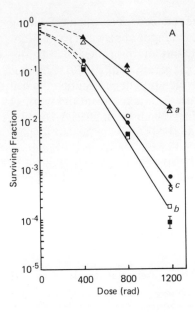

Figure 3.2. Dose response curves of two cell lines irradiated immediately before or after heating. Chinese hamster cells (HA–1, panel A) or mouse mammary sarcoma cells (EMT6, panel B) were exposed to the radiation dose indicated on the abscissa. Curve a: X ray only; curve b: X ray followed by 43°C, 60 min; curve c: X ray preceded by 43°C, 60 min. Note that treatment c is more effective against Chinese hamster cells, while (b) is more effective against the EMT6 cells. Two types of experiments were performed: cells were irradiated as single after trypsinization (open symbols) or in reverse order (closed symbols). Data from Li and Kal (1977), with permission.

The experiments become more difficult when the time of exposure is fixed and the temperature is increased. At the higher temperatures, cell killing by heat alone can become very appreciable and the shape of the X-ray curve becomes hard to establish with certainty. Hence, a comparison of slopes becomes equally difficult. Nevertheless, the results of Sapareto *et al.* (1979) do indicate that the amount of sensitization achievable is limited in this type of experiment also.

3.2.2. The Survival Surface

The survival analysis of heat–X ray interactions always involves three independent variables: X-ray dose, temperature, and duration of heat exposure. To accommodate at least two of these on one graph, Loshek *et al.* (1977a) define a survival surface. Duration of heat at fixed temperature is used as one axis, radiation dose as the other. Isosurvival values are plotted and connected, yielding a series of curves (e.g., Figure 3.4) whose general shape immediately indicates whether interactions do or do not occur and over what range of exposure durations or X-ray dose. By generating a survival surface at several different temperatures, presumably a survival "volume" could be developed, though I for one would not want to be the one to have to obtain all the data necessary for its construction!

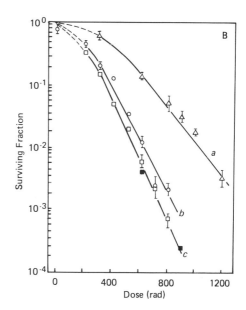

Figure 3.2. (*continued*)

3.2.3. X-Ray Sensitivity and Thermosensitization of Thermotolerant Cells

As discussed in the last chapter, an initial heat exposure causes cells to become resistant to subsequent heat exposures. Do these cells also then become resistant to X irradiation? Is the degree to which they are heat sensitized to X rays affected by the earlier heat dose? Obviously the answers to these questions are of great importance for the clinical use of hyperthermia during a course of fractionated radiotherapy. Somewhat surprisingly, to date these questions are not completely answered.

Nielsen and Overgaard (1979) examined the thermal enhancement of the radiosensitivity of L182 cells under two sets of conditions. In one set of experiments, cells were exposed to graded doses of X rays either at room temperature or halfway during a 90 min exposure at 42°C. The unheated cells had a D_0 of 117 rad, while for the heated cells this was reduced to 79 rad, for a TER of 1.5. In a companion experiment, this procedure was repeated, but the cells at risk had been exposed to 90 min at 42°C 10 hr earlier. These cells were demonstrated to be heat resistant. For these thermotolerant cells, the X-ray D_0s measured were 142 and 96 rad, respectively, yielding again an enhancement of 1.5. While it would appear that this study showed that thermotolerant cells are somewhat more resistant to X irradiation than unheated cells (D_0s of 142 *vs.* 117

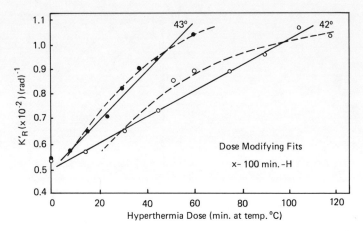

Figure 3.3. Radiation and heat (42 and 43°C) interaction; indication of saturation. V–79 Chinese hamster cells were irradiated to graded doses of 250 kV X rays at room temperature. 100 min later the cells were exposed to either 42 or 43°C for the durations shown on the abscissa. The "interaction coefficient" K'_R, i.e., the change in slope of the X-ray survival curve resulting from the heat exposure, is plotted on the ordinate. The data seem to be more consistent with the assumption that the coefficient approaches a maximum value as the exposure time increases (dotted line) (i.e., saturation) than with the assumption that the value of K'_R increases linearly with duration of the exposure. Data from Loshek *et al.* (1977b), with permission.

rad) this need not be the case. The first heat shock may have induced a partial synchrony among the surviving cells that may have caused cells 10 hr later to accumulate primarily in an X-ray-resistant compartment of the cell cycle, e.g., early G1. Since only the 10-hr point was examined, this remains an open question. The study did show clearly that the thermotolerant cells were sensitized to X irradiation by the second heat exposure, and that the degree of sensitization was the same as for the control cells.

Pertinent here are data presented by Miyakoshi *et al.* (1979). In this interesting work the interactions of 42, 44°C, and X irradiation were examined, using various sequences of exposures. Cells exposed to 42°C for 60 min, then to 44°C for 50 min, and finally X irradiated were slightly more resistant to the action of the ionizing radiations than were cells in which the order of heating was reversed. Now, 42°C is permissive for the development of thermotolerance, while 44°C prevents its occurrence for up to several hours (Li and Hahn, 1980b), even for cells transferred to 37°C. Thus, this experiment compares the X-ray sensitivities of tolerant and normal cells. Again it appeared that the thermotolerant cells were slightly more resistant than their unheated counterparts (change in D_0 of

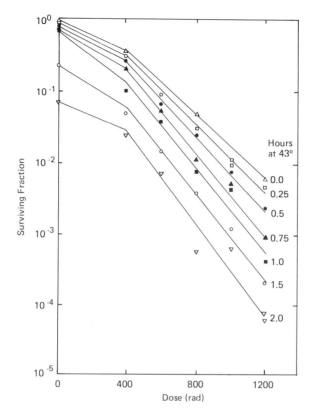

Figure 3.4. X-ray survival curves of cells exposed to 43°C. HA–1 cells were irradiated to the dose indicated on the abscissa and then immediately exposed to 43°C for the durations indicated. These results are also consistent with the assumption that the amount of sensitization that heat can effect approaches a maximum value. Data from Li and Hahn (unpublished).

~10%). However, the difference in X-ray sensitivities between normal and thermotolerant cells in both studies was small, certainly not mirroring the difference in heat response.

Finally, Henle *et al.* (1979) suggest that both radiosensitivity and thermal radiosensitization are affected in a major way by prior heat treatment. Cells (CHO) were heated (10 min, 45°C) and then returned to the 37°C incubator for 24 hr. At that time they were either immediately given graded doses of X ray or else heated (10 min, 45°C) and then X irradiated. The cells were more resistant to X irradiation than cells that had never been heated, and the degree of sensitization provided by the second heat pulse was reduced. This last study also suffers from the problem that only one time point was chosen, and therefore, the problem remains that heat-induced partial synchrony may have affected the results. It does seem likely from the results of these three studies that indeed heat can provide either sensitization or some protection against X irradiation, depending upon the time interval between the application of the two modalities, and perhaps depending upon the cell line examined.

The implications for therapy, assuming these conclusions are valid, are twofold. For multiple fractions in which both normal tumor and tissues are heated and irradiated to the same extent, the results indicate that an appropriate dose-modification factor must be chosen. Law *et al.* (1979) have shown that at least some heated and X-irradiated normal tissues behave very much the way cells do *in vitro*. Secondly, by clever preferential heating (to nontoxic levels) of critical normal tissue, it is quite conceivable that advantage can be taken of this phenomenon to provide a gain in relative tumor–normal tissue damage, i.e., in the therapeutic gain factor (TGF), not only for heating but also for X irradiation. The possible advantageous utilization of thermotolerance for the preferential protection of normal tissue is discussed more fully in Chapter 7.

3.2.4. Thermal Enhancement of the X-Ray Response of Normal and Malignant Cells

There is no reason *a priori* to assume that heat can make malignant cells more responsive to X irradiation than normal cells. Hope springs eternal, however, and in view of the greater heat sensitivity of malignant cells reported by some investigators, the possibility of greater X-ray enhancement seemed worth examining. Two studies show conflicting results. Kim *et al.* (1974) examined the thermal enhancement of "normal" 3T3 cells (a mouse fibroblast line cultured specifically in such a way as to show "contact inhibition" of mitosis) and HeLa cells, i.e., malignant cells of human origin. The X-ray response of the HeLa cells was appreciably enhanced by a 3-hr exposure at 42°C, while an equivalent treatment of 3T3 cells did not significantly modify their X-ray survival kinetics. However, 3T3 cells are not normal (e.g., their chromosome complement is quite different from that of normal mouse cells), and they are not human cells. This comparison of TERs is therefore not very meaningful. The other study (Harisiadis *et al.*, 1975), perhaps more relevant, involved a comparison of the enhancement by heat of X-ray sensitivities of normal rat liver cells *vs.* those of rat hepatoma cells. Heating was for 20 min at 43°C and was carried out before irradiation. The degree of sensitization observed for normal cells was not significantly different from that for the hepatoma cells.

While one can never completely rule out the possibility that heat can preferentially sensitize malignant cells, such a result would seem to be very fortuitous indeed. In any case, more studies are required before conclusions can be drawn.

3.2.5. Oxygen Enhancement Ratios

One of the most encouraging aspects of early reports on the hyper-thermic enhancement of X-ray responses involved hypoxic cells. It was suggested that hyperthermia sensitized such cells preferentially. Hypoxic cells are very resistant to X irradiation, and as many as 30% of cells of untreated murine tumors may be hypoxic. Poorly oxygenated cells are also thought to be responsible for many failures in radiotherapeutic treat-ments of human neoplasms. Elaborate schemes for dealing with these *bêtes noires* have been suggested and, at times, tried: placing the patient in hyperbaric chambers; having patients breathe 95% oxygen–5% CO_2 mixtures; using densely ionizing (high LET) radiations, particularly neu-trons; and finally, employing electron-affinic drugs, currently in clinical trials, that act perhaps by mimicking the electron-acceptor role played by oxygen during X irradiation. None of these attempts have, until now, been entirely successful. Therefore, the suggestion that heat could reduce the oxygen enhancement ratio was very exciting.

Robinson *et al.* (1974b) exposed mouse bone marrow cells *in vitro* to 37.5, 42.5, and 43°C for 1 hr. X irradiation was carried out so that the durations of heat exposure before and after the X ray treatment were equal. The cells were either oxic, or made hypoxic by passing a mixture of high-purity nitrogen and 5% carbon dioxide over the cell suspensions, which were agitated periodically to assure gas equilibriation. Gas flow was maintained over the entire course of the experiment. Dramatic changes in OER were observed: 2.5 at 37.5°C, 1.7 at 42.5°C, and finally 1.4 at 43°C. Needless to say, these results were normalized for any killing due to heat alone.

A somewhat similar result was found by Kim *et al.* (1975a). These investigators used HeLa cells, which were also irradiated while in sus-pension. Heavily irradiated feeder cells were used to produce hypoxia. To each milliliter of medium containing cells whose colony-forming ability was to be assayed, the investigators added 3×10^6 dead cells. The hypoxia resulted from the metabolic utilization of available oxygen by the feeder layer cells during a 2-hr incubation at 37°C. (Oxic controls were treated in the absence of a layer of feeder cells.) Heating reduced the OER from 2.9 at 37°C to 1.6 at 42°C.

The results of these early optimistic studies have now been questioned by a very careful study by Power and Harris (1977). Both V-79 Chinese hamster cells and EMT6 mouse tumor cells were irradiated under precisely controlled conditions. The cells were made hypoxic using a technique initially described by Koch and Painter (1975); it involved careful degassing. The degree of hypoxia was labeled as "extreme." Both temperature and pH were monitored carefully. Hyperthermia was 43°C for 45 min, either before or after irradiation. Experiments were performed with cells either in suspension or in monolayers. The OER did not change for EMT6 cells; it *increased* (from 3.0 to 3.9) for the heated Chinese hamster cells. Another study, though not done with mammalian cells, is of interest here. Kiefer *et al.* (1976) examined the OER of X-irradiated diploid yeast over a wide range of temperatures and found no dependence of OER on irradiation temperature.

The discrepancy between these results is not easily resolved. To be sure, the experiments of Kim *et al.* (1975a) involved modification of pH and the cells' nutritional status, as well as of degree of oxygenation, and one might attribute the results obtained to these factors. But this is not true of the data of Robinson *et al.* (1974b); although pH was not monitored, there is no reason to assume a temperature-associated systemic change in proton concentrations. I suppose I can only offer the lame comment that we really need more studies on this important point. Of particular use would be a careful study that examines the role pH and nutritional factors play in possibly modifying the temperature dependence of the OER.

3.2.6. Hyperthermia and High LET Radiations

Gerner *et al.* (1976) and Gerner and Leith (1977) exposed CHO cells to 4 MeV X rays and to accelerated carbon and helium ions at the University of California Bevelac Facility. Heating (41, 42, and 43°C, usually 1 hr, though in some experiments 30 min) was carried out before irradiation. The results showed that, in contrast to the synergistic effects of heat and low LET radiation, the effect with high LET radiation was additive. This is shown in Figure 3.5. The survival curves in that figure illustrate the effect of a 60-min exposure at 43°C on X-ray and on carbon-ion cytotoxicity. What is somewhat curious is that at 37°C the relative biological efficiency (RBE) of these two radiations is very dependent upon the survival level at which it is measured. For example, at 80% survival it is about 3; 100 rad of ^{12}C ions kill the same number of cells as 300 rad of 4 MeV X rays. However, at a survival level of 1%, 500 rad of ^{12}C ions are equivalent to approximately 850 rad of X ray, an RBE of about 1.7. This difference disappears almost entirely at 43°C; the RBE is probably not

Figure 3.5. Comparison of interactions of low and high LET irradiations with 43°C. Chinese hamster (CHO) cells were exposed to either 37°C (closed symbols) or 43°C (open symbols) for 60 min. At the completion of the heat exposure, they were then irradiated to the dose shown on the abscissa, with either 4 MeV X rays (circles) or accelerated carbon ions (squares) (obtained from the Bevelac Facility at the University of California, Berkeley). Note that while the RBE for carbon ions was approximately 2 at the 10% survival level for the 37°C treated cells, the RBE was essentially 1 for the cells treated at 43°C. Data from Gerner and Leith (1977), with permission.

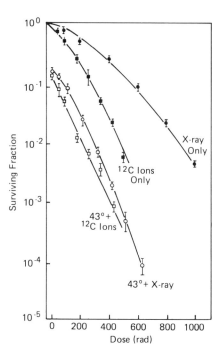

statistically different from 1.0 at any survival level. These results could suggest that the difference in RBEs at 37°C relates to repair processes operative at 37°C but not at 43°C.

Parenthetically, the interaction of hyperthermia with fast neutrons on local tumor response was investigated by Hahn *et al.* (1976). Their *in vivo* results essentially agree with the *in vitro* results presented here and are discussed in Chapter 5.

3.2.7. Sequencing and Timing

The simultaneous application of X irradiation and hyperthermia may not always be feasible in a clinical setting. Several investigators, therefore, have examined the question of how survival is modified when a time interval at 37°C is allowed to elapse between the applications of the two modalities (Li and Kal, 1977; Joshi *et al.*, 1978; Sapareto *et al.*, 1979). A more or less representative finding is that of Li and Kal (1977) for exponentially growing EMT6 cells (Figure 3.6). In this experiment, cells were heated to 43°C for 60 min. At various times either before initiation or after completion of heating, they were also exposed to an X-ray dose

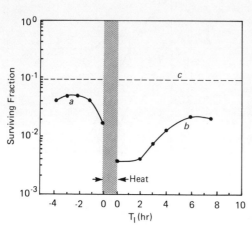

Figure 3.6. Effect on survival of exponentially growing cells of an interval at 37°C between exposures to X rays and 43°C (or 43°C and X ray). EMT6 cells were exposed to 43°C for 1 hr. X irradiation (600 rad) was administered either before initiation of the heat treatment (curve a), or after its completion (curve b). The time interval at 37°C between treatments is shown on the abscissa. Curve (c) shows the expected survival in the absence of interaction. The finding that this level of survival was not reached by either curve a or curve b probably reflects cell-cycle-associated events. Data from Li and Kal (1977), with permission.

of 600 rad. The left half of Figure 3.6 demonstrates how X irradiation sensitized cells to a subsequent heat dose, while the right hand portion shows how heat similarly modified a later X-ray response. What is apparent from the figure is that the radiation-induced heat sensitization disappears quite rapidly, probably with a halftime of about 1 hr. On the other hand, heat-induced X-ray sensitization has a slower decay, with little or no change in survival values over the first 2 hr. The fact that neither of these curves approaches the additive survival value, i.e., the value to be expected in the absence of interaction, most likely reflects radiation- (or heat-) induced changes in proliferation kinetics. That this interpretation is likely to be correct is shown in Figure 3.7, where a similar set of experiments was repeated utilizing plateau phase HA-1 cells. In this system, about 90% of the cells are in a G1-like part of the cell cycle and remain there for several days (Hahn and Little, 1972). When measured in this system, which does not suffer from the complication of cell proliferation, both curves tend to approach the "no interaction level," though again with different temporal kinetics.

3.2.8. Hyperthermia, Radiation, and the Cell Cycle

At least two studies have examined survival of cells exposed to hyperthermia and x irradiation as a function of position of the cell in the mitotic cycle at the time of application. Kim *et al.* (1976) synchronized HeLa cells utilizing the shakeoff procedure developed by Terasima and Tolmach (1963a,b). In this technique, mitotic cells are preferentially dis-

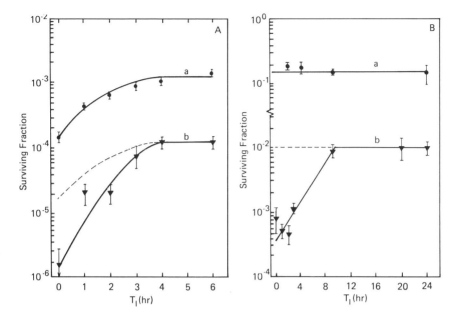

Figure 3.7. Effect on survival of plateau phase cells of an interval at 37°C between exposures to X rays and 43°C (or 43°C and X ray). HA–1 cells were grown to plateau phase and exposed to 43°C for 45 min. Either before initiation of heating (A) or after completion of heating (B), these cells were irradiated to a dose of 1000 rad (curve b). Explant was immediately after the second treatment. The duration of the interval at 37°C in Hanks's Balanced Salt Solution is shown in the abscissa of both panels. Curve (a) is a control exposed to either X rays only (A) or heat only (B). The increase in survival of curve a, panel A, represents recovery from X-ray-induced potentially lethal damage. The absence of such an increase in panel B shows the absence of recovery, in the balanced salt solution, from heat-induced potentially lethal damage. The dotted line represents the survival expected in the absence of an interaction of heat and X rays. In plateau phase cells, particularly if they are placed in balanced salt solutions, there is little or no proliferation. Compare Figure 3.6. Data from Li *et al.* (1976), with permission.

lodged from their growth surface by mechanical agitation. The investigators then treated cells at various times after harvest with heat only (43°C for 30 min), radiation only (400 rad), or with radiation followed by heat (Figure 3.8). The small heat dose killed, on the average, only about 30% of the cells, and there was little variation over the cell cycle. The age response for X rays was very similar to that obtained by Terasima and Tolmach, namely sensitive mitotic cells, resistant early G1 cells, another sensitive compartment at the G1/S interphase, and finally highly resistant late S phase cells.

The response to the sequential treatment is illustrated in the bottom

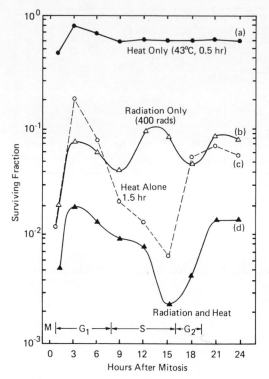

Figure 3.8. Age response of cells sequentially exposed to 43°C (30 min) and X rays (400 rad). HeLa cells were synchronized with the mitotic shakeoff technique. Cells were exposed at various times after harvest to either: 43°C for 30 min, (a); 400 rad, (b) or the sequential treatment of radiation followed by heat (d). Shown for comparison is also an age response of cells exposed to 43°C for 90 min. The sequential treatment is most effective against the radiation-resistant late S phase cells. Note the similarities in the shapes of curves (c) and (d). Data from Kim *et al.* (1976), with permission.

(solid) line. I have also shown, in Figure 3.8, the age response to a more severe heat treatment, namely 1.5 hr at 43°C (dashed line). The reason I have included this graph is to point out an interesting feature of the combined response. The response to heat followed by X irradiation seems to mimic much more closely that of heat only, rather than the response seen following an X-ray treatment in the absence of heat. In other words, operationally it appears as though the initial X-ray treatment sensitized cells to the subsequent heat effects. Most hyperthermia experiments were performed by radiation biologists, and it has, therefore, become customary to think of heat as a modifying factor for X irradiation. But here the data indicate the reverse. Another feature of the combined response is that the radiation-resistant G2 cells become very sensitive when exposed to the sequential exposure of heat and X rays.

In another study, Ben-Hur *et al.* (1974) compared responses of V-79 Chinese hamster cells synchronized with hydroxyurea. Cells were irradiated at a dose rate of 12 rad/min at temperatures of 0, 37, and 42°C. The doses chosen, 947, 664, and 385 rad, respectively, yielded equal survival in asynchronous populations. The age response of cells irradiated at the lower temperature or at 37°C were very similar; however, at the elevated temperature, 42°C, a very different response resulted (Figure 3.9). These results again emphasize that heat does not simply amplify X-ray effects.

3.2.9. Proliferation Kinetics

Modifications by various treatments of the normal rates at which cells traverse the cell cycle are of considerable importance, particularly when assessing the effects of multiple doses of X rays and heat on survival. The effect of possible induction of partial synchrony has already been mentioned several times in connection with the interpretation of data obtained in experiments involving two or more treatments (e.g., see section 3.2.3.).

Current methodology of analyzing proliferation kinetics involves primarily the use of microfluorometry. The approach is to obtain and then analyze distributions of the DNA contents of individual cells of normal or perturbed populations. One technique involves the exposure of cells to RNase, followed by staining with a fluorescent dye that binds specifically and quantitatively to the remaining double-stranded nucleic acid, DNA. Two dyes used frequently are acridine orange and ethidium bromide. By exciting the bound dye molecules and measuring the emitted

Figure 3.9. Age responses of Chinese hamster cells irradiated at various temperatures. Chinese hamster cells (V–79) were synchronized with hydroxyurea (HU). The abscissa represents the time of initiation of the exposure after completion of the drug treatment; 0´hr corresponds to the G_1/S interface. The treatments were chosen so that the effect on survival of asynchronous cells was always about 8%. The shape of the age responses of cells irradiated at 37°C or at 0°C is not too different and is not greatly affected by dose rate. However, at 42°C the age response function changes substantially. Data from Ben Hur *et al.* (1974), with permission.

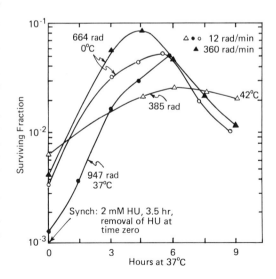

fluorescence in a flow cytofluorometer, the relative amount of DNA of the individual cell can then be measured. Histograms from normal and perturbed populations, each usually consisting of at least 10^5 cells, are shown in Figure 3.10. From these histograms, the percentage of cells in the various compartments of the cell cycle can be estimated. An example of such an estimate performed on populations obtained at various times after heating of EMT6 cells is shown in Figure 3.11. There are several caveats that one should keep in mind when examining data obtained by this technique. Analysis is on the amount of DNA per cell; hence a cell in early or late G1 will give a similar signal. No distinction can be made between G2 or M cells; more importantly, none between live and dead cells. This last limitation means that if the perturbing treatment is toxic to a large percentage of the cells exposed, the data may not be a measure of the behavior of the remaining live cells. Finally, the conversion of DNA histograms (Figure 3.10) to kinetic data (Figure 3.11) involves some arbitrary assumptions; hence, the absolute values of the occupancy numbers are uncertain. However, the changes (with time) of these numbers will be more or less similar irrespective of the particular model used to calculate the conversion.

Kal *et al.* (1975) and Kal and Hahn (1976) compared the kinetics of cell cycle progression after three different treatments: 300 rad X ray, 1 hr at 43°C, and 300 rad followed by 1 hr at 43°C. The results after X irradiation show a familiar pattern: an induced mitotic block (3 hr) and

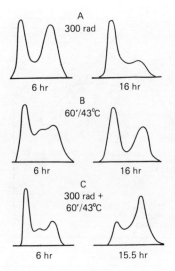

Figure 3.10. DNA distributions of cells after treatments with heat and X rays. EMT6 cells, growing exponentially at the time of exposure, were treated with: 300 rad, line A; 43°C, 60 min, line B; and 300 rad followed by 43°C, 60 min, line C. DNA distributions shown were obtained by cytofluorometry at 6 hr and at 16 hr after completion of the treatments. In each histogram, the first peak is a measure of the number of cells in G_1, the second of cells in $G_2 + M$; cells with intermediate DNA content are in S phase. Abscissa: DNA/cell (arbitrary units); ordinate; number of cells (arbitrary units). Data from Kal and Hahn (1976), with permission.

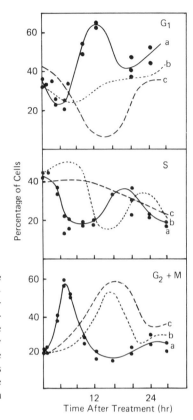

Figure 3.11. Percentages of cells in G_1, S, and G_2 + M phases after treatments with heat and X ray. DNA distributions such as those illustrated in Figure 3.10 were obtained at various times after treatments of EMT6 cells with 300 rad of X ray (curve a), 43°C, 60 min (curve b), or 300 rad followed by 43°C, 60 min (curve c) and then converted to the indicated percentages of cells. The top panel shows cells in G1, the center panel, cells in S, and the bottom panel, cells in G_2 + M phases. Data from Kal and Hahn (1976), with permission.

an associated accumulation of cells in G2 + M, followed by the appearance of a parasynchronous cohort of cells moving through the cell cycle at a rate not very different from that of controls. For cells exposed to heat alone there was not only a mitotic block (~9 hr), but also an accumulation of cells in S, which continued for about 6 hr; cells then moved into G2 + M. After the combined exposure, the mitotic block lasted about 18 hr and the S phase disturbance 10–12 hr; in other words, the sequential treatment accentuated the heat (rather than the X-ray) effects.

In an interesting study, Lücke-Huhle and Dertinger (1977) looked at the effects of hyperthermia and X irradiation on the kinetics of V-79 cells growing as spheroids (Sutherland and Durand, 1976). By a fractionated method of trypsinization of these spheroids, these authors were able to distinguish between the behavior of cells at the outer layer of the spheroids, *versus* those existing in the center of the three-dimensional cell aggregates. Cells were heated for 4 hr at 42°C, and the DNA distributions of the outer and inner cells were examined separately by cytofluorometry. The outer cells behaved very similarly to the EMT6 cells just described, with a sharp G2 peak reflecting the mitotic block occurring at about 12 hr. The inner cells showed very different behavior, with a reduction in the G1 complement beginning at about 8 hr; this was exactly compensated for by an increase in the number of cells in the S phase. The results are consistent with the interpretation put forth by the authors, that the hyperthermic exposure induced proliferation in the noncycling cell compartment at the center of the spheroids. In this connection it is interesting to note that Dickson and Calderwood (1976) have reported that hyperthermia can induce nonproliferating Yoshida sarcoma cells treated *in vivo* to enter the cycle.

3.2.10. Recovery Phenomena: X Irradiation and Heat

The two types of recovery phenomena discussed in the radiobiological literature, recovery from sublethal and from potentially lethal damage, were defined in section 2.6.1. When two modalities are involved, conceptual and experimental complications arise. First, let me take up recovery from sublethal damage as measured by two-fraction or by low-dose-rate experiments. One question that can be asked is: "How does giving each dose at elevated temperatures affect this type of recovery?" At high dose rates, the possible introduction of new and different lesions could be reflected in the lower survival measured. Such lesions, resulting from the simultaneous application of the two insults, might not be reparable. Alternatively, the damage might be similar, but the repair enzymes might be modified so that their rate of repair at 37°C is changed. At low dose rates, reduction of survival could imply either of these possibilities and additionally the possible inability (or reduced ability) of enzymes to function, even without permanent modification, at the elevated temperature. Applying heat before the first X ray treatment tests for possible permanent damage to enzymes. While no complete analysis of this phenomenon has been undertaken, the work of Ben-Hur *et al.* (1972; 1974) goes a long way toward answering some of these questions. In one set of experiments, V-79 Chinese hamster cells were irradiated at a dose rate of 3.3 rad/min at various temperatures. Increasing temperatures progressively from 34 to 41°C also increased the cytotoxic efficiency of low-dose-rate (3.3 rad/min) X irradiation (Figure 3.12). But the maximum sensitization observed did not exceed that seen if irradiation was carried out at 0°C. At the latter temperature repair is known to be inhibited. The authors also carried out a two-fraction experiment. If cells were incubated at 41°C for 2 hr after an initial X-ray dose, given at a high dose rate, the sparing

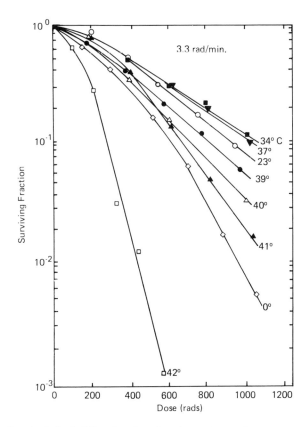

Figure 3.12. Survival of cells X irradiated at a low dose rate at various temperatures. Chinese hamster cells (V–79) were X irradiated at 3.3 rad/min while suspended in medium at the indicated temperature to the dose shown on the abscissa. Between 23 and 37°C, cells recover from sublethal damage during irradiation and hence survival is high. At 0°C, such recovery is inhibited and survival is low. Increasing temperatures from 37 to 41°C causes survival curves to shift progressively from the 37 to the 0°C survival levels, indicating that elevated temperatures may also inhibit such recovery. At 42°C, cytotoxicity is more severe than at 0°C, suggesting that at that temperature sensitization occurs in addition to possible inhibition of recovery. Data from Ben-Hur *et al.* (1974), with permission.

effect of fractionation disappeared. These results strongly suggest that heat causes damage to repair enzymes responsible for effecting recovery, but an alternate explanation, namely the conversion by heat of X-ray-induced repairable lesions into irreparable lesions, cannot be excluded.

That the substrate, presumably DNA, is directly affected in the modification by heat of recovery from potentially lethal damage was suggested by experiments of Li *et al.* (1976). Plateau phase HA-1 cells were irradiated with 1000 rad. Heat (43°C, 0 to 1 hr) was applied either directly before or after X irradiation. The cells were then either explanted immediately, or returned to a 37°C incubator for various lengths of time. The recovery patterns observed are shown in Figure 3.13. Heating before X irradiation (panel A) did not inhibit recovery, although it did certainly modify the kinetics by slowing the rate of recovery. Heating for increasing durations at 43°C after irradiation (panel B) progressively reduced the magnitude of recovery, until at 1 hr no recovery was observed. If damage to enzymes had been responsible, heating before or after irradiation would have been expected to have similar effects. Hence, the most likely explanation for these results is that heating after irradiation modified the damage so that enzymes could then not deal with the lesions.

Finally, it should be pointed out that the interaction experiments such as those described in Figures 3.6 and 3.7 also constitute recovery from damage, though in a different, perhaps more complicated way than those discussed here. For example, consider an experiment in which an X-ray dose is given at various time intervals after a heat dose. What is measured in that experiment is the rate of repair of that component of heat-induced damage specifically capable of interacting with subsequent X-ray-induced lesions (Gerweck et al., 1975). It may very well be true that this type of repair is different from that involved in the experiments that were discussed in the previous two paragraphs.

3.3. ENHANCEMENT BY HYPERTHERMIA OF DRUG CYTOTOXICITY

The study of how drugs kill cells at elevated temperatures is interesting for a variety of reasons. Obviously there is an important possible clinical application. If the efficacy of the drug against a tumor could be enhanced without a concomitant and equivalent increase in critical normal tissue toxicity, then either chemotherapy could be made more efficient or the usual severe side effects could be reduced by an appropriate reduction in drug dose. Because of the variety of side effects that are treatment limiting, depending upon the particular agent used, this is not an altogether unlikely prospect. Then the simultaneous use of chemotherapy and whole-body hyperthermia against generalized cancers would become attractive. In the absence of such results (and to date no such data have been reported), the combination of localized hyperthermia and chemotherapy offers interesting possibilities. The ability to localize heat should make particularly dangerous or painful tumors more tractable to treatment by chemotherapy. Combinations of heat–drug exposures then might be useful for palliative treatments. On the biological side, studying the in-

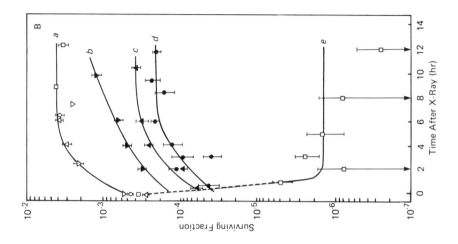

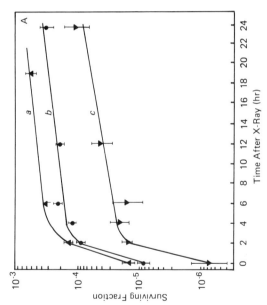

Figure 3.13. Inhibition by heat of recovery from X-ray-induced potentially lethal damage. Chinese hamster cells (HA–1) were grown to plateau phase. A: Cells were heated to 43°C for (a) 15, (b) 30, or (c) 60 min and then exposed to 1500 rad of X irradiation. At the time after X-ray exposure shown on the abscissa, they were trypsinized and plated for colony formation. B: Cells were heated to (a) 0, (b) 15, (c) 30, (d) 45, or (e) 60 min after X irradiation. Heating before irradiation slowed, but did not stop recovery from sublethal damage. Heating for 60 min after X-ray exposure completely inhibited recovery. Data from Li et al. (1976), with permission.

teraction of drugs and heat may shed light on how the drugs kill cells and perhaps also on how heat kills cells. In the rest of this chapter, I will concentrate on summarizing the existing descriptions of drug–heat interactions. There are now literally hundreds of experimental anticancer drugs, only a few of which have been examined in terms of their cytoxicity at elevated temperatures. Furthermore, there is essentially an infinite number of others whose anticancer activity at 37°C is essentially nil, but that do have considerable activity at higher temperatures. These "thermic sensitizers" might have considerable clinical use, since their biological actions could be limited to the heated tumor volume, and no whole-body toxicity need be associated with their use.

The task of summarizing available knowledge on heat–drug interactions is much simpler than that of summarizing radiation–heat interactions, simply because very little work has been done to date. Much of the work has been done in my laboratory, and of necessity most of the data quoted will be from our results.

3.3.1. Classification of Interactions

Based on a phenomenological analysis of the type of their interaction with heat, drugs can be ordered into several classes. Such an arbitrary ordering does not necessarily imply a commonality of mode of action within any group. For some agents, the slope of the survival curve changes smoothly with continuously increasing temperature. Another group of drugs shows distinct threshold effects: little or no sensitization below about 42°C, with marked sensitization occurring at 43°C or higher. Then there is another group of agents that shows essentially no cytotoxicity between 37 and 42°C; these are agents that currently have no function in chemotherapy. However, above 42°C some become highly cytotoxic, and these offer considerable promise. Finally, there is a miscellaneous group of drugs whose modes of action do not fall into any clear category and that I have, for lack of anything better, combined into a category called "other agents showing hyperthermic interactions."

3.3.2. Technical Aspects of Drug Studies In Vitro

A word of caution with respect to technical aspects of drug studies. These involve specific problems usually not associated with X-ray experiments. Some drugs bind to dishes, both glass and plastic, and upon release, may continue to kill cells (Elkind et al., 1969; Hahn, 1978). Furthermore, drug-killed cells themselves may release drug upon lysis and thereby contribute to cytotoxicity. Some agents are not or are only partially soluble in water, and organic solvents are then required. These themselves may kill cells, particularly at elevated temperatures (Li *et al.*, 1977a). Unless all necessary control experiments are performed, the data on cell survival after drug exposure may be contaminated with artifactual results. A final caution is that drugs may be unstable, either during long-term storage, or during the experiment, even during one exposure. This latter possibility may require a careful definition of dose in terms of the active moiety capable of continuous inactivation of cells. For example, if the active material remaining in the medium behaves according to $c(t)$, then instead of the usual concentration–time product, the dose is replaced by the effective dose, $\dfrac{1}{t_f} \displaystyle\int_0^{t_f} c(t)dt$, where t_f is the duration of exposure. If the drug decay follows first order kinetics, the effective dose is proportional to $c(0)(1 - e^{-t_f\gamma/\gamma})$, where $c(0)$ is the drug dose at the initiation of exposure, and γ the decay constant in the medium and at the particular temperature of the experiment. The temperature dependence of decay of a nitrosourea, BCNU (1-(2-chloroethyl)-3-cyclohexyl-1-nitrosourea), is illustrated in Figure 3.14.

3.3.3. Drugs Showing No Threshold Effects

Most prominent among these are the bifunctional alkylating agents, the nitrosoureas, and cis-platinum. The alkylating agents have been stud-

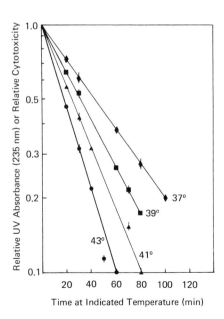

Figure 3.14. Temperature dependence of the decay of drug activity. BCNU, freshly dissolved to a concentration of 100 μg/ml, was added to media at the temperature indicated, to yield a final concentration of 10 μg/ml. After the time indicated on the abscissa, the active amount of drug remaining in the medium was monitored spectrophotometrically, and, at a few points, these results were verified by testing the cytotoxicity of the material at 37°C against Chinese hamster cells (HA–1) (slashed symbols). Possible decay of drug toxicity should always be determined and, if need be, taken into account when testing for the temperature dependence of drug efficacy *in vitro*. Data from Hahn (1978), with permission.

ied most extensively (Woodhall *et al.*, 1960; Suzuki, 1967; Giovanella *et al.*, 1970; Dickson and Suzanger, 1974; Johnson and Pavelec, 1973; Hahn, 1974; Kaufman and Davidson, 1976; Goss and Parsons, 1977; Van Den Thillart and Modderkolk, 1978; Vig, 1979). Perhaps the most thorough study is that of Johnson and Pavelec (1973), who have examined the cytotoxicity of thio-TEPA over the temperature range of 37 to 43°C (Figure 3.15). This drug has a long half-life, so that hydrolysis is not a problem over the 60 min of exposure. The investigators performed survival experiments over the temperature range of 39 to 43°C. The Arrhenius plot constructed from these data yielded an activation energy consistent with that for an alkylating reaction. Survival results for several nitrosoureas as well as for cis-platinum are shown in Figure 3.16. In all these studies the cells used were Chinese hamster cells. Very marked heat sensitization is observed for these agents.

Other alkylating agents studied include alkane, cyclophosphamide (Dickson and Suzanger, 1974), and peptichimeo (Djordjevic *et al.*, 1978). All except cyclophosphamide exhibited increased action at elevated temperatures. Data on this latter drug are hard to interpret. It needs activation by liver enzymes in order to show cytotoxicity and the reference is un-

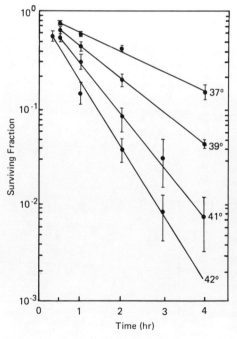

Figure 3.15. Survival of cells exposed to an alkylating agent at temperatures between 37 and 42°C. Chinese hamster cells (V-79) were exposed to thio-TEPA (5 μg/ml) at the indicated temperatures and for the times shown on the abscissa. No corrections for possible drug decay were made. "Activation" energies calculated from Arrhenius plots indicate that the increased cell killing at elevated temperatures reflects increased rates of alkylation (presumably of DNA). Data from Johnson and Pavelec (1973) with permission.

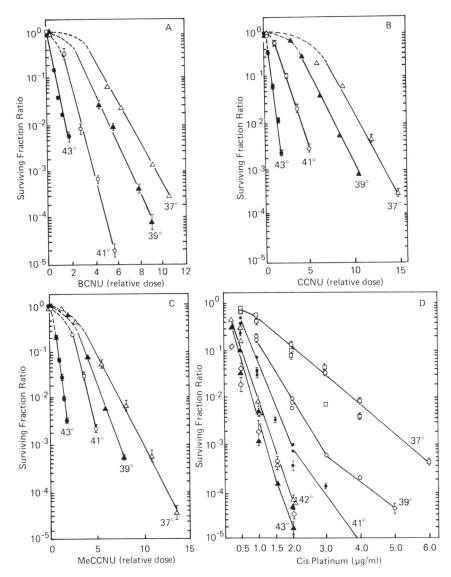

Figure 3.16. Dose response curves of cells exposed to nitrosoureas or to cis-platinum at various temperatures. Exponentially growing Chinese hamster cells (HA–1) were exposed to the drug indicated in the panel at the temperatures shown and at the concentrations marked on the abscissas. Because the activity of the nitrosoureas decays with time (Figure 3.14), the doses on the abscissas of panels A, B, and C are presented in units of relative dose. These units represent the average (over the exposure period) of the active material present in the medium. Cis-platinum is stable over the temperature and time range of interest. Its concentration is therefore presented in μg/ml. The last graph also indicates that results are highly repeatable: multiple points indicate results from different experiments. Open triangles and closed triangles (43°C) are from experiments performed 24 months apart. All survival values are corrected for cell killing by heat alone. Data from Hahn (1978), with permission.

fortunately not clear on how activation was achieved *in vitro* and if the temperature dependence of activation was measured. Thus, I cannot judge the validity of these results.

3.3.4. Drugs Showing Marked Threshold Effects

Of primary interest here are the two antibiotics bleomycin and adriamycin (Figure 3.17). These drugs both show a similar behavior, with a marked threshold for the interaction with heat at or near 43°C, although as discussed in Chapter 5, the nature of the thermal modification of the cytotoxicity of each agent may be very different.

3.3.5. Thermosensitizers

These drugs are characterized by an almost complete lack of cytotoxicity at 37°C over the dose interval of interest. However, at elevated temperatures they act as potent cell inactivators. A good example of these

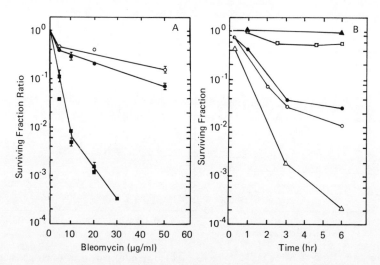

Figure 3.17. Survival of cells exposed to bleomycin or adriamycin: temperature threshold effects. In panel A, Chinese hamster cells (HA–1) grown to confluence without medium change, and then exposed to graded doses of bleomycin for 1 hr at 37°C (open circles), 41°C (closed circles), and 43°C (closed squares). The cells were then trypsinized and plated for colony formation. In panel B, exponentially growing EMT6 cells were exposed to a dose of 0.5 μg/ml of adriamycin at temperatures of 37°C (open triangles), 41°C (open circles), or 42°C (closed circles) for the times indicated on the abscissa. Also shown are cell killing due to heat alone at 41°C (closed triangles) and 42°C (open squares). Note the drastic change in cytotoxicity occurring at about 42°C. Data from Hahn *et al.* (1975), with permission.

is the sulfhydryl-rich compound cysteamine (Kapp and Hahn, 1979). Survival curves of Chinese hamster cells exposed to a fixed concentration (16 mM) of cysteamine at temperatures of 37, 41, 42, and 43°C for various lengths of time are shown in Figure 3.18, panel A. Up to 100 min, there is essentially no killing by this agent if the incubation temperature is 37°C, and there is only very limited killing up to 42°C. However, a marked increase in the efficiency of cysteamine is noted between 42 and 43°C. For example, 90 min at 42°C leave 20% of the cells capable of proliferation, but increasing the incubation temperature by only one more degree reduces the surviving fraction to 10^{-3}. Qualitatively similar results are obtained for other sulfhydryl-rich compounds, including ΛET (2-amino-ethylisothiourium bromide) and cysteine, but the degree of cytotoxicity

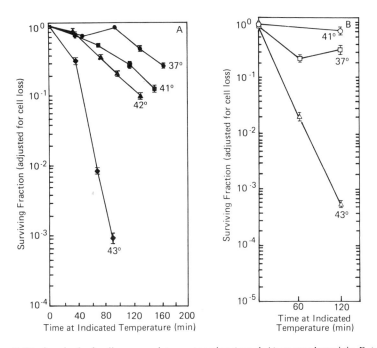

Figure 3.18. Survival of cells exposed to cysteamine (panel A) or amphotericin B (panel B), thermic sensitizers. Chinese hamster cells (HA–1) were exposed to a fixed dose of cysteamine (16 mM) or amphotericin B (10 μg/ml) at temperatures between 37 and 43°C. Both drugs are stable at these temperatures and for the time periods of interest. Even at doses that cause little if any killing at 37°C, these drugs become efficient cytotoxic agents at elevated temperatures. Note, however, that the temperature threshold to cause this conversion is at about 42 to 43°C. Data from Kapp and Hahn (1979) and Hahn *et al.* (1977), with permission.

is very different for the various compounds. Another group of drugs, all of which greatly increase the action of heat, are the naturally occurring polyamines putrescine, spermidine, and spermine (Gerner and Russell, 1977). Addition to the medium of as low as 10^{-5} M spermidine or spermine measurably enhances the killing of Chinese hamster cells (Gerner *et al.*, 1980). These agents are very likely not of clinical interest, but their study may reveal information about the mechanisms of the action of heat itself (Ben-Hur and Riklis, 1978; 1979; Ben-Hur *et al.*, 1978), and possibly about the development of thermotolerance. The latter suggestion arises from the fact that the polyamines are claimed to both prevent the occurrence of thermotolerance during heating as well as reverse its effect in cells made thermotolerant by previous heating (Gerner *et al.*, 1980).

Another drug whose thermal enhancement is phenomenologically not too different from that of cysteamine is the anti-fungal agent amphotericin B. Dose-dependent survival curves of Chinese hamster cells exposed to this agent at temperatures between 37 and 43°C are shown in Figure 3.18,

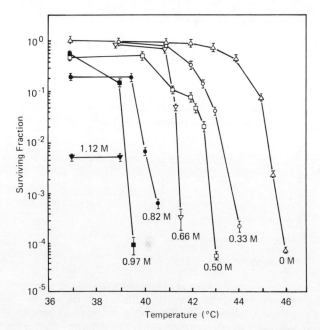

Figure 3.19. Survival of cells exposed to ethanol: temperature threshold and sensitizing effects. Chinese hamster cells (HA–1) were exposed for 30 min to the indicated doses of ethanol at the temperatures shown. Ethanol appears to shift both temperature threshold and the efficacy of heat in killing. Data from Li and Hahn (1978), with permission.

panel B. Again, at a dose level where there is essentially no cytotoxicity at 37°C and perhaps none even at 41°C, marked cytotoxicity is shown at 43°C. Both the sulfhydryl drugs and amphotericin B can be considered to modify the cytotoxic action of heat. At at any one temperature, they reduce the amount of time required to achieve a given level of damage. Since there is very little killing by heat alone at 41 or 42°C, the effect of these agents at these temperatures is also minimal. However, at 43°C cell killing becomes appreciable.

There is another group of thermosensitizers that behaves differently. These drugs seem to effect temperature shifts. The amount of the shift is determined by the amount of agent present in solution. This is shown most clearly in Figure 3.19 for ethanol, the only agent that has been examined in detail. The threshold temperature, i.e., the temperature at which the cytotoxicity increases sharply, is seen to be a function of alcohol concentration. Very striking also is the similarity between the action of ethanol and that of heat in conjunction with many of the agents described in this section (Hahn, 1980; Li et al., 1980b). Very likely similar behavior will be observed for a variety of drugs, all showing the properties of local anesthetics, e.g., lidocaine and procaine. For these agents a concentration can be found that is the equivalent of a one-degree rise in temperature. For example, for ethanol, one degree of heat is approximately the equivalent of the presence of 1% of ethanol in the medium (Li et al., 1980b). In this sense ethanol, and perhaps the other agents, mimic heat effects.

3.3.6. Modification of Drug–Heat Interactions

There are certainly important gaps in our knowledge about how factors such as pH, nutritional milieu, thermotolerance, or recovery factors modify heat–X-ray interactions. However, when compared to our state of knowledge about the effects of similar factors on heat–drug interactions, the X-ray situation is infinitely better. In fact, there are only about five reports on this vast subject that are worth discussing. Braun and Hahn (1975) have shown that a 1-hr heat pulse at 43°C after bleomycin exposure, but not before, inhibits subsequent recovery of potentially lethal damage. This is exactly analogous to similar findings by Li et al. (1976) for inhibition of recovery from X-ray induced potentially lethal damage. Hahn and Strande (1976) have demonstrated that a time interval of a few hours between heating and exposure of Chinese hamster cells to adriamycin causes them to become refractory to cell killing by the drug. Somewhat similar results are seen for actinomycin D (Donaldson et al., 1978). Interestingly, studies by Morgan et al. (1979) indicate that the adriamycin tolerance just described probably has different kinetics than does the development of thermotolerance. For example, after a 3-hr pulse of preheating at 40°C, a permissive temperature, thermotolerance was at a maximum but adriamycin tolerance (at 43°C) had not as yet developed. A similar treatment offered the cells a slight degree of protection against BCNU and against bleomycin, as determined during a 1-hr exposure at 43°C. In contrast, if the preheating was 1 hr at 43°C, cells were sensitized to BCNU and bleomycin but protected against adriamycin. Obviously, this whole area is one where considerable work needs to be done. To what extent, if any, are drug and heat tolerance related? Are these permeability modifications or do the results describe other aspects of heat-modified cell physiology? And, of course, are any of the findings of use in the clinic?

Furthermore, no studies exist on a wide range of other topics. These include effects of pH, nutrition, hypoxia, etc. on drug–hyperthermia interactions. It is a commentary on the parochialism of cancer research that the cytotoxicity of drugs against hypoxic cells has not been studied in detail. Obviously, the addition of hyperthermia would add another dimension to such endeavors.

These data also point up the necessity for additional large-scale trials of studies before the combined use of drugs and heat in whole body hyperthermia is initiated. Then, because of the relatively low temperature and long durations of exposure, development of drug tolerance, both in tumor and in normal tissue, will have to be examined with some care. Otherwise a situation might occur in which protection develops in tumor, and normal tissue toxicity is either unaffected or accentuated. Particularly for drugs such as adriamycin and bleomycin for which cardiac or lung toxicity are treatment limiting, such considerations must be kept in mind. The situation is not nearly as complicated or dangerous if localized heating is utilized. Exposure times are relatively short and temperatures are high. Hence, drug tolerance probably does not develop during treatment. And, since the dimension of heated volumes can be controlled, particularly sensitive tissue can be kept at normal temperatures.

3.3.7. Negative Studies

Not all drug actions are modified by temperature changes in the 37 to 45°C range. Cell killing by the thymidine analog 5-fluorodeoxyuridine is stable, as is the cytotoxicity of the folic acid analog methotrexate. The vinka alkaloids, vinblastine and vincristine, continue to inactivate cells at similar rates at 37 or at 45° C. Without question there are many other agents whose rate of action is affected only minimally in the range of temperatures of interest here.

3.4. SUMMARY

Heat modifies the cytotoxicity of many, though not of all, anticancer agents. If X irradiation is carried out at high dose rates and at temperatures above 41°C, the TER observed is a function of temperature and duration of treatment. The maximum TER measured is about 1.5. Heating immediately before or after the radiation also results in increased toxicity, though the TER is reduced. For some cell lines, heating before X-ray exposure is more effective; for others the reverse is true.

Cells made thermotolerant by earlier heat exposures may have a somewhat reduced X-ray sensitivity; however, a second heat treatment still sensitizes thermotolerant cells to X ray. The degree of sensitization either is that of normal cells or may be slightly reduced. There is no reliable evidence that the TERs of normal and malignant cells differ.

The OER may not be reduced by the effects of heat alone; in one study it actually increased. However, an environment of poor nutrient supply, low pH, and chronic hypoxia apparently does lead to a reduced OER; in one study it was reduced from 1.9 to 1.6. Hyperthermia does not increase the cytotoxicity of high LET radiations; combining heat and ^{12}C radiation resulted in additive killing.

Introducing of an interval at 37°C between heat and X irradiation (or X irradiation and heat) reduces the effectiveness of the interaction; when the sojourn at 37°C exceeds about 8 hr, cell killing becomes additive, though in exponentially growing cells, cell cycle effects may modulate the survival measured.

Studies employing synchronized cells show that heat sensitizes cells to X irradiation in all parts of the cells cycle but that the major effect is on the radiation-resistant late S phase cells. The age response function following sequential heat and X-ray treatments closely resembles that of cells treated with heat alone. Proliferation kinetics are modified by heat, which introduces a block in cell cycle traverse both in the S and in the G_2 phases. Combining heat with X-ray exposure increases the duration of both blocks. Heat, as well as heat and X ray, may also induce proliferation in cells out of cycle at the time of exposure.

Finally, the recovery from X-ray-induced sublethal and potentially lethal damage is reduced or abolished by heating. Effects of the former are most clearly seen in low dose rate studies, where even at temperatures below 41°C the cytotoxicity of the irradiation is enhanced substantially. At 43°C, a 1-hr exposure after X-ray treatment is required to abolish recovery from potentially lethal damage.

Drug–heat interactions fall into several classes. Potentiation may be observed as a continuous change with increasing temperatures of the rate at which cells are killed by the drugs (alkylating agents, nitrosoureas, and cis-platinum), or there may be a threshold temperature that must be exceeded (bleomycin, adriamycin). Compounds that are nontoxic at low doses at 37°C, but at similar concentrations become effective killers at elevated temperatures, include sulfhydryl-rich compounds, amphotericin B, and alcohols and other "fluidizing" agents. No interaction is seen for most analogs (methotrexate, 5-fluorodeoxyuridine), nor for the vinka alkaloids. Thermotolerant cells are protected against adriamycin and actinomycin D.

4

Mechanisms of Heat Action

4.1. INTRODUCTION

In the last two chapters I have portrayed various ways that mildly elevated temperatures modify survival kinetics of mammalian cells. Environmental factors were shown to have considerable influence in determining cell death. Ionizing radiations, as well as many drugs, become more effective in inactivating cells when exposures are carried out at hyperthermic temperatures. Now I will describe some of the known or suspected mechanisms underlying the phenomenological descriptions. Specifically, I will sequentially address the following questions: Are there specific critical "targets," i.e., subcellular organelles or molecules, that are particularly heat sensitive and hence responsible for cell death? If so, what are these likely to be? What is the cause of thermotolerance? What are the mechanisms of accentuated X-ray cytotoxicity at elevated temperatures? Finally, I will look at some of the mechanisms likely to be responsible for heat–drug interactions.

4.2. HEAT DEATH OF CELLS

4.2.1. Definition of Heat Dose

Before beginning any discussion of mechanisms, I need to consider the definition of heat "dose." Quantitation of dose in a biologically meaningful way is not easy. For example, in the case of ionizing radiations, dose is measured in terms of absorbed energy, one rad being defined as 100 erg/gm of tissue. If different radiations are compared, say protons and X rays, it is found that biological effects are not necessarily proportional to this quantity. An important auxiliary concept is "relative biological effectiveness" (RBE*). RBE needs to be invoked because the

$$*RBE = \frac{\text{Dose of 250 kVP Xrays}}{\text{Dose of other ionizing radiation}}$$

spatial statistics of energy deposition as well as the total absorbed energy influence biological responses. Even RBE cannot be defined without specifying the exact application; the endpoint (or the assay used) can greatly influence its value.

It is not easy to translate radiobiological dosimetry ideas directly to hyperthermia, as suggested, for example, by Dietzel (1975). This point is perhaps most easily appreciated by considering a simple example, the comparison of the inactivation of cultured cells by heat or by X rays. I'll start by mentally "heating" a thermally insulated tissue culture dish containing cells in 5 ml of medium initially at 37°C. I do this by "opening" this system for a short time, say 1 min. During that time, I allow energy to enter the dish (for example *via* conduction from a hot water bath or by absorption of microwave energy) so that the final temperature is 43°C. The "heat dose", if we were to use the X-ray analogy, is approximately 6 cal/g, the dose rate, 6 cal/g/min. However, during the period the system is thermodynamically open, no cells are killed; one minute at 43°C, as I illustrated in Chapter 2, kills no mammalian cells. After I close the system again, the "heat dose" remains at 6 cal/g, but now the "dose rate" returns to zero; no additional energy is admitted nor does any leave. Yet it is only well after the reinsulation of the system that cell killing starts. The fraction of cells surviving treatment is not only a function of the "heat dose", but equally important, of the duration during which the culture is maintained at the elevated temperature. I reemphasize: once the absorption of energy is stopped and an equilibrium temperature established, cell survival is determined by the time the cells had spent at that temperature (and perhaps by the cells' ability to adapt to that temperature).

Contrast this to the X-ray case. Much less energy is required to inactivate cells; 6 cal/g is equivalent to approximately 10^5 rad, a dose sufficient to kill most if not all the mammalian cells on earth. But more important, from my immediate viewpoint, is that cell inactivation occurs only during the period of energy absorption; the cell's ultimate survival level, in the example that I discussed, is established by the events of the first hour. I am neglecting the role of repair processes, which influence this discussion in a negligible manner. The X-ray dose rate describes the space-averaged pattern of energy absorption. The quality of irradiation dose affects the efficiency of cell inactivation, but only in a relatively minor way; once RBE is specified or measured, it is the dose in rads that is the all-important quantity. Heat dose, on the other hand, depends both on temperature and on the time at that temperature. While temperature does depend on absorbed (or retained) energy, duration of exposure obviously does not. These relationships are illustrated in Figure 4.1.

Therefore, absorbed energy is not a satisfactory or meaningful defi-

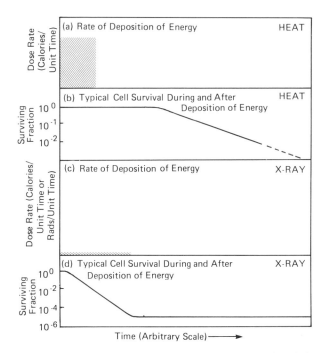

Figure 4.1. Deposition of energy and cell survival during heating or X irradiation of cultures. For heat killing, energy deposition and cellular inactivation are not necessarily correlated. Thus, in panels a and b, energy deposition during 5 min raises the temperature to a nominal value, say 43°. During this time interval, no cells are killed; cell death is only measurable if the culture remains at the elevated temperature for longer periods of time. On the other hand, it is only during X irradiation that cells are killed; once the deposition of energy, and hence the ionization, ceases, no additional cell inactivation occurs (panels c and d). The amount of energy required to kill cells with heat tends to be much larger than that needed to inactivate cells with ionizing radiations; this is indicated by the larger shaded area in panel a when compared to that of panel c.

nition of heat dose. Other attempts to formulate a definition have not been too successful and have not enjoyed general acceptance. The most reasonable of these, from an operational point of view, is that of Atkinson (1977), who suggested that heat dose be defined with respect to a standard survival curve of heat-exposed mammalian cells. Then one unit of heat dose, for example, could be any combination of time and temperature that would lead to 90% cell inactivation. But we have already seen in Chapter 2 that the heat response of cells can be changed drastically by relatively minor modifications of their environment. Owing to the sigmoidal shape of the survival curves, this definition of unit of heat dose would depend both on the shoulder and on the slope of the "standard" curve. These limitations make the value of such an *ad hoc* definition somewhat questionable. Until something better comes along, the slightly cumbersome specification of time–temperature profiles is appropriate; at least in the near future we will have to forego the luxury of a precise and concise definition of heat dose. Nevertheless, I will continue using this term, but in a colloquial sense, as describing a specific time–temperature combination. Another complication occurs in practical use. If the time required to reach the final temperature is an appreciable fraction of the total heating time, particularly if it may involve induction of thermotolerance, a complete time–temperature profile may need to be specified (Henle and Roti Roti, 1980).

4.2.2. A Nonspecific Model of Heat Inactivation

How is it possible that heat can continue to kill cells in the absence of additional energy deposition? Increasing the temperature from 37°C to a clinically meaningful hyperthermic temperature raises the average kinetic energy of cellular molecules by only a small amount. For example, a rise in temperature of 6°C corresponds to only about a two-percent increase in the average kinetic energy of each molecule. However, such a small energy change can lead to large changes in the rates of many biochemical reactions. The temperature dependence of enzymatic activities regulating rates of biosynthetic synthesis is certainly not uniform. Hence, small temperature changes could bring about a situation of "unbalanced growth," i.e., a state of the cell in which some molecules have been produced in excess, while others are in critically short supply. This situation is known to cause cell death under certain conditions (Cohen and Barnes, 1954). If unbalanced growth is indeed the mode of heat-induced cell death, a search for specific "targets" may turn out to be a wild goose chase. The various correlations that have been reported to exist between heat-induced cell death and damage to specific organelles would then simply be a consequence of unbalanced growth, rather than an indication of any causal connection. This is a consideration to keep in the back of one's mind when reading the somewhat bewildering array of correlations between heat killing and heat-induced modifications of the state of cellular organelles that will be summarized in this chapter.

From an experimental viewpoint, the unbalanced growth hypothesis is neither profitable nor satisfying. It is nearly impossible to test, and I do not find it intuitively appealing. Cellular inactivation by modalities other than heat, for example X rays or ultraviolet radiation, results from damage to specific molecules or organelles, and it seems appropriate to hypothesize that such putative intracellular "targets" also exist for heat killing. Suppose I start with such a hypotehsis, and without in any way specifying these objects, see what implications that proposed mode of cell death has with respect to the shape of the survival curve. My analysis follows the classical target-theory approach (Lea, 1947).

The observation that cell death is not exclusively determined by the amount of energy deposited within the cell surely implies that the average kinetic energy of the critical molecules is not the sole or even the primary quantity that determines the life or death of the individual cell. The experimental fact that cell killing is a function of the duration of exposure at the elevated temperature suggests that it is the temporal statistics of energy distribution that are at least equally important and that cell death is associated with one or more relatively rare molecular events. I suggest that an individual target (molecule or organelle) becomes inactivated when its instantaneous kinetic energy exceeds a critical value (E_c) at any time during the exposure time, t. Since the event is rare, $E_c >> E_{AVE}$ where E_{AVE} is the average kinetic energy of the target molecules. If $P(E)$ is the energy distribution, then the probability that the instantaneous kinetic energy of a molecule exceeds E_c during unit time is

$$P(>E_c) = \int_{E_c}^{\infty} P(E)dE / \int_{0}^{\infty} P(E)dE = \int_{E_c}^{\infty} P(E)dE \qquad (4.1)$$

If I assume $P(E)$ to follow the Maxwell–Boltzman distribution, then

$$\int_{E_c}^{\infty} P(E)dE = e^{-E_c/RT}$$

a quantity that is small compared to unity.

Then the probability that the molecule is not inactivated in that time interval is given by $1 - e^{-E_c/RT}$. For t time intervals, $P(>E_c)$ is $(1 - e^{-E_c/RT})^{t/\tau}$, where τ is an appropriate scaling constant. If we have K identical targets, all of which need to be inactivated before the cell dies, then $P_c(S)$, the probability that the cell survives during the time interval t at temperature T is:

$$P_c(S) = 1 - [1 - (1 - e^{-E_c/RT})^{t/\tau}]^K \qquad (4.2)$$

It is not difficult to demonstrate that an approximate form of equation (4.2) is:

$$\log P_c(S) = \log K - (t/\tau)e^{-E_c/RT} \qquad (4.3)$$

This equation is similar in form to those frequently employed to describe cell killing by ionizing radiation. When log $P_c(S)$ is plotted against t/τ, the shape of the resulting survival curve is governed by a shoulder whose width is determined by K, followed by a linear region whose slope is $e^{-E_c/RT}$. Thus K is analogous to the extrapolation number, while $e^{E_c/RT}$ is equivalent to D_0. For temperature changes that are small compared to the absolute temperature, T, D_0 decreases approximately linearly with temperature. Both the predicted shape of the survival curve and the temperature dependence of D_0 are consistent with experimental findings.

Equation (4.3) can be used to derive a useful relationship. Suppose we know that a time t_1 at temperature T_1 leads to a given survival, and we ask what is the time t_2 at a different temperature, T_2, to achieve a similar level of cell killing? Then from equation (4.3):

$$t_1 e^{-E_c/RT_1} = t_2 e^{-E_c/RT_2} \tag{4.4}$$

let $T_2 - T_1, = \Delta T$, so that

$$t_2/t_1 = e^{-(E_c/R)\,(\Delta T/T_1 T_2)} \tag{4.5}$$

which is of the form $t_2 t_1 = \alpha^{\Delta T}$
an equation deduced empirically by Dewey et al. (1978). The value of α can be determined experimentally.

Indeed, many estimates of α have been made, not just for cell killing in vitro, but also for a variety of other heat inactivations of biological systems. Probably the first of these estimates was by Pincus and Fischer in 1931. These workers quantified the growth inhibition suffered by cultured chick embryo fibroblasts after exposure to elevated temperatures. They noted no effects below 44°C (the normal temperature of a chicken is about 41 to 43°C), while above that temperature the time required to completely inhibit growth dropped by a factor of 2 for each degree of temperature increase. Thus, their estimate of α was 0.5. Pincus and Fischer took the calculation a step further. They assumed that the conversion from growing cultures to completely inhibited cultures could be described by a rate constant, and in that sense was similar to a chemical reaction whose rate is governed by one specific, rate-limiting step. Under such conditions, according to Arrhenius, the reaction rate constant, k, is given by $k = Ae^{-\Delta H/RT}$. In this equation, ΔH is the energy of activation. It can be determined by plotting $\ln k$ against $1/T$. If this plot yields a straight line, ΔH is proportional to the slope of that line. Arrhenius analysis is meaningful only if the measurements are made under quasi-steady state conditions; the slope of the Arrhenius plot results in a straight line only if the same chemical step remains rate limiting over the temperature range of interest. If either of these requirements is not met, ΔH becomes a function of temperature, and the Arrhenius plot does not yield a straight line. In the experiments of Pincus and Fischer, a straight line was found, that is to say, ΔH had a constant value, at least between 44 and 47°C. Its magnitude was determined to be 149 kcal/mole. This is a very high value for any chemical reaction, but according to earlier work by Brown and Crozier (1927), this value is consistent with the "thermodestruction" of proteins.

Since 1931, many investigators have found activation energies of similar magnitudes for induction of thermal damage to biological systems. Henriques (1947) showed that 150 kcal/mole was appropriate for causing the appearance of necrotic foci in the skin of pigs. A value of 141 kcal/mole was obtained by Westra and Dewey (1971) for the inactivation of mammalian cells at temperatures between 43 and 47°C; below that temperature, a "break", i.e., a change in the slope of the Arrhenius plot, was seen, indicating that perhaps a different enzymatic reaction became rate limiting, or that the quasi-steady state assumption was no longer valid. Values of 100 to 200 kcal/mole are consistent with those required for the denaturation of proteins, and it is not unreasonable to hypothesize that proteins are the molecules at risk, a suggestion made in one form or another by all the workers who have measured these activation energies. This working hypothesis would provide a clear hint on how to proceed to determine the actual, heat-sensitive target: identify the proper protein. Fluctuations in protein energies have been evaluated by Cooper *et al.* (1979), allowing one to estimate E_c directly. The values suggested by him lead to estimates of ΔH in line with the experimental values measured by various workers. Thus, so far at least, all the available data are consistent with the protein hypothesis.

The simple reaction scheme adopted by Pincus and Fischer, in which the cells' only possible states are either alive or dead, may not be adequate. Landry and Marceau (1978) suggest that survival data for HeLa cells are more consistent with a process involving one or two intermediate states. This complicates the analysis, since two or three different reaction constants have to be considered, but does not materially change the conclusion regarding the role of proteins. At temperature above 47°C, however, Landry and Marceau (1979) show that inactivation energies as low as 20 to 30 kcal/mole may describe the cell killing by heat. This suggests that at the higher temperatures the nature of the cell killing mechanism may be fundamentally different. This last conclusion is based on a series of ingenious survival experiments in which a CO_2 laser was used to heat cells to temperatures as high as 167°C and for periods as short as 10 msec. The 10-msec minimum was not owing to technical problems (the pulse length of the laser was 70 nsec!) but resulted from an inability of the cells to dissipate heat at a more rapid rate. In other words, no matter how quickly cells are exposed to this temperature, the limited cooling causes the time–temperature profile to become lethal. Based on this observation one can define a true "death point" for cells and tissue (i.e., a temperature above which the survival of cells or tissue cannot be sustained for any length of time), i.e., ~170°C. Below that temperature limit, the probability of survival at any fixed temperature is a function of the duration of exposure, though of course toward the upper limit of this range cells tend to survive for only very short times.

There remains a serious problem, however, even below 47°C: if equation 4.3 is correct, then not only E_c but also K, the number of "targets," should be meaningful. An analysis of the survival curves of Chapter 2 shows that this number ranges from 1 for HeLa cells to perhaps 10–20 for some heat-resistant lines and even larger values for cells heated in close contact with other cells (W.C. Dewey, private communication). These are *very* small numbers, and it is difficult to conceive of a class of protein molecules playing such a critical role in the cell's life so that the inactivation of a few copies could lead to cell death. Of course it is quite possible that the model I have presented is entirely wrong and that the correlation between predicted and measured shape of the survival curves is accidental. I am reluctant to accept this because of the generality of the approach. Another suggestion appears more palatable. It is possible to bypass the "target" number difficulty by invoking cooperative phenomena. If these were involved in cell death, then damage to one molecule, or a few molecules, would greatly increase the probability of damage to an entire class of similar molecules. The low value of K would then not be unreasonable. Cooperative phenomena have been observed when dealing with cells; they usually involve protein–lipid interactions, although other purely protein-related events cannot be ruled out. Another possiblity of dealing with the target number difficulty relates to repair mechanisms. If there is a systematic method that the cell has evolved to repair heat-induced damage, the value of K implied by extrapolation of the survival curve does not give a realistic measure of "target number" (although in most models it overestimates the true "target number"). Of course, until we know what the "targets" are, any discussion of putative repair systems is academic.

4.2.3. Macromolecules as Heat "Targets"

4.2.3.1. Proteins or Protein Synthesis

The evolutionary process has provided thermophilic bacteria with proteins of remarkable thermal stability. For example, an aldolase isolated from *Thermus aquaticus* (a thermophile, as its name implies) can be kept at 97°C for at least 30 min, and it fully maintains its activity at that temperature. On the other hand, a similar enzyme isolated from *Bacillus stearothermophilus,* a moderate thermophile, is readily inactivated at 75°C. Aldolases isolated from mesophiles are activated at even lower temperatures (Brock, 1978). This subject is discussed in considerable detail by Alexandrov (1977) and in a review by Hazel and Prosser (1974). It is doubtful that evolutionary pressures have selected for heat-resistant enzymes in mammalian cells. It is therefore not unlikely that enzymes of mammalian origin are denatured somewhere in the neighborhood of 50°C, or at even lower temperatures. In addition to the thermodynamic arguments presented in the previous section, a variety of other experimental data is consistent with the view that one or more cellular proteins are critical elements at elevated temperatures. Cells incubated in the presence of sulfhydryl-rich compounds become very heat sensitive (Kapp and Hahn, 1979) (Figure 3.18a). Similarly, many enzymes lose activity at a much higher rate if, at elevated temperatures, cysteine is added to the buffer in which the activity determination is made. Cells can be protected against heat by the substitution, during heating, of deuterium oxide (D_2O) for H_2O in the medium (Fisher *et al.,* 1982) (Figure 2.10). By the same token, a similar substitution allows enzymes to maintain activity at higher temperatures (Hermans and Scheraga, 1959). Two mechanisms have been postulated to explain the stabilizing action of D_2O. First, it has been suggested that the direct substitution of deuterium for hydrogen would lead to the strengthening of hydrogen bonding; an alternate explanation is that the additional solvent action presented by D_2O would stabilize macromolecules whose higher order structure depends primarily upon weak bonding. Both of these suggestions would certainly apply to proteins. Alexandrov (1977) suggests that glycerol may play a similar role. Finally, Minton *et al.* (1980) has recently shown that hydrostatic pressure can reverse, at least partially, the cytotoxic effect of elevated temperatures. Again, this could result from a stabilization of the structure of proteins, though stabilization of lipids or lipid–protein interactions is also possible.

There are, however, serious problems associated with assuming that generalized denaturation of proteins is responsible for cell death. Although several studies have shown that protein synthesis is almost completely inhibited by the exposure of cells to 43°C or higher (McCormick and Penman, 1969; Mondovi et al., 1972; Fuhr, 1974; Bleiberg and Sohar, 1975; Henle and Leeper, 1979), these studies also clearly demonstrate that some time after the return of the cells to 37°C, protein synthesis resumes. The rate of synthesis in cells that have been heated approaches and sometimes even exceeds that in unheated controls. Protein synthesis resumes even in those cells still capable of division, but whose progeny at a later time will express their inability to proliferate indefinitely (Bleiberg and Sohar, 1975). For these reasons it appears unlikely that it is the inhibition of gross protein synthesis that is related to cell death. It also makes questionable the suggestion by Strom et al. (1977) that it is polyribosomal RNA aggregation or maturation that is at fault, since any major, irreversible disruption of the integrity of polyribosomes might be expected to interfere permanently with protein synthesis.

Instead of looking at gross protein synthesis, it seems more profitable though obviously also more difficult, to examine whether a specific individual protein is unusually heat sensitive so that its inactivation would lead to cell death. But here one quickly encounters a conceptual problem. It is difficult to see how inactivation of specific enzymes could result in cell death (leaving aside the possibility of such inactivation leading to unbalanced growth); presumably individual proteins could be resynthesized after the cell had returned to its normal temperature, provided the DNA template had not been damaged excessively so that appropriate RNA species could be resynthesized at 37°C. It would seem that hyperthermic destruction of enzymes could only be lethal if it were coupled with the inactivation of one or more early steps in protein syntehsis. More plausible is the hypothesis that damage occurs to structural proteins associated with chromosomes or proteins that are constituent elements of other organelles. The resynthesis of such molecules might be insufficient or proceed too slowly to restore functional integrity to the cellular structure.

Protein stability may be involved in the frequently voiced claim that malignant cells are more heat sensitive than are their normal counterparts (Chapter 2). Pertinent here is an interesting study by Langridge (1968). This investigator isolated fifty-two variants of the enzyme β-galactosidase and measured the temperature dependence of their ability to release 0-nitrophenol from 0-nitrophenyl-β-galactoside. The mutant enzymes differed from the normal type in the substitution of one single serine for another amino acid, and from each other only in the place of that substitution. Langridge measured inactivation curves of the various enzymes by plotting enzyme activity vs. time; he used the half-time for reduction of activity as a measure of the thermal stability of the protein. Between 10 and 20°C, the mutants demonstrated the same activity as did the wild type, but fully 60% of the altered proteins were less able to retain activity at 57°C. Whether or not any of the mutants were more stable at the higher temperatures than the normal enzyme was not determined. Another interesting finding of that study was that enzyme–substrate complexes were more heat-stable than free enzymes.

From Langridge's data it can be inferred that mutations are more likely to lead to thermosensitivity than to thermostability. If, and this is by no means established fact, malignant transformation is necessarily a result of one or more specific mutations, then by analogy, a transformed cell is more likely to be thermosensitive than thermoresistant. A sensitive cell mutation would result whenever the most thermosensitive component of the transformed cell became more likely to be heat inactivated than the most sensitive component of the normal cell. The important point is that these two "targets" would not have to be the same. A different molecule could be at risk in the normal cell than in the malignant one.

This is most easily seen by appealing to the "weakest link" analogy. A chain with one particularly weak link can be made more vulnerable in one of two ways: either by making that same link even weaker or by modifying any one of the other links to the extent that it now becomes the weakest link. On the other hand the only way to strengthen the chain is to improve the weakest link. Buttressing any of the other elements has no effect on system stability. This line of reasoning would suggest that mutations have a reasonable probability of leading to increased heat sensitivity but that the finding of heat-resistant mutants would be rare. But it must be remembered that no data exist to lift such a hypothesis from the level of speculation.

4.2.3.2. RNA or RNA Synthesis

In the temperature range of major interest, 43 to 47°C, it is very unlikely that RNA species themselves are the "targets" responsible for the cells' heat death. Measurements of temperature stability of various functions of RNA lead to inactivation energies of between 20 and 30 kcal/mole (Bacher and Kauzmann, 1952, Ginoza, 1958). These values are very different from those discussed earlier for cell killing. Above 47°C, however, destruction of specific RNAs might become important, since Landry and Marceau (1979) suggest that at high temperatures inactivation of HeLa cells may be governed by a process whose activation energy falls into that range.

Many studies have shown that heat affects the synthesis of RNA (Simard *et al.*, 1969; Warocquier and Scherrer, 1969; Palzer and Heidelberger, 1973; Strom *et al.*, 1973; 1975; Nilsson, 1975; Kumar *et al.*, 1976; Henle and Leeper, 1979). A step in the synthesis or the maturation of ribosomal RNA appears to be particularly sensitive. Warocquier and Scherrer (1969) showed that in HeLa cells heated to 42°C the synthesis of messengerlike RNA is hardly affected. The 45S precursors to ribosomal RNA are still formed, but their normal metamorphosis to functional ribosomal RNA is blocked. They suggest three possibilities to explain this finding: (1) formation, in the nucleolus, of altered 80S preribosomal particles. The change in these subunits, either as a consequence of faulty structure of 45S pre-RNA or of protein associated with this precursor, could prevent them from proceeding to correct maturation; (2) thermosensitivity of some enzyme required for correct maturation; or (3) thermosensitivity of some step in the process of correct methylation of pre-RNA. However, more recent studies by Kumar *et al.* (1976), who examined ribosomal metabolism in temperature-sensitive mutants of BHk (baby hamster kidney) cells, suggest another possibility. In these cells, protein synthesis is markedly reduced after only a short exposure to the nonpermissive temperature. Associated with the reduction of protein synthesis is the increased degradation of an 18S precursor of ribosomal RNA. Kumar *et al.* suggest that considerable protection against the effects of heat is afforded those ribosomes actively participating in protein synthesis. This would be analogous to the increase in thermal stability of enzyme–substrate complexes over that of free enzymes (Langridge, 1968), as discussed in section 4.2.3.

This last finding raises the point that most of the studies discussed did not look at RNA synthesis after protein synthesis had resumed. It may very well be that once the specific enzymes necessary for RNA maturation are resynthesized normal RNA development can again proceed. It would seem to be essential to carry out such studies before reaching conclusions about the role of ribosomal RNA in determining heat death (Overgaard, 1977; Strom *et al.*, 1977). This view is reinforced by the finding of Simard and his group (Simard and Bernhard, 1967; Simard *et al.*, 1969), who demonstrated a heat-sensitive lesion in the nucleolus (presumably, the site of ribosomal assembly) but showed no difference in the rates of induction of this lesion in heat-resistant or in heat-sensitive cells. The one thing that can be concluded from these studies is that heat interferes with specific aspects of ribosomal RNA assembly. The major problem appears to be an imbalance in synthesis of the two ribosomal subunits (45S and 80S), both of which act in a functionally coupled manner during messenger RNA translation. It is possible that this imbalance results from the lower heat stability of the 80S subunit, if that subunit is not engaged in protein synthesis during heating. But, in view of the massive resumption of protein synthesis some time after heating, it seems difficult to assign a primary role in cell death to ribosomal RNA sensitivity without invoking the concept of damage to specific genes involved in RNA synthesis.

4.2.3.3. DNA or DNA Synthesis

It is very unlikely that the DNA molecule itself is the direct target for heat inactivation. *In vitro*, the melting temperature of DNA is around 87°C. At that temperature, mammalian cells would be inactivated in a fraction of a second. Of course, other damage to DNA, not nearly as drastic as melting, could result in a cellular inactivation. DNA loses its transforming ability as a result of depurination at temperatures somewhat below melting (Ginoza and Giold, 1961). For example, at 86.9°C DNA obtained from a pneumococcal strain lost its transforming ability very slowly. After 200 min at that temperature, only about 20% of the transforming ability had been lost in DNA that had been extracted using a phenol technique. DNA isolated utilizing chloroform isoamyl alcohol showed much more rapid loss of transforming ability. But even DNA so extracted still maintained 1% of its transforming ability after 200 min at 86.9°C. Interestingly, the difference in inactivation rates between these two preparations was ascribed by Ginoza and Giold (1961) to contamination in the alcohol-extracted DNA by small amounts of protein. The possible role of protein–DNA binding in determining heat sensitivity will be discussed in section 4.2.4.1. These authors also calculated the activation energy required for depurination and concluded it to be 28 kcal/mole, a value not too different from that reported by other authors (Greer and Zamenhof, 1962; Lindahl and Nyberg, 1972). This is of course, again, appreciably less than the 100 to 150 kcal/mole that has been demonstrated to be associated with heat inactivation of mammalian cells. A possible exception to this statement comes from the work of Wong and Dewey (cited by Dewey *et al.*, 1980), who demonstrate that the elongation of at least some replicons results from the interruption of DNA synthesis. Such elongation could lead to chromosomal aberrations.

Just as there is little evidence to indicate that the DNA itself is the target of heat damage, so there is equally little evidence to implicate DNA synthesis. Although, to be sure, DNA synthesis is depressed dramatically after exposing the cells to elevated temperatures (Nilsson, 1975; Henle and Leeper, 1979), this inhibition is reversible, and DNA synthesis proceeds within a few hours after returning the cells to normal temperatures, albeit at a somewhat lower rate (per cell).

4.2.4. Cellular Organelles as Heat "Targets"

In the last paragraphs I have indicated that it is unlikely, although certainly not impossible, that inactivation of a class of macromolecules is responsible for heat death, or that the apparatus required for the regeneration of such molecules is permanently damaged. It seems reasonable to extend the search for heat "targets" to specific organelles. The involvement of molecules in specific organelles was suggested early by Mondovi *et al.* (1969b). Disruption of the complicated structure of some organelles such as chromosomes or membranes appears particularly attractive since here cooperative processes are of considerable importance.

4.2.4.1. Chromosomes

There are three distinct pieces of evidence for the role of chromosomes in heat death. In both yeast (Wood, 1956) and Chinese hamster cells (Lücke-Huhle, 1978), polyploidy has been found to be associated with increased heat resistance. Nevertheless, ploidy does not seem to regulate heat responses, and certainly does not do so exclusively. I have pointed out many times that minor modifications of the cellular environment, such as pretreatment of cells with a very modest heat dose, can dramatically and within a few hours change the cells' response to heat. Obviously, this treatment does not involve chromosomal modifications. Furthermore, the heat-resistant mutant Chinese hamster cell isolated by Harris (1980) has a modal number of 23, not too different from its parent line. Harris did not perform any karyotyping, and it is therefore conceivable that the heat-resistant mutant contained a small amount of DNA that coded for one or more proteins foreign to the wild type. These might be able to confer heat resistance.

A more direct implication of the role of chromosomes is the finding by Dewey *et al.* (1971) that S phase cells heated to 45°C developed chromosomal aberrations. The number of chromosomal aberrations correlated very well with cell death. A heat dose that reduced survival by e^{-1} (D_{37}), produced, on the average, one aberration per cell. According to target theory, an exposure of cells to a D_{37} should inflict one lethal "hit" per target. Heat-induced chromosomal aberrations could be manifestations of such "hits," and the induction of even one such aberration might be lethal to the cell. The same study showed, however, that neither G1 nor M phase cells sustained any visible chromosomal aberrations at heat exposure well above the D_{37}. This greatly complicates the picture, since these cells must have been killed by another mechanism. Of course, it is possible to postulate that S phase cells are killed by heat in a manner different from cells in other parts of the cell cycle. But then survival curves of asynchronous cultures might be biphasic: one slope accounting for the cell killing of S phase cells and another for the killing of cells not synthesizing DNA. As has been shown in Chapter 2, survival curves of mammalian cells heated above 43°C have characteristics more consistent with a uniform mechanism for cell killing. It seems more likely that the chromosomal aberrations in S phase cells are a consequence of some primary damage, and that the initial lethal lesion is common to all cells; although it must be pointed out that if the D_0's of the two putative modes are not too different, the biphasic nature of the survival curve might not be discernable.

Perhaps the strongest evidence for the role of chromosomes comes from quantitative comparisons of protein–DNA binding in cells exposed to various heat treatments. Two studies (Roti Roti and Winward, 1978; Tomasovich et al., 1978) have shown that DNA isolated from heated cells is coated with nonhistone proteins, and that the amount of bound protein is a function of the thermal dose. Certainly a close association of protein to DNA could interfere permanently with transcription, and thereby sterilize cells just as Ginoza and Giold (1961) demonstrated that a protein–DNA complex induced by the alcohol extraction procedure reduced the transforming ability of bacterial DNA. Furthermore, selective coating of DNA could still permit resumption of macromolecular synthesis, but might interfere with synthesis of specific messenger RNA species. In an analysis of the increased chromatin protein content of heated cells, Roti Roti et al. (1979) demonstrated that at a heat dose equivalent to the D_{37}, there was an increase in the protein–DNA ratio, and that this increase was the same, independent of the exact temperature–time profile used to achieve this level of cell killing. As I have just pointed out, target theory implies that at a D_{37} exposure there is approximately one lethal event per cell. Therefore, these results strongly suggest a role or chromosomal protein binding in cell killing.

Roti Roti's findings were further strengthened by thermodynamic analysis of his data. The activation energy for the binding event was somewhat lower than that for cell killing, but that associated with protein–DNA binding had a Gibbs free energy that was almost identical to the

Gibbs free energy calculated for cellular inactivation. (Although, obviously, if protein–DNA association only mirrored cell death, such a correlation would hardly be surprising.) More puzzling was the demonstration that the heat dose varied linearly, rather than logarithmically, with the normalized protein-to-DNA ratio. Survival varies logarithmically, and it might have been expected that if protein–DNA binding is the lethal event it would show a similar dose dependence.

Where did the excess protein come from? If it came from within the nucleus, then the effect of heat is specific in modifying the rate of protein-to-DNA binding. Such evidence would further strengthen the suggestion of a direct involvement of this phenomenon in cell killing. However, if the protein came from the cytoplasm, the binding might simply reflect the increased availability of protein and hence an increased probability of protein–DNA interaction, without implying any causative relationship. Furthermore, if the extra protein did not come from the nucleus, the primary event would not be the binding itself, but modification of the nuclear envelope, or some other extranuclear event. Changes in the order parameter of the nuclear membrane could lead to permeability changes, and these could easily result in an increased protein content of the nucleus. This possibility was examined by Blair et al. (1979), who utilized both cytofluorometric techniques and standard biochemical assays to measure the quantity of protein in nuclei of heated and unheated cells. Isolated nuclei from heated cells were found to contain a larger amount of protein. As these researchers point out, the difference in protein content could result from the isolation procedure. Proteins of nuclear origin might be soluble in unheated cells and therefore lost during centrifugation; these same proteins might form insoluble complexes in heated cells. The additional proteins could also arise from the influx of cytoplasmic proteins (or newly synthesized proteins) into the nucleus in response to a heat-induced modification of cellular membrane physiology. To me it seems that the latter explanation is more plausible, and that therefore the data of Blair et al. reduce the probability that protein–DNA binding has any causal relationship to cell inactivation.

Coating of chromatin by "heat shock proteins" has been reported in Drosophila (Mitchell and Lipps, 1978). These proteins, not normally found in any large amount in the insects' cells, are synthesized in response to heat exposure, as well as in response to a variety of other stresses (Ashburner and Bonner, 1978). Some of them may concentrate in the nucleus shortly after their synthesis. Whether these proteins, which have also been found after heating mammalian cells (Kelley and Schlesigner, 1978), play any role in determining heat sensitivity remains to be seen. This subject will be discussed somewhat more fully in the section on thermotolerance (4.2.5).

4.2.4.2. Intracellular Membrane Systems

Of the effects of heat on various intracellular membrane structures, those on mitochondrial, lysosomal, and nuclear envelopes are of particular interest, although as was pointed out by Wallach (1977), damage to the endoplasmic reticulum is also of concern. The latter could very well lead to disassociation of membrane-bound polyribosomes, resulting in a permanent inhibition of protein synthesis. Heat-induced damage to mitochondrial membranes should result in measurable changes in cellular respiration rates. These would be of particular interest, as malignant cells seem to have fewer mitochondria than do normal cells (Pedersen, 1978). Unfortunately, data in the literature concerning rates of both respiration and glycolysis of heated cells are quite contradictory. For example, in two reviews in the same volume, Strom et al. (1977) and Dickson (1977) arrive at almost opposite conclusions. In all the tumors examined by Strom's group (Novikoff rat hepatoma, Morris 5123, minimal deviation rat hepatoma, Yoshida rat sarcoma, Ehrlich ascites mouse carcinoma, seven different human melanomas, three different human osteosarcomas, one human rectal carcinoma), glycolysis was unaffected by the exposure of cells from these tumors to temperatures up to 44°C. Von Ardenne and Reitnauer (1976) reported that glycolysis in heated Ehrlich ascites tumor cells was inhibited slightly, but this inhibition occurred only as a relatively late event.

On the other hand, Dickson and Suzanger (1974; 1976) found that the same process in human tumors is relatively easily inhibited by temperatures as low as 42.5°C. They proposed that the measurement of glycolysis as well as of oxygen uptake should be utilized as a routine assay procedure to quantify the effectiveness of heat treatment or as a predictor of the sensitivity of cell cultures from human tumors.

The situation with respect to respiration is equally controversial. Strom et al. (1977) maintained Novikoff hepatoma cells at 43°C for up to 4 hr. The cells were then transferred to 38°C, and the oxygen uptake was determined. Incubation times extending to 1.5 hr after treatment did not affect oxygen uptake; even after 6 hr, cells incubated earlier at 43°C showed oxygen uptake rates reduced only by about 40% from control values. Based on these results, and also on data showing that mitochondria retained their morphological integrity upon heating (Heine et al., 1971; Levine and Robbins, 1970), Strom et al. (1977) concluded that mitochondria are not sensitive targets of heat inactivation. On the other hand, a later study by Durand (1978) utilizing V-79 Chinese hamster cells showed markedly different results. Cells incubated at temperatures above about 42°C showed an initial but short-lived increase in oxygen uptake. This was followed by a precipitous decline in respiration; the duration of increase and the subsequent rate of decline were temperature dependent. It is interesting to plot respiration data such as those obtained by Durand on the same time scale as survival data of cells exposed to the same temperature. This has been done in Figure 4.2. As can be seen, the precipitous decline in respiration precedes by a few minutes the initiation of cellular inactivation. The reduced mitochondrial activities therefore do not simply reflect a general state of cellular disintegration resulting from cell killing. On the contrary, Durand's results suggest that cells become extremely heat sensitive once their metabolic rate and, hence, presumably their rate of ATP production are diminished. Unfortunately, no studies exist that examine cellular respiration under conditions that are known to enhance or reduce cell death. Such studies might demonstrate a direct link between the absence (or the greatly reduced rate) of ATP production (or levels) and cell cytotoxicity.

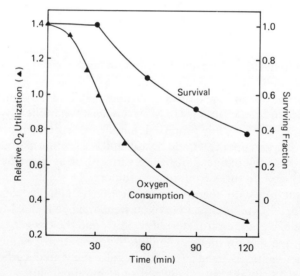

Figure 4.2. Temporal relationship between cell inactivation and respiration. Oxygen consumption of V–79 cells at 43°C (lower curve, left ordinate) starts at 1.4 times the level of unheated controls; 15 min after initiation of heating it drops precipitously. Survival (upper curve, right ordinate) remains high for 30 min and only then proceeds to drop, indicating that inhibition of respiration may lead to cell death. From Durand (1978), with permission.

Several studies, carried out at temperatures between 15 and 30°C, have examined possible relationships between respiration rates and membrane compositions. Arrhenius plots of respiration rates were constructed over the temperature range of interest. Three studies have shown that when the ratio of saturated to unsaturated fatty acids making up membranes is varied, transition temperatures of thermotropic phase changes in mitochondrial membranes are shifted, and simultaneously the "breaks" in Arrhenius plots of respiration rates are translated equally (DeKruyff et al., 1973; Janki et al., 1975; Watson et al., 1975). It is therefore not inconceivable that membrane changes introduced by elevated temperatures could result in changes of the structures of membrane-bound enzymes, and these in turn could then change respiration rates. A recent work tried to examine this possiblity by studying the respiration of goldfish acclimated to different temperatures. Changes in the fatty acid composition of membranes accompanied adaptation to new temperatures. Activation energies of respiration were compared with the ratio of saturated to unsaturated fatty acids of mitochodrial membranes from various organs of the fish. No consistent correlations were found. Mitochondrial membranes obtained from liver, white muscle, and red muscle showed large differences in the degree of unsaturation of the lipids, without any associated measurable changes in respiration rates. This study therefore did not support the hypothesis that respiration rates are influenced greatly by the physical characteristics of mitochondrial membranes.

Just as is the case for glycolysis, no studies exist that examine respiratory rates of mammalian cells under conditions that are known to change survival parameters. For example, the effect of variations of extracellular pH on respiratory rates at mildly elevated temperatures has not been examined; neither do studies exist that look at changes in respiratory rates in the presence of heat-protective agents such as deuterium oxide. These same criticisms apply to the suggested connection between effects on lysosomal membranes and mammalian cell death. These organelles, through release of their acid hydrolases, could certainly bring about irreparable cell damage. A study by Allison and Paton (1975) describes chromosomal damage in human diploid cells following activation of lysosomal enzymes. Thus, even the findings of Dewey and Sapareto (1978) implicating chromosomal aberrations might be related to damage to lysosomes. Heat is claimed to affect the lysosomal membrane (Von Ardenne et al., (1969), to increase lysosomal enzyme activity (Overgaard, 1975; Hume and Field, 1977), and to increase the total number of lysosomes (Heine et al., 1971; Overgaard and Overgaard, 1974).

Von Ardenne (1975) suggests that differential heat sensitivity of tumors compared to normal tissue results from an increase of lysosomal membrane lability in tumors. In the presence of high concentrations of glucose, he argues, intracellular pH would be decreased in all cells, but this decrease might be accentuated in cells that utilize anaerobic pathways for glycolysis. Low intracellular pH would labilize lysosomal membranes and this would make cells more heat sensitive. Unfortunately for this hypothesis, there is little evidence that intracellular pH, as opposed to extracellular pH, can be increased by the availability of excess glucose (Dickson and Oswald, 1976; Spencer and Lehninger, 1976; Haveman, 1981).

Data of Spencer and Lehninger (1976) have been used by Wallach (1977) to show that intracellular acidification by lactate production could only occur in cells that lack a proton export system; to my knowledge no such mammalian cells exist. Hence the hypothesis that glucose induces intracellular acidification, which in turn increases lysosomal activity appears not to be backed by any experimental results. A primary role of lysosomes in thermal cytotoxicity would imply that cells showing a large number of lysosomes would be heat sensitive; by the same token cells having few lysosomes should be heat resistant. This possibility has been examined only in one system. Fajardo *et al.* (1980) showed that in EMT6 tumor cells there are very few lysosomes. Yet this tumor is particularly heat sensitive, as demonstrated by the finding that 100% cure rates can be achieved by single heat doses of 43°C for 1 hr (Marmor *et al.*, 1978a). Furthermore, EMT6 cells *in vitro* also do not display any particularly heat-resistant features (Gerner *et al.*, 1979).

The evidence for the involvement of the nuclear envelope in heat death is even scantier than that implicating other intracellular membrane structures. I have already discussed the work of Blair *et al.* (1979), who showed that the increased protein content in nuclei harvested from heated cells could be interpreted as resulting from the transfer of proteins from the cytoplasm into the nucleus, secondary to the hyperthermic modification of nuclear membrane permeability. Also cited in support of the involvement of the nuclear envelope could be the evidence shown by Dewey *et al.* (1978), also previously discussed, that only in S phase cells is the primary heat lesion translated into chromosomal damage. Since DNA synthesis (or DNA repair) may very well occur in sites directly connected to the nuclear membrane, this evidence might be used to reinforce suggestions that this organelle plays an important part in the cells' heat death. Quite clearly both these pieces of evidence are subject to alternate interpretations, and hence I conclude that at this time we simply are unable to make any meaningful statements about the possible role of the nuclear envelope in cellular inactivation.

4.2.4.3. Plasma Membrane

By far the greatest number of studies attempting to elucidate heat effects on mammalian cells have shown some modification of membrane structure and/or function (Bowler *et al.*, 1973). Before I go into the details about how exposures to elevated temperatures affect the membrane, it may be useful to describe very briefly the currently accepted model of membrane structure and outline some critical membrane functions. The plasma membrane consists primarily of an asymmetric lipid bilayer. The structural phospholipids are oriented with their hydrophilic polar heads to the outer surfaces and the hydrocarbon tails in the membrane's interior, forming an ordered structure. Saturated phospholipids are highly "ordered", while hydrocarbon chains with unsaturated bonds introduce some measure of disorder or "fluidity." Phospholipids in artificial bilayers undergo phase changes, frequently near 20°C. Below that temperature the lipids are in a solid state, while at a higher temperature the bilayers have properties of fluids. In mammalian cell membranes, phase changes are masked by the presence of cholesterol and proteins. Cholesterol acts as a buffer of fluidity, stiffening the membrane at temperatures above the phase transition and fluidizing it below that temperature. At 37°C the average viscosity of the mammalian cell plasma membrane resembles that of mineral oil.

The presence of proteins, however, makes the concept of a uniform membrane viscosity rather questionable. Protein–lipid interactions introduce what may well be fluid "islands" into the semisolid structure. The analogy has been made to icebergs in a sea that is itself at the freezing temperature, though in the case of the membranes there may be more ice than water. The relative proportion of liquid and solid phase microregions appears to depend upon a variety of factors, including the amount of cholesterol present, the ratio of saturated to unsaturated fatty acids making up the membrane, and even the cells' position in the cell cycle. Dynamic aspects of membrane structure largely involve membrane proteins and glycoproteins, which may be either loosely associated, peripheral membrane components or integral macromolecules that sometimes span the membrane. The protein–lipid interactions depend on secondary and higher order structures of the proteins and on the physical makeup of the membrane. Proteins are involved in active (and perhaps passive) transport phenomena and in "recognition." By recognition I mean formation of bonds between individual cells, and the binding to the plasma membrane of small molecules (lectins and hormones). These govern the interactions of the cell with its surroundings.

The evidence indicating that the membrane is indeed a major heat target has been reviewed by Strom *et al.* (1977) and by Wallach *et al.* (1979). These two reviews, separated by only a few years, come to exactly opposite conclusions. Although Strom *et al.* cite a variety of data that indicate that a correlation exists between membrane damage and heat inactivation, they conclude that, "It appears that although heat treatment of tumor cells brings about modification of the cell at the membrane level, these cannot be considered as the primary effect of thermal exposure, but rather a consequence of previous cellular lesions." On the other hand Wallach's conclusion is that, "The results suggest an important and testable mechanism, namely tumor membrane proteins may modify the collective thermotropic behavior of membrane proteins and membrane lipids, in the process making the tumor cell plasma membrane inherently thermal sensitive." He therefore proposes that not only is the membrane the primary target, but that specific tumor membrane proteins are responsible for the heat sensitivity of tumor cells. Let us look at what constitutes the evidence either way.

A variety of reports have shown that bacteria modify their membrane composition in response to changes in environmental temperatures. These membrane changes are then accompanied by changes in heat resistance. This literature is extraordinarily rich and interesting. Here I will cite only a few studies (Cullen *et al.*, 1971; Esser and Souza, 1974; Huang *et al.*, 1974; Miller and Koshland, 1977; Yatvin, 1977; Yatvin *et al.*, 1979). In general, these investigators show that bacteria attempt to maintain a constant "fluidity" of their membrane independent of the environmental temperature. This they achieve by varying the ratio of unsaturated to saturated fatty acids comprising the phospholipid component of their plasma membranes. Under isothermal conditions, an increased ratio of unsaturated to saturated fatty acids brings about increased membrane fluidity. Since elevated temperatures increase fluidity, the organisms' adaptive response to being placed at higher temperature is to substitute lipids with a reduced ratio of unsaturated to saturated fatty acids in the membrane. Not only is that a short-term adaptive process, but it is also found on an evolutionary scale. Animals living at low temperatures appear to evolve a lipid metabolism designed to produce a membrane whose fluidity is consistent with function at the environmental temperatures (Cossins and Prosser, 1978).

In the studies cited, fluidities were measured either by monitoring a spin-label probe such as Tempo (Hubbell and McConnell, 1971) utilizing electron spin resonance (ESR) techniques, or by measuring the rotational mobility of a fluorescent probe such as diphenylhexatriene (DPH). Both ESR and particularly fluorescent polarization techniques have been criticized. It is suggested that neither technique provides an unequivocal measurement of fluidity, and even more importantly, it is questioned whether fluidity is a meaningful parameter in heterogeneous systems such as membranes (Wallach *et al.*, 1975). The arguments are technically complex, but there is very little question that it is a long step to extrapolate from fluorescence polarization data to actual fluidity measurements (e.g., "microviscocity," measured in poise). This extrapolation is made difficult by the shape of the probe, its location, and the question of whether a single decay constant determines the relaxation of the molecules. Other difficulties relate to the possible asymmetry in the distribution of membrane lipids within the bilayer, and above all, to the presence of proteins. The measured behavior of any probe is therefore an average over several parameters, which are determined by the lipids involved, by protein–lipid interactions, and by the location of the probe. Nevertheless, it is clear that changes in ESR spectra or in fluorescence polarization ratios reflect some changes in the biophysical makeup of the membrane. The problems are not the measurements, but their precise interpretation.

Not all membrane functions are affected by fluidity. To quote Miller and Koshland (1977), "Some steps involved in growth or maintenance of viability must depend strongly on a large amount of membrane fluidity, whereas the sensory and motility functions do not." Among the processes dependent on fluidity are, interestingly enough, many transport processes and respiration as well as the activities of certain membrane-bound enzymes (Kutchai *et al.*, 1976). Not only in bacteria, but also in yeast (Hagler and Lewis, 1974), and perhaps in mammalian cells there is good indication that fluidity is related to heat sensitivity. As discussed earlier, in eukaryotic cells the fluidity of membranes is modulated not only by proteins but also by cholesterol content. In general, the higher the cholesterol content the lower the fluidity (Kapitulnik *et al.*, 1979). Cress *et al.* (1980) have indicated that in several cell lines examined there is an inverse correlation between the cholesterol–phospholipid ratio of the cells' membranes and heat sensitivity, although a more recent work has failed to confirm this finding (R.L. Anderson and S.B. Field, private communication).

In another study, Li and Hahn (1980b) have demonstrated that it is possible to adapt Chinese hamster cells whose usual surroundings are at 37°C to grow at 32, 39, and 41°C. In parallel with this adaptation, cells grown at 32°C become more heat sensitive, while those grown at 39 and 41°C become more heat resistant. Anderson *et al.* (1981) have shown that when Chinese hamster cells so heat adapted reach confluence, membrane fluidity, cholesterol–phospholipid ratios, and heat sensitivity are all correlated. The 32°C-grown cells, when examined at 37°C, had more fluid membranes and a lower cholesterol–phospholipid ratio than did the controls. On the other hand, the cells adapted to 41°C had stiffer membranes and higher cholesterol–phospholipid ratios. These correlations did not extend to exponentially grown cultures. The reasons for that may be that cells grown at 32°C grow very slowly, while at 38°C growth rate is at a maximum. Distribution of cells in various parts of the cell cycle may well have been different in these populations, and cell cycle effects may have been dominant. On the other hand, almost all the cells in confluent cultures are in a G1-like part of the cell cycle (Hahn and Little, 1972).

The possible importance of fluidity is accentuated by the finding that a variety of fluidizing agents are able to mimic the behavior of heat to a surprising degree. A variety of molecules whose only common denominator, as far as is known, is their ability to fluidize membranes, elicit similar behavior. Perhaps of particular interest are experiments involving a series of alcohols. As has been described earlier, the addition of ethanol and several other alkanols to growth media acts to lower the temperature threshold required for cellular inactivation. The molarity needed to achieve a given temperature shift depends upon the alcohol's carbon number. This may be important, because it has been shown by Jain *et al.* (1978) that the molar equivalent needed to achieve a given change in membrane properties depends on the alcohol involved and on the partition of the alcohols between the lipid and aqueous regions within the cell. If the actual molarity of each alcohol is corrected according to its lipid–water partition coefficient so that only the number of molecules within the lipids is considered, the efficiency of aliphatic alcohols in changing membrane fluidity changes linearly with carbon number, and the differences between adjacent carbon numbers are small. In Figure 4.3, I show how straight-chain alcohols in the carbon number range of 2–5 inactivate Chinese hamster cells, either at 35 or at 43°C. The abscissa of that figure is in moles of the alcohol, which are seen to vary by a factor of about 20 (to achieve a given level of cell inactivation). However, concentrations in the aqueous phase vary by better than 100:1, while in the lipid-rich regions the variations are greatly reduced. This makes it most likely that the alcohols exert their cytotoxic action within the only lipid-rich regions of the cell, namely the membranes (Hahn and Li, 1981).

A comparison of Figures 4.3a and 4.3b shows that at the elevated temperature (43°C) the minimum concentration required for each alcohol to become cytotoxic is reduced. These results imply either that heat and alcohols act independently but have a common site of action, or that heat simply increases the efficiency of alcohols perhaps to induce "disorder" in the membrane. In the latter case, heat killing in the absence of alcohols might have no relationship to killing in their presence. Several pieces of evidence favor the first hypothesis. Ethanol can induce thermal tolerance,

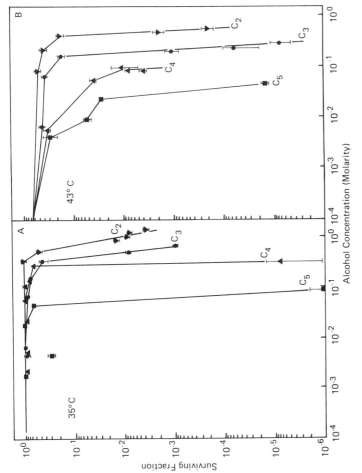

Figure 4.3. Survival of Chinese hamster cells (HA–1) exposed to aliphatic alcohols. The lengths of the carbon chains is indicated by C_i, i.e., C_2 is ethanol, C_5 is n-pentanol. Exposures were for 30 min at 35°C (panel a) or 43°C (panel b). Note the threshold effect for each alcohol, and that the magnitude of the threshold is a function of both carbon number and temperature. Data from Hahn and Li (1982), with permission.

and heat can induce tolerance to ethanol. As shown in Figure 4.4, both modalities can induce a temporary resistance to adriamycin (Li and Hahn, 1978). In neither of these cases is there any possibility that heat might be potentiating an ethanol effect. Additionally, ethanol and heat behave similarly over a range of interactions with several probes. In the presence of either heat or ethanol, deuterium oxide protects against cell killing, while cysteine sensitizes; low pH (<7.0) enhances both heat and ethanol toxicity (Li et al., 1980b). Cells either heated or exposed to ethanol show more rapid agglutination by the plant lectin concanavalin A (conA) (Hahn and Li, 1981), but reduced capping ability (Stevenson et al., 1981). Examples of the correlation of survival and capping ability are shown in Figure 4.5. Finally, several scanning electron microscopic studies have demonstrated directly that heating modifies the plasma membrane structure (Rockwell and Rockwell, 1976; Bass et al., 1978; and Lin et al., 1973).

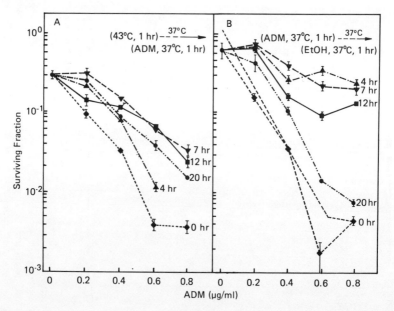

Figure 4.4. Induction of adriamycin tolerance by heat and by ethanol. In panel A, Chinese hamster cells (HA–1) were exposed to 43°C for 1 hr, and adriamycin (ADM) dose response curves were obtained at time intervals of between 0 and 20 hr later; panel B depicts results from similar experiments, but the initial exposure was to 6% ethanol (37°C, 1 hr). Panel B also shows the survival of cells exposed to adriamycin only (line originating at 0 dose—10^0 survival point); these results are included to demonstrate that true tolerance is involved, rather than the disappearance of heat- (or ethanol-) induced sensitization. Data from Li and Hahn (1978), with permission.

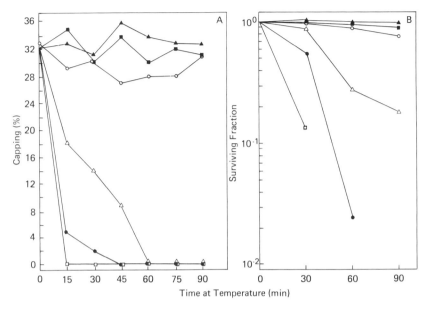

Figure 4.5. Comparison of capping and survival of heated cells. Chinese hamster cells (HA–1) were exposed to various temperatures for the time indicated on the abscissa, and capping ability (panel A) and cloning ability (panel B) were measured. Loss of capping ability appears to precede cell death. Solid triangles, 37°C; solid squares, 41°; open circles, 42°; open triangles, 43°; closed circles, 44°; open squares, 45°. From Stevenson *et al.* (1981), with permission.

Further direct evidence for plasma membrane involvement comes from studies involving the antibiotic amphotericin B, already mentioned in the previous chapter. The antibiotic binds to cholesterol. In mammalian cells this sterol is concentrated almost exclusively in the plasma membrane. Cholesterol–amphotericin B complexes form channels, and presumably when too many of these channels are formed, the cell dies. When Chinese hamster cells and EMT6 mammary sarcoma cells were exposed to graded doses of amphotericin B, which at 37 or 41°C killed few if any cells, at 43°C substantial cell killing was observed. This increased effectiveness at 43°C may result from the availability of an additional number of cholesterol binding sites, or an increased lateral mobility of cholesterol–amphotericin B complexes to form the necessary aggregates for transmembrane channel formation, or it may reflect the temperature sensitivity of the process of channel formation. Whatever the mechanism, the results imply that between 41 and 43°C a thermotropic event takes place in the plasma membrane.

In experiments on whole cells, Mikkelsen and Wallach (1977) demonstrated that the transmembrane electrochemical potential of glucose-deprived erythrocytes shows an abrupt decrease with increasing temperature, with a midpoint at 38°C. Glucose-supplemented cells exhibit a somewhat similar "transition," except that the temperature midpoint is shifted to 41°C. The permeability of cells to adriamycin (Hahn and Strande, 1976), polyamines (Gerner et al., 1980), and small ions (Strom et al., 1977) is modified by hyperthermia. In a human T-lymphocytic leukemia line (Molt 4), Kwock et al. (1978) have shown that sodium-dependent amino acid transport is partially inhibited by an exposure of cells to 43°C for 1 hr or longer. After 4 hr of continous exposure, transport was reduced by about 40% of the control value; clearly transport is not inhibited completely even in heat-inactivated cells.

Finally, several experiments have been done on purified membrane fractions that specifically demonstrate modification of membrane structure resulting from an exposure to elevated temperatures. Results from these studies are discussed in some detail in the review by Wallach (1977). Briefly, Raman spectroscopy data have shown that although lipids in erythrocyte membranes show only a very broad transition from crystalline to fluid structure at a temperature less than 5°C, all membranes exhibit two distinct transitions. These are centered at −4 and +17°C, respectively. At a physiological pH (between 7.0 and 7.5), there is an abrupt, large change in the methyl-residue environment that can be seen between 38 and 45°C. Verma and Wallach (1976) interpret this as very likely resulting from changes in membrane protein structure. Reinforcing this interpretation, Bieri and Wallach (1975), utilizing the technique of paramagnetic quenching of erythrocyte membrane tryptophase fluorescence, showed a sharp change in apolar lipid–protein association between 38 and 45°C. Relatively small changes in pH, from a value of 7.0 to 6.5, reduced the transition temperatures by about 16°C. The Raman spectroscopy data and those from experiments involving paramagnetic quenching techniques suggest that there are hyperthermic effects on cell membrane proteins or on protein–lipid interactions. Whether these are direct effects, or secondary to possible heat-induced changes in the physical state of the lipids, is not known.

The data presented in the last few paragraphs amply demonstrate that mammalian cell membranes undergo major changes upon being heated. Several of these changes mirror changes in survival parameters. Most of the observed modifications, in part because of the measurement techniques, refer specifically to the plasma membrane. This comment obviously applies to all the data obtained on plasma membrane fractions, to the data involving agglutination and capping by conA, and also to the amphotericin B results. Some of these results may be modulated by the availability of ATP or by effects on cytoskeletal elements. Furthermore, if indeed the intracellular pH of mammalian cells is kept relatively constant over changes in the extracellular pH, the pH sensitivity of thermal inactivation, detailed in Chapter 2, would also suggest that the plasma membrane is a primary traget of heat inactivation. In this sense, my conclusions would certainly be in concordance with those of Wallach, as well as those of Bowler *et al.* (1973).

My personal view is that the plasma membrane is in fact the initial and perhaps even the primary target of heat inactivation. Making the plasma membrane the major traget would make it relatively simple to explain the shape of the survival curves, and in particular the low extrapolation numbers observed, as discussed in the beginning of this chapter. The complex lipid, protein, and sterol structure that constitute this membrane makes it an ideal place for cooperative phenomena to take place. They can occur in relatively small domains and thereby escape detection by many techniques (Shinitzky and Barenholz, 1978).

In spite of all the evidence involving membranes, at present I cannot exclude the possibility that other organelles may prove to be more important than the plasma membrane. In particular, chromosomal structures, mitochondria, lysosomes, ribosomes, and components of RNA synthesis remain as possible competitors. Some other structures, for example the cytoskeleton, have not been examined in great detail. Finally, one always has to keep in the back of one's mind the possibility that many "targets" may be of approximately equal heat sensitivity, and that heat death is determined primarily by the environmental parameters of the particular experiment, or involves different organelles or macromolecules depending upon the particular cell line examined.

4.2.5. Thermotolerance

The transient resistance to heat observed in cells heated previously and called thermotolerance has been discussed several times. Its study is merited for several reasons. In the clinic, scheduling of fractionated hyperthermia with respect to tolerance of tumor and normal tissue may well spell the difference between tumor eradication and treatment failure. Seen through the eyes of a biologist, tolerance presents an unusually interesting example of a cellular adaptive process, and as such may have evolutionary and ecological implications. Were this not enough, a thorough understanding of thermotolerance would very likely provide insight into the mechanism(s) of heat-induced cell death. I have pointed out earlier that in order to make a cell more heat resistant, it is the cell's most heat-sensitive subunit that must be stabilized. Understanding thermotolerance might therefore help in identifying the heat "target."

Needless to say, the precise molecular mechanisms responsible for thermotolerance are not known. A virtue of the model of thermotolerance presented in section 2.6.2. is that it permits analysis of the induction of thermotolerance in terms of at least two constituent processes, namely triggering and development. Triggering occurs at all supranormal temperatures, but development is restricted to a permissive range, 42.5°C or lower for most cell lines. For the cell to change its heat response, development must have been permitted to occur.

The kinetic experiments of Li *et al.* (1981) place specific limits on the molecular events of triggering. These are based on an Arrhenius analysis of these results as shown in Figure 4.6. To obtain the data illustrated in that figure, the time to reach 50% of maximum tolerance (as measured on a plot of log-survival vs. duration of exposure to the trigger signal) was plotted against T^{-1}. The two clearly observable features of the Arrhenius plot are: (1) There is a clear and very sharp transition in triggering

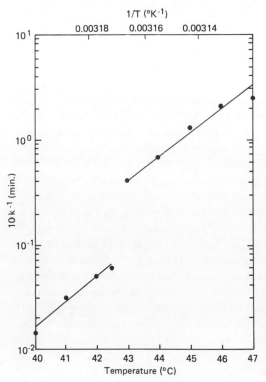

Figure 4.6. Arrhenius plot for the initial event ("trigger") in the induction of thermotolerance. The kinetics of the triggering of thermotolerance were obtained for Chinese hamster cells (HA–1) over the range of 41 to 47°C, and from these results the Arrhenius plot shown was constructed. The rate constant (k), plotted on the ordinate, is a measure of the duration of the initial treatment required to induce maximum tolerance. The abscissa is in units of Celsius degrees and (absolute temperature)$^{-1}$. The sharp transition between 42.5 and 43°C is indicative of the occurrence of a thermotropic cooperative process. Data from Li *et al.* (1982b).

kinetics that occurs between 42.5 and 43°C. Below 42.5°C, half-times are measured on a time scale of hours; above that temperature the scale is better expressed in minutes. (2) The slope of both segments of the Arrhenius line is the same (at least within experimental error). The activation energy obtained from the slope is about 120 kcal/mole, not significantly different from the 125 kcal/mole required for the killing of HA-1 cells.

The sharpness of the transition is very unusual. For example, phase changes of lipids, even in homogeneous systems, take place over a temperature range of several degrees. Thus, the change in triggering kinetics observed between 42.5 and 43°C is very likely a reflection of a phenomenon involving a high degree of cooperativity. The data in Figure 4.6 suggest a marked modification, within a half-degree temperature range, of a complicated structure that depends for its function on the structural integrity of a great majority of its subunits. The value of the activation energy involved suggests that the damaged subunits may be proteins, although this is not necessarily the case. There is not much else that can be said with any certainty, other than to point out that the possible structures involved are not too many. Purely speculatively, a plausible scenario might be that the target proteins are intramembrane proteins and that the structure affected by the thermal treatment is the cytoskeleton. As long as the latter is intact, protein inactivation is a very rare event; hence long times are required for triggering. However, after the putative collapse of the cytoskeleton, inactivation would become more probable and triggering would proceed more rapidly. The activation energy required would stay constant, but the average kinetic energy of the protein molecules would increase appreciably after the collapse of the structural support. Again I point out that the suggestion is speculative and that no data exist that implicate cytoskeleton collapse at or near 43°C.

The mechanisms governing the second part of tolerance induction, namely development, are also not understood. Protein synthesis appears to be involved, as shown by the finding of Palzer and Heidelberger (1973) that the addition to the growth medium of cycloheximide, a potent inhibitor of protein synthesis, tends to protect cells against heat death. In a similar vein, McCormick and Penman (1969) demonstrate that pretreating cells with this drug before heating tends to reduce the subsequent heat effects on protein synthesis. A direct connection between thermotolerance and protein synthesis is suggested by the work of Henle and Leeper (1979). Chinese hamster cells exposed to 45°C for either 10 min or 17.5 min showed precipitous reduction in protein synthesis immediately after heating; however, synthesis recovered, and this recovery took place at just about the same time that the cells developed thermotolerance. Furthermore, incubation of cells at 0°C after heating, the addition of cycloheximide, or the replacement of H_2O by D_2O in the medium inhibited the induction of resistance to a second heat exposure. All these procedures are accompanied by the reduction or total inhibition of protein synthesis. Thus, these results are quite consistent with the view that protein synthesis is a requirement for the development of thermotolerance.

Interestingly, placing cells at 41°C only partially inhibits their protein synthesis (Fuhr, 1974), and this temperature is "permissive" for the development of thermotolerance, i.e., thermotolerance develops during heating. Evidence exists that questions the need for protein synthesis, at least on a massive scale, in the development of thermotolerance. Li and Hahn (1980a) demonstrated that cells placed in a balanced salt solution develop heat resistance at the same rate and to the same extent as do cells in a nutrient-rich environment. Yet protein synthesis is greatly reduced in the salt solution (Hahn *et al.*, 1973). Therefore it may be the synthesis of only very specific proteins that is involved in the development of thermotolerance. Such synthesis could proceed under conditions that inhibit large-scale productions of the macromolecules. It is tempting to equate the so-called heat shock proteins (hsp's) with the putative proteins capable of protecting the cell. Hsp's are a heterogeneous class of proteins that appear to be synthesized preferentially by many organisms including mammalian cells in response to a variety of stresses. Included among them are: exposure to heat, cold, anoxia, ethanol, vinblastine, etc. (reviewed by Ashburner and Bonner, 1978). Suggestions have indeed been made that in both yeast and *Drosophila* synthesis of hsp's may confer protection against heat damage (Mitchell *et al.*, 1979; McAllister and Finkelstein, 1980). Recently Li *et al.* (1982b) demonstrated that the kinetics of the development of tolerance correlate well with the synthesis of hsp's but correlate poorly with the resumption of synthesis of actin, a structural protein. Chinese hamster cells were exposed to 45°C for 20 min and then returned to 37°C. At various times later, survival was assayed after a second test exposure. Other cells were pulse-labeled with [^{35}S] methionine, and then the proteins were separated on acrylamide gels. Rates of synthesis of 59K, 70K, and 87K hsp's as well as that of actin, were estimated from autoradiographs by densitometer tracings. While the rates of synthesis of the three hsp's correlated well with the development of tolerance, the rate of synthesis of actin recovered in a manner that seemed not related to the kinetics of tolerance development.

While these results are certainly interesting, not all is peaches and cream. The induction of hsp's follows several stresses, but only two of these (heat and ethanol) have been reported to result in the induction of tolerance. Either hsps have nothing to do with tolerance, or else only a subset of hsp's is involved in heat protection, and this subset is not produced in response to the other stresses. Furthermore, hsp's within the cell are ubiquitous once they appear, and do not provide specific hints as to "target" location. Thus, only the identification of the appropriate subset responsible for heat tolerance (if indeed such a subset exists) and perhaps the isolation of monoclonal antibodies against the specific hsp's responsible for protection, will lead to important new information regarding cellular "targets." Since experiments along these lines are beginning to proceed, interesting results should soon appear.

4.3. HEAT-ENHANCED X-RAY CYTOTOXICITY

There is no question that heat increases the efficiency of X rays to kill mammalian cells. An obvious question to be asked is: Is the mode of heat death the same as that responsible for this enhanced cytotoxicity of X rays? The last sections have been devoted to pointing out that, on the biochemical level, we really don't know what constitutes the lethal action of hyperthermia. Thus, obviously this question cannot be answered with an absolute yes or no. On the other hand, considerable evidence indicates that important differences must exist. Raaphorst et al. (1979) found only a mild correlation between hyperthermic sensitization and heat sensitivity in seven cell lines examined. A variety of agents that protect against X irradiation (SH compounds, ethanol, dimethylsulfoxide, etc.) are potent heat sensitizers. Thus, if heat killing and heat-induced radiosensitization do have some overlapping mechanism, they cannot be exclusive. In fact, the data seem to suggest that if an overlap exists it is not the major mechanism involved. The strong suggestion that the modes of the two processes are different, however, does not necessarily imply that the "targets" are different.

Most radiobiologists would agree that ionizing radiations kill cells largely by damaging the cells' reproductive apparatus. However, as pointed out by Hall (1978), "Accumulated evidence does not by any means prove conclusively that the DNA of the chromosomes constitutes a primary target for radiation-induced lethality." Alper (1974) has presented considerable evidence that membrane damage may be of considerable importance. Nevertheless, it is not surprising that investigators have looked at various aspects of DNA damage and repair to see if the influence of elevated temperatures can be detected and if correlations can be found between the frequency of observed DNA lesions and heat potentiation of X-ray killing. Conceptually, there are several ways in which amplification by heat of either immediate or residual X-ray damage could occur. First of all, heat could increase the efficiency by which X rays cause all types of DNA damages, such as single-strand and double-strand breaks and base damage. Secondly, repair of lesions could be affected, since heat might induce differential changes in the rates of recovery vs. fixation of damage. Heat might also cause a direct conversion of reparable into irreparable lesions. Finally, the probability of misrepair could be increased, for example by increasing the rate of base repair. This would lead to a larger number of lethal mutations.

Let's look at the experimental data for each one of these possibilities. Increased X-ray-like damage resulting from heat exposure has only been reported in one study. Corry et al. (1977) point out that although the frequency of double-strand break induction remains unaffected by heat treatment, there does appear to be a 10 to 20% increase in the frequency of single-strand break induction. In this study cells were exposed to 43°C for 30 min prior to being irradiated with either 35 krad for the determination of the number of double-strand breaks introduced, or with 3 krad for single-strand breaks. Strand breakage was assayed in alkaline or neutral sucrose gradients.

The rate of rejoining of single-strand breaks in DNA from cells heated and X irradiated was measured by several investigators. In one group of experiments, radiation of cells was at 37°C (or lower), followed by incubation at hyperthermic temperatures (42 to 43°C). No reduction in the rate of rejoining was seen by Ormerod and Stevens (1971), nor by Weniger et al. (1979), while Ben-Hur and Elkind (1974) actually measured an increased rate of rejoining at 42°C when compared to 37°C controls. Dikomey (1978) investigated the rejoining of double-strand breaks and saw no effect from the heat dose.

In other experiments, heating preceded irradiation, and very different results were seen. Both Corry et al. (1977) and Clark and Lett (1978) found that the cells heated before irradiation were significantly less efficient in effecting repair than were unheated controls. The same proved to be the case for the rejoining of double-strand breaks. Here an exposure of cells to 43°C for 30 min resulted in a reduction by 50% of the rate of rejoining.

Two other pieces of data might be relevant here. Dewey et al. (1980) examined the effect of heat on the priming ability of β-polymerase; this enzyme has been reported as playing a role in the repair of DNA (Bollum, 1975; Bertazzoni et al. 1976). The ability of this enzyme obtained from several sources (Novikoff hepatoma, calf thymus DNA, or DNA from human placenta) to initiate DNA repair was severaly impaired after incubation at 45°C for as little as 10 min. For example, the incubation at 45°C of Novikoff hepatoma cells reduced the activity of β-polymerase to about 15% of that obtained from unheated controls. On the other hand, the work of Weniger *et al.* (1979) indicated that the same enzyme obtained from pig thymus maintained full activity over the temperature range of 37 to 43°C. Even a 2-hr exposure at 45°C reduced the rate of polymerization only by about 25%. Unfortunately, no survival studies were done with this same cell line; it would certainly be interesting to know if pig thymus cells were not sensitized to X irradiation by heat. Ben-Hur and Elkind (1974) describe the effects of combined heat and X-ray treatments on the restoration of a DNA–lipid "complex." They also find a close correlation between heat sensitization to X irradiation and the inability of the complex to reform itself at 37°C.

Finally, I come to the possibility that heat modifies the rate of misrepair. By misrepair I mean production of "repaired" DNA whose fidelity is compromised so that a cell carrying it would have a lower probability of completing a successful cell division, but an increased probability of producing progeny with heritable defects. One could, for example, envisage that heat would convert a relatively error-free repair system to an error-prone one. Increased cell killing would result from the production of an increased number of lethal mutations. Any heat-induced excess rate of error-prone repair can be measured by quantifying changes in X-ray-induced rates of mutations or of oncogenic transformation, since the latter are thought to be expressions of one or more specific mutations. Very few such studies exist.

Heat, without X irradiation, can amplify mutation rates. For example, Mittler (1979) showed that a 1-hr exposure to 38°C increased the production of recessive lethal mutations in *Drosophila*, normally grown at 25°C, by a factor of about 2 over the spontaneous rate. Many other studies have shown similar effects in *Drosophila*. In human lymphoblasts, Gilman and Thilly (1977) measured resistance to mutation by the purine analog 6-thioguanine. In their hands, a 10-min exposure to 45°C approximately doubled the mutant fraction. They commented that 45°C heat behaved like a strong chemical mutagen, when comparisons of mutant fractions were made at similar levels of cell survival. Mittler (1979) also examined the effect of X irradiation on normal or preheated *Drosophila*. The same 38°C, 1-hr treatment increased the percent of X-ray-induced recessive, sex-linked lethal mutations by the same factor of 2. The effects of inverting the order of treatment were not examined.

Two studies have been performed, each of which examines the induction of oncogenic transformations by X rays and heat. Clark *et al.* (1981) and Harisiadis *et al.* (1980) used very similar techniques. Individual transformations are recognized as the growth of aberrant clones seen superimposed on a background of confluent "normal" fibroblasts. Cells from the transformed clones can be shown to be capable of producing tumors in appropriate hosts, while the "normal" cells are incapable of doing so (Section 2.4.3.). Clark *et al.* demonstrated that the frequencies of radiation-induced oncogenic transformations of 10T1/2 cells could be increased or decreased by heat, depending upon the sequencing of the two treatments, i.e., exposures of 15 and 60 min at 45 or 43° respectively before irradiation resulted in 3.5-fold increases in the mean transformation rate induced by 1000 rad. Similar heating apparently reduced the frequency two-fold if it followed the X-ray treatment. This latter finding was also demonstrated by Harisiadis *et al.* (1980), who examined temperatures from 40°C (2 hr) to 45°C (20 min). The calculated "thermal inhibition of transformation," i.e., the ratio of the transformation with heat to that without heat, ranged from a low of 1.2 to a high of 2.8. In most experiments the thermal inhibition of transformation was greater than the thermal enhancement of all killing. Neither of these groups found any transformations induced by heat alone.

The lack of correlation between the mutation and the transformation data with respect to the effects of heat alone is somewhat difficult to explain. Perhaps the locus determining 6-thioguanine resistance is particularly heat sensitive or else those loci governing transformation are heat resistant. More likely is the possibility that spontaneous transformation frequencies are so low that doubling or even quadrupling them does not raise them to a measurable level. In any case, the effects of sequencing treatments on radiation transformation rates are more intriguing. The transformation rate found if heating precedes irradiation likely reflects increased damage (and its repair) resulting from the interactions of heat and X rays. The reduction of transformation rates by the reversal of the sequence suggests that heat reduced the amount of error-prone repair. Increased cell killing is also explainable on this basis as resulting from a similar interaction. I should point out that this viewpoint requires the implicit hypothesis that heat alone causes sublethal damage to the "target" at risk during X irradiation. An alternate hypothesis that would explain both increased cell killing and increased transformation rates is that enzymes responsible for error-free repair are affected by heat so that the rate of error-free repair is reduced. More error-prone repair would result, leading to the observed effects. This suggestion is consistent with the finding by Li *et al.* (1978) that the rate of recovery from potentially lethal damage was lower in irradiated plateau phase cultures of HA-1 cells that had been preheated (43°C) than in unheated controls, although the total amounts of recovery were similar.

Heating after irradiation appears to interfere preferentially with error-prone repair. As a result, cell killing is increased, but the transformation rate may be reduced. The data on plateau phase cultures are consistent with this view. Repair of potentially lethal radiation damage is associated with the enhancement of malignant transformation (Terzaghi and Little, 1976). Heating cells to 43°C (1 hr) after X irradiation inhibits recovery from potentially lethal damage (Li *et al.*, 1976). Therefore a partial inhibition of error-prone repair is not surprising. This need not result from modification of enzyme activity; alteration of the X-ray-induced lesions by the subsequent heating might equally be responsible. The binding to DNA of nonhistone proteins (Tomasovic *et al.*, 1978; Roti Roti and Winward, 1978; Roti Roti *et al.*, 1979), for example, might modify the stereochemical structure of DNA so that the appropriate enzyme system could not function to effect repair.

Perhaps the strongest evidence implicating DNA and chromosomes in determining survival after combined treatments of heat and X ray comes from a study by Dewey *et al.* (1978). This group had previously presented some convincing evidence that chromosomal aberrations could quantitatively account for cell killing by X irradiation (Dewey *et al.*, 1971). When these workers plotted the logarithm of the survival of cells exposed to graded doses of X rays against aberration frequency, they found that 37% survival corresponded to approximately one aberration per cell. When either S phase or G1 phase cells were heated for short periods of time (11 min or 7 min respectively) and then exposed to X irradiation, a similar relationship was obtained: in either case the 37% survival level corresponded to approximately 0.9 aberrations per cell (Figure 4.7). The important point here is that according to target theory, the 37% survival level should correspond to approximately one critical lesion per cell. It is not difficult to suggest from such results that chromosomal aberrations are responsible for X-ray-induced lethality, and that this holds true both for heated and for unheated cells.

Not all studies implicate DNA. A transient effect of moderate hyperthermia (less than 42°C for 1 hr) on the activation of a lysosomal enzyme (acid phosphatase) in the mouse spleen was shown by Hume and Field (1977). The increase in enzyme activity found as a function of temperature was approximately equal to the heat potentiation of radiation damage. Also, the time course of enzyme activation and its subsequent decay were more or less similar to the time course and decay of the interaction of the elevated temperature and X irradiation. In a later study (Hume *et al.*, 1978), it was found that in thermotolerant cells the rate of enzyme activation was not affected by a similar thermal exposure, i.e., lysosomes in thermotolerant cells were also heat resistant. Of course the usual question is unanswered: is the enzyme activation merely a reflection of cell death, or is it a primary event?

As discussed in Section 3.2.3, Nielsen and Overgaard (1979) have

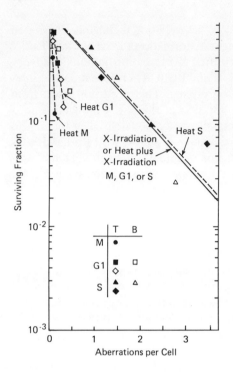

Figure 4.7. Survival vs. chromosome aberrations for heat-treated Chinese hamster cells. Synchronized cells were exposed to thymidine (T) or bromodeoxyuridine (B), and heated at 45.5°C to yield the indicated survival. Cell killing by X irradiation or by heat followed by X irradiation during S, G1, or M, or by heating during S phase all correlated well with the induction of aberrations. However, cells heated during G1 or M showed a very different pattern. For cells heated during the latter phases of the cell cycle, the low aberration frequency observed could not account for cell killing. Data from Dewey *et al.* (1980), with permission.

indicated that the ability of heat to sensitize cells to X irradiation is not affected by the thermotolerant state. Therefore, the data on lysosomal enzyme activation and those on survival do correlate. Furthermore, it is even conceivable that the chromosomal data and acid phosphatase data are connected, because Allison and Paton (1975) have indicated that chromosomal damage could result from the activation of lysosomal enzymes. The major problem with this line of reasoning is that in the absence of radiation, heat by itself does not introduce chromosomal aberrations in G1 cells (Dewey *et al.,* 1971). As pointed out by these authors, a close correlation between chromosomal abnormalities and cell killing has only been shown for one sequence of heat and radiation interactions. Thus, one can hardly claim that the mechanism for the heat-induced radiosensitization has been established.

Whatever the mechanism of the interaction, there is good evidence that it differs from that of cell killing by heat. Two additional relevant pieces of data have been mentioned in the previous paragraph: the finding that G1 cells do not evidence chromosomal aberrations when exposed to a heat exposure that allows only a fraction of these cells to divide (Dewey *et al.,* 1971), and the indication that cells that have been made heat tolerant by a previous exposure to elevated temperatures do not always show a concomitant resistance to X irradiation or to heat-induced sensitization to X irradiation. In addition, Loshek *et al.* (1977b) showed that the activation enthalpy required for heat sensitization is appreciably lower than that required for heat inactivation. Finally, the X-ray saturation data (Section 3.2.1) are also consistent with the view that the two mechanism are different; the amount of sensitization becomes independent of the duration of heating, and no saturation exists for killing by heat alone.

4.4 DRUG CYTOTOXICITIES AT ELEVATED TEMPERATURES

I have remarked earlier on the remarkable paucity of data on drug–heat interactions. While this comment applied to the phenomenological studies, the observation is even more striking when it comes to describing studies on the mechanisms of potentiation by heat of drug cytotoxicity. The reports can be counted on the fingers of one hand.

4.4.1. Alkylating Agents

Almost all the existing papers deal with alkylating agents. Investigators have directed their attention primarily to the effects of heat on the rejoining of single-strand breaks or on the rates of nonconservative DNA synthesis (i.e., repair). Two of these studies (Bronk *et al.*, 1973; Ben-Hur and Elking, 1974) examine the effects of the monofunctional alkylating agent methylmethanesulfonate (MMS). In the DNA of Chinese hamster and human skin cells treated with this drug, a dose-dependent number of single-strand breaks was found (Bronk *et al.*, 1973). The number of breaks caused per milligram of the drug was greater at 42°C than at 37°C. Rejoining of single-strand breaks was observed at 37°C, but if the postexposure incubation temperatures was 42°C, rejoining was completely inhibited. The maximum time interval examined by these authors was 3 hr after treatment; data on the recovery from MMS-induced potentially lethal damage indicate that observation over a 12 to 24-hr interval might have been more convincing (Hahn, 1976). The Arrhenius plot for break induction was nonlinear, as was the Arrhenius plot for cell killing by MMS (Hahn, 1976). These findings were interpreted to imply that only part of the increased cell killing at the higher temperature could be attributed to the increased rate of drug action; Bronk *et al.* suggested that the remainder was likely to be a result of the inhibition of repair of single-strand breaks. In the second study on MMS, very similar observations were made (Ben-Hur and Elkind, 1974), except that at elevated temperatures repair was not inhibited but only slowed down. Ben-Hur and Elkind (1974) also demonstrated that the rejoining process of MMS-induced single-strand breaks had a half-time of several hours; this is in marked contrast to the half-time of perhaps 30 min for irradiation. In this connection it may be noted that very different half-times for the repair of potentially lethal damage have been measured after the exposure of cells at 37°C to X rays and to MMS (Hahn, 1976). The relationship between the rejoining of single-strand breaks caused by the alkylating agents and increased survival remains to be established with certainty.

Two other studies can be mentioned. Djordjevic *et al.* (1978) examined the temperature dependence of the ability of the drug peptichemio (a multipeptide unit of mi(di) 2-chloroethyl(-amino)-L-phenylalanine) to induce single-strand breaks into DNA and of their subsequent repair. If exposure to the drug was at 37°C, no single-strand breaks were observed; if incubation took place at 42°C, however, a large number of such breaks were seen. Those breaks that were induced at 42°C could be rejoined if subsequent incubation took place at 37°C, but not if incubation was at 43°C. Cells were killed more efficiently at the elevated temperatures, as was also true in the earlier studies cited.

Djordjevic *et al.* attributed the increased cell killing to changes in membrane permeability allowing more drug to enter the cell. This explanation is a little difficult to reconcile with the fact that at 37°C no single strand breaks were seen. If the observation could be attributed entirely to increased drug entrance, one would expect to see a dose-dependent, fractional change in the number of single-strand breaks, but hardly a change from zero to a measurable quantity. Finally, Osieka *et al.* (1976) used bromodeoxyuridine (BUdR) to investigate nonconservative repair replication in human malignant cells exposed to the alkylating agent N-acetoxy-2-acetyamino-fluorene. A cesium chloride gradient technique was employed that measured the ability of BUdR (which is heavier than the thymidine for which it substitutes) to shift the peak of BUdR-substituted DNA from its normal position. Conditions of the experiment were such that semiconservative DNA replication was largely inhibited. Cells were incubated with drug before the addition of either tritiated thymidine or BUdR at either 37 or 43°C. Little if any effect on repair synthesis was seen at the higher temperature, although semiconservative synthesis was essentially blocked. It should be pointed out that of all the alkylating agents that have been examined, recovery from potentially lethal damage is of importance only in the case of survival after exposure to MMS (Hahn, 1976). For all other agents, such as, for example, thio-TEPA (Johnson and Pavelec, 1973), nitrogen mustard, and the nitrosoureas, increased cytotoxicity at elevated temperatures can simply be considered as resulting from the increased rate of alkylation of DNA as predicted by Arrhenius theory. The Arrhenius plots in the cases of these drugs are linear, and the activation energies obtained are consistent for alkylation reactions (Johnson and Pavelec, 1973; Hahn, 1976).

4.4.2. Bleomycin and Adriamycin

As suggested by Braun and Hahn (1975), the increased cytotoxicity of bleomycin might result from the inhibition of the recovery from potentially lethal damage. The exact way this agent kills cells at 37°C has not been completely determined. Biochemical studies of cytotoxicity at elevated temperatures have therefore not been performed. At high doses, adriamycin is able to enter the cell more readily at elevated temperatures than at low temperatures. For Chinese hamster cells, this has been shown at concentrations of 100, 50, and 30 g/ml; at lower doses the technique used for the measurement, fluorescence of the drug as measured by a flow cytofluorometer, was not sufficiently sensitive (G. M. Hahn, unpublished data). Nevertheless, a plot of average cellular fluorescence vs. drug dose when extrapolated to zero dose intercepts the origin. Assuming a linear dose relationship at low doses, this finding suggests that even at physiologically meaningful doses (e.g., approximately 1 g/ml), permeability may be the determining factor in the drug's effectiveness.

4.4.3. Cis-Diamminedichloroplatinum(II)

Meyn *et al.* (1980) showed that increased killing of CHO cells by cisplatinum at 43°C reasonably matched increased DNA cross-linking (Figure 4.8). Cross-linking is generally accepted as the mechanism by which this compound kills cells. In these experiments, cross-links were quantified using an elutriation technique. Over the dose range examined, a 1-hr exposure to the drug was 10 times as efficient in killing cells at 43°C as at 37°C, while the ratio of cross-links was 6.5. As the authors point out, the additional cross-linking observed at the higher temperature might have resulted from changes in membrane permeability, or might reflect increased accessibility of DNA to the drug. Alternatively, it might simply reflect elevated binding kinetics resulting from the higher temperature.

4.5. SUMMARY

Heat "dose" is a concept very different from radiation dose; the former requires specification of temperature and duration, the latter only

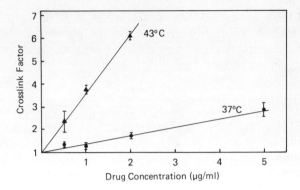

Figure 4.8. Correlation between "cross-link factor" and concentration of cis-Diammine-dichloroplatinum(II) (cis-DDP). Chinese hamster cells (CHO) were exposed for 1 hr at 37 or 43°C to the dose of cis-DDP indicated on the abscissa. The cross-link factor was determined from alkaline elutriation of DNA from appropriately treated cells. This factor is defined as the ratio of log of the fraction of DNA retained on the filter using a radiation standard (400 rad) to the log of the fraction of retained DNA from a radiation-plus-drug-treated sample. The increased cross-linking observed at the higher temperature may be responsible for the increased cell inactivation at the higher temperature. From Meyn *et al.* (1980), with permission.

of absorbed energy. Heat dose more closely resembles drug dose, and indeed a simple model of cell inactivation based on the distribution of molecular energy states yields the correct shape of the survival curve at a fixed temperature as well as the observed dependence of survival parameters on temperature.

Thermodynamic analysis of thermic data of wide origins indicates that the activation energy for cell killing or other thermic injury is large (100–200 kcal/mole), consistent with an assumption that configuration changes in proteins are responsible for cell death. Considerable evidence other than thermodynamic analysis implicates the role of proteins. However, protein synthesis resumes in cells following even fairly severe heat shocks; therefore, generalized protein denaturation is unlikely to be responsible for cell death.

It is possible that individual, specific proteins are at risk, but no data exist identifying them. Some thermally sensitive mutants are known to contain one or more heat-sensitive enzymes, while heat-resistant bacteria contain heat-stable proteins.

Neither RNA or its synthesis nor DNA *per se* or its synthesis are likely candidates as "targets" for heat killing, at least in the temperature range of 43 to 47°C. At higher temperatures the possible primary involvement of some nucleic acids cannot be dismissed.

Quite likely, heat damage to cellular organelles, rather than inactivation of molecular species, determines the cells' death. Chromosomes are possibly implicated. Ploidy changes, binding of nonhistone proteins to DNA, and chromosome aberrations (at least in S phase cells) have been correlated with thermal inactivation rates. A priori, intracellular membrane appear as likely targets, but evidence of correlations is far from clear. Mitochondrial function may be correlated with heat killing, though evidence suggesting the opposite also exists. Certainly cells deprived of exogenous energy sources become very heat labile. Lysosomal membrane integrity is correlated with cell survival. Heat damage to other intracellular membranes has as yet not been associated with cell killing.

Many studies deal with heat effects on the plasma membrane, perhaps because it is relatively easily studied. Correlations between changes in membrane morphology, capping ability, permeability, etc., on the one hand and cell survival parameters on the other hand have been established. Cellular heat sensitivity is said to correlate with membrane composition and with membrane "fluidity."

The results of these studies show an array of correlations, but no clear understanding of what is cause and what is effect. No doubt many other correlations will be found. Whether or not these by themselves can ever pinpoint the cause of heat-induced cell death is questionable.

Thermal tolerance is an interesting phenomenon whose induction involves at least two processes. The temperature-dependence of the first of these, "triggering," is characterized by an Arrhenius plot consisting of two linear, parallel segments. For Chinese hamster cells, the transition between these segments occurs between 42.5 and 43°C, suggesting a cooperative phenomenon involving a very highly organized structure, such as the cytoskeleton. The second process, development requires protein synthesis; whether protein synthesis in general or of specific proteins is involved is currently under active investigation.

Heat sensitizes cells to X rays, but the mechanism of interaction may well be different from the mechanism of heat killing. DNA damage and probably inhibition of repair have been assumed to be responsible for additional cell killing; the data, however, are still not conclusive. Heat introduces delays in DNA synthesis (initiation and elongation of replicons) and delays the excision of base damage. The enzyme β-polymerase, reported to be a repair enzyme, may be particularly heat sensitive. Mutation and transformation studies suggest that the amount of error-prone repair may be increased if cells are heated before X-ray exposure, but reduced if heating follows irradiation.

The rates of strand breakage and strand rejoining in cells treated with heat and alkylating agents does not seem to reflect all of the additional killing involved, though data here are far from completely convincing. Damage to the DNA "complex" may be involved. Bleomycin–heat interactions may also partly result from repair inhibition, although the data here are purely inferential. Adriamycin is able to enter heated cells more readily, at least for a short period following (or during) exposure. In cells exposed to cis-platinum(II) at either 37 or 43°C, the rate of cell killing correlates moderately well with DNA cross-linking.

5

Responses of Murine Tumors and Normal Tissues

5.1. INTRODUCTION

The data presented in Chapters 2 and 3 amply demonstrate that mild heating can kill cells and also that such heating accentuates the cytotoxicity of many anticancer agents. But it is a long way from experimental results on cell systems to the clinical use of hyperthermia. The next step in the usual hierarchy of experimental escalation is a demonstration that heat, either by itself or in cooperation with the more classical modalities, has beneficial effects against transplanted tumors in murine systems. By beneficial effects I do not only mean that tumors can be caused to regress or to be sterilized, but that this can be done without causing excessive damage to appropriate critical normal tissue. In this chapter I am going to provide evidence that demonstrates conclusively that some murine tumors can be eradicated by time–temperature profiles that cause only minimal normal tissue damage. The finding is not universal: other murine tumors appear to be more heat resistant, and their sterilization by heat alone can only be accomplished at the cost of considerable and perhaps excessive local tissue damage. I will also present data on combined heat–X-ray and heat–drug treatments; some of the heat-resistant tumors can be controlled effectively by these. There is, however, some dispute as to whether or not the combined X-ray and heat treatments necessarily result in therapeutic benefits because normal tissue effects may be magnified to the same extent as are antitumor effects. In my view, many of these discussions are misdirected. They usually involve the wrong normal tissue, namely skin, and they frequently ignore the possibility of heating the tumor to higher temperatures than much of the normal tissue. For drug–heat combinations the data are too fragmentary to allow any definitive or even tentative statements to be made regarding eventual clinical applications.

5.1.1. Model Systems

5.1.1.1. Localized Heating

The mechanics of locally heating murine tumors are quite simple—too simple in many ways to have clinical relevance. The investigator can choose the anatomical site where he wants the lesion to grow; tumor implants can be made in the animals' flanks, thighs, feet, etc. Dimensions of tumors to be treated can be chosen so that heating equipment can provide uniform temperature distributions within the lesions. Tumor responses to treatment can be assessed by a variety of techniques. The most obvious is by determining tumor cure rates; but in the absence of cures, the progression of the lesions can be followed by caliper measurements. In some tumor systems, the treatment's effectiveness can be evaluated by determining the colony-forming ability (*in vitro*) of cells obtained from tumors treated *in situ*. Many murine tumors differ greatly from spontaneous human neoplasms in degree of antigenicity, in growth rates, and in other cell-kinetic parameters. For these reasons, the question is raised periodically, and with some justification, whether the data obtained from murine neoplasms have any predictive value for human treatments. Giovanella *et al.* (1979) and Osieka and Maginiera (1978) currently use human heterotransplants in nude mice (i.e., thymus-deficient) and suggest that these constitute a more realistic model. Certainly this system bypasses some of the problems associated specifically with mouse tumors. Murine cells may be more or less heat sensitive than human cells, and therefore, the heat response of the former may not accurately reflect what would be seen in cells from human tumors. Antigenicity is surely less of a problem in animals defective in one of their major immune systems. It seems to me, though, that to some extent new problems supplant those avoided. This is particularly true if heating techniques are utilized that depend for heat generation upon the deposition of energy within the tumor and its surrounding tissue. The exact temperature distribution generated by these heating techniques depends strongly on blood flow rates in tumors as well as in surrounding normal tissue. Thus, in the case of hyperthermia for the heterotransplant system to have any real predictive value, a demonstration seems to be required showing that the relative blood supply to the transplanted tumors is more or less equivalent to that found in human tumors, and, furthermore, that normal mouse tissues have blood flow rates closely matching those of humans. In the absence of such data, it is not clear to me that the limited extra amount of information that can be derived from working with such genetically immune depressed animals warrants the additional experimental difficulty and expense involved.

In order to avoid completely the problems associated with transplanted tumors in mice, several groups have elected to use large outbred animals such as dogs and cats as experimental subjects (Connor *et al.*, 1977; Gillette, 1979; Marmor *et al.*, 1979). Sizes and anatomical distributions of tumors in such animals closely match those found in man. The growth rates of the spontaneous tumors, particularly in dogs, as well as the histologies seen, tend to mirror the human clinical situation. For the testing of heating equipment particularly, the normal tissue–tumor combination of large animals is much more satisfactory than that of mice. This must be balanced by the disadvantages of having to work with what is obviously an uncontrolled population. Among outbred animals there is a wide distribution of tumor sizes and stages, and the number of tumors of any one histology is limited. Frequently the dogs and cats obtained for treatments are pets, and many times these are still under the control of their current or former owners. This relationship must be treated with the proper respect. Even for localized treatments the animals must be anesthetized, while humans treated with localized hyperthermia do not require anesthesia. Finally, the treatment of pets can be expensive and time consuming, and therefore, the possible amount of information to be gained from utilizing outbred animals should be carefully evaluated before large-scale experiments are started. Nevertheless, because of the proven predictive value of these studies (Marmor *et al.*, 1979), large-animal treatments have found strong advocates. Experiments with outbred animals are really preclinical studies and have more in common with phase I human trials than with the usual mouse experiments. For this reason I will postpone their description to Chapter 7.

5.1.1.2. Whole-Body Heating

The physics of whole-body heating certainly presents no big difficulties. Unfortunately, no one has as yet reported an adequate animal model for whole-body heating, and the absence of such a model seriously retards biological research in this area. The problem is that neither mice nor rats seem to be able to stand exposures to temperatures exceeding 41 or 41.5°C for periods of longer than a few minutes; even at the quoted temperatures, the maximum treatment time is of the order of 1 hr. This is in contrast to the human situation where exposures at 41.8°C lasting several hours appear to be well tolerated.

Whole-body heating of dogs is probably feasible and perhaps warranted. Because of the expense involved, experiments should be designed to answer questions of particular clinical importance. A good example here might be normal tissue effects of drug–hyperthermia combinations.

Dog studies are only mentioned briefly in clinical papers (e.g., Storm *et al.*, 1979) and no detailed normal tissue studies have been carried out on these animals.

5.2. RESPONSES OF MURINE TUMORS TO HYPERTHERMIA ALONE

Murine tumors in inbred strains do represent systems where a large number of identical "patients" can be treated with a variety of regimens, and comparisons can then be made as to their relative antitumor effects. The assay to determine results of treatments can be one of several: (1) tumor cure, usually expressed as the dose (heat, X ray, drug, etc.) required to cure 50% of the animals and usually written as TCD_{50}; (2) tumor regrowth, frequently measured as the time required for a tumor to reach a specific size or to double in volume; (3) cell survival, assayed either *in vitro* or *in vivo*. Cell survival (colony formation) can be measured *in vitro* for a limited number of tumors whose cells have been adapted to growth both in the animal and in tissue cultures. The survival assay *in vivo* consists of the injection of graded and known numbers of treated cells into appropriate hosts and subsequent examination for the number of tumors observed. Although a useful and precise technique, it is slow and requires many animals and therefore is rarely used today. Each of the assays mentioned measures a different combination of factors, such as cellular cytotoxicity and recovery phenomena, and possible host responses. Therefore, very different results may be obtained from the individual assays, depending upon the particular experimental procedures selected. This is true for all neoplasms, but *a fortiori* so for highly antigenic tumors. An excellent discussion of some of the problems associated with interpretation of data obtained from tumor experiments is that of Brown (1979).

5.2.1. Methodology of Heating Murine Tumors

Techniques used for heating mouse tumors range from immersion of limbs with tumors into hot water baths, to current or microwave heating, to ultrasound. The particular method used as well as the anatomical location chosen for implantation may profoundly influence the temperature distribution both in the tumor and in normal tissue. The degree of uniformity achieved may, in turn, modify the response to treatment. Robinson *et al.* (1978) illustrated how difficult it is to use water baths to achieve uniform temperature distributions, and how uniformity can be improved by a clever microwave technique. Mouse tumors of mammary origin were implanted in the legs of syngeneic mice. The tumors were then heated either by immersion of the legs into hot liquid baths or by such immersion combined with simultaneous exposure to 2.54 GHz microwaves. The microwave irradiation was carried out with the legs in a liquid whose composition was such that the electrical characteristics matched those of tissue. This liquid "bolus" was arranged so that it and the mouse leg formed a slab with parallel sides. Two opposed, parallel microwave applicators were then used to provide uniform deposition of energy. Heating could be achieved two ways, either by having the liquid at a predetermined temperature, or by additionally irradiating with microwaves. The thermal profiles obtained either with or without microwaves are shown in Figure 5.1. The bolus material was maintained at 42.9°C. In the absence of microwave power, the intratumor temperature varied between 42.8 and 41.9°C, with the coldest spot near bone. When the microwave power was turned on, the variation was reduced to 0.3° and the cold spot near the bone was eliminated. A difference of 1.0° intratumor temperatures may not sound impressive, but to compensate for a 1.0° cold spot would require an increase of about 100% in heating time in order to achieve an equivalent level of cell killing. Furthermore, a comparison of cure rates of tumors

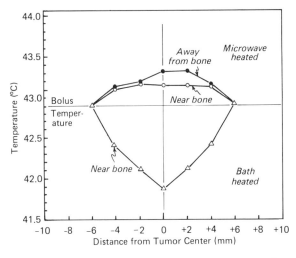

Figure 5.1. Temperature distributions in murine tumors. Mammary carcinomas, implanted in the legs of syngeneic hosts, were heated either with a liquid bath alone or with the addition of 2.54 GHz microwaves. A "cold spot," 41.9°C, was seen near the center of the tumor and close to the thigh bone. The temperature difference, approximately 1%, between the cold spot and the surroundings was reduced to 0.3° with the addition of microwaves. Data from Robinson *et al.* (1978), with permission.

treated with the two modalities indicated that it is the lowest temperature measured within individual tumors that correlates with the cure rate (Hahn *et al.*, 1980). Therefore, uniformity of heating and specifically the elimination of cold spots is a problem of considerable concern.

To demonstrate the role anatomical location plays in influencing temperature distribution, Robinson *et al.* (1978) implanted the same tumor into the flanks of the hosts. In that location the intratumor temperature varied only by about 0.1° even without the use of microwaves.

Water-bath heating depends upon conduction for heat transfer. When heating with such a technique, it is inevitable that the maximum temperatures will always be found on that surface that is in direct contact with the water—that is to say, the skin. Therefore, if tumor response is compared to that of the skin overlying the tumor (as an example of normal tissue response), water-bath heating invariably results in data prejudicial to the normal tissue if the appropriate temperature correction is not made. Furthermore, water-bath heating *per se* may involve damage not seen with dry heating techniques (Martinez *et al.*, 1980). Of course, water-bath heating is considerably simpler than that employing other modalities, and therefore it is used in many studies, but great care must be taken in evaluating results based on such experiments. The anatomical location of either the tumor or normal tissue may very well influence response to therapy in another way. In the extremities, both the tumor and some normal tissues may be at a temperature well below that of the core of the animal; this is true even in mice not under anesthesia. As a result, the cells may be adapted to low temperatures (e.g., ~30°C in the ear of the mouse). Such cells show a heat response somewhat different from that seen in tissue existing at the usual 36 to 38°C body temperature (Li and Hahn, 1980b).

5.2.2. Tumor Cures and Survival of Tumor Cells

An initial look at only tumor cure data yields some interesting observations. Single, moderate exposures of tumors to heat generated by any of the modalities discussed can lead to tumor cures. For example, Westermark (1927) showed that the Jensen sarcoma in the rat can be cured efficiently by immersing the region containing the tumor into hot water baths at temperatures between 41 and 45°C. Furthermore, he demonstrated that the time required to obtain 50% cures was a function of the temperature of the water bath. Similar results were later obtained by Goetze and Schmidt (1931), who extended the temperature range to 48°C. It appeared that in order to cure 50% of treated animals in the range of 43 to 48°C, each additional degree corresponds to approximately a 50%

reduction in the time required to heat the tumor. Below 43°C, approximately each ½ degree requires a doubling of the exposure time. Very similar results were also obtained by Overgaard (1934; 1935), Overgaard and Overgaard (1972; 1977), and Overgaard and Suit (1979). In the last group of experiments cited, diathermy was used to elevate tumor temperature. Another study where water baths were used to heat tumors, that of Crile (1963), not only demonstrated similar temperature–time relationships, but also showed that some tumors could be cured by heat without doing permanent damage to critical normal tissue.

The relationship between temperature and time of exposure to effect tumor cures was very similar to that found for cell killing by Westra and Dewey (1971), and for the inhibition of cellular growth by Pinkus and Fischer (1931). While this does suggest that these three examples of heat inactivation of biological tissue have a similar origin, it does not necessarily imply that all cell killing in tumors is governed precisely by the same mechanisms as cell killing *in vitro*. Tumor cures result from the elimination not only of the majority of the cells, but particularly from the elimination of the most heat-resistant cells. The tumor cure data may, therefore, reflect only the behavior of the most resistant subpopulation. Nor should it be concluded from these results that all murine tumors have the same heat sensitivity. Far from it. The results quoted only imply a similar temperature dependence of the rate constant governing inactivation of those cells most resistant to heat. An example of the wide range of tumor sensitivities comes from my laboratory. We have examined the heat sensitivities of four tumors, designated EMT6, KHJJ, KHT, and RIF. These tumors were all heated with identical instruments, the lesions were of identical size at the time of treatment, and they were implanted in the same location (in each case in syngeneic hosts). The EMT6 tumor proved to be exquisitely sensitive to hyperthermia; a 20-min exposure at 44°C cured 100% of the animals so treated. The KHJJ was somewhat less heat sensitive; a similar exposure only cured 50% of the treated animals (Marmor *et al.*, 1977). However, 20-min exposures at this temperature of the KHT and RIF tumors did not measurably affect the growth rates of these lesions, much less lead to tumor cures. Even a 60-min exposure at 44.5°C cured no animals. These results are summarized in Figure 5.2. These data are in marked contrast to those reported for human heterotransplants in nude mice. For these it has been stated that, "At the temperature achieved (43°), the antitumor effect obtained does not seem to vary much from tumor to tumor" (Giovanella *et al.*, 1979). As we shall see in Chapter 7, the heat responses of spontaneous tumors in patients vary considerably.

Do the tumor cure data exclusively reflect hyperthermic responses

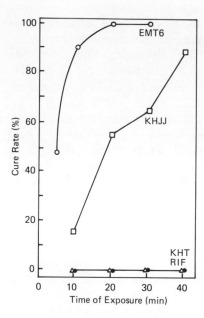

Figure 5.2. Cure rates against four murine tumor systems treated under standardized conditions. All tumors were grown from tissue culture cells implanted intradermally into the flanks of syngeneic hosts. Tumors were treated at a nominal weight of 100 mg. Heating (to 44°C) was accomplished with an RF system operating at 13.56 MHz. Tumor temperature was monitored throughout the treatment; measurements are estimated to be reliable to ± 0.3°C. Tumor cure was defined as the absence of palpable tumor 30 days after treatment. Data from Marmor *et al.* (1976), with permission.

of tumor cells or are other factors involved? To examine this question we need to look not only at tumor cure results, but also at tumor regrowth and cell survival data. One of the most striking phenomena observed *in vitro* is that of thermotolerance, i.e., the ability of an initial heat dose to make cells more resistant to subsequent heat exposures (Section 2.6). Does this also happen in tumors? Initially Crile (1963) indicated that previously heated tumors were more difficult to eradicate than unheated ones, suggesting a similar behavior of tumor cells *in vivo*. In Figure 5.3, I show growth delays of RIF tumors exposed to 44°C for 30 min at various times after a ''conditioning'' dose; the latter given at 41°C (15, 30, or 60 min). A reduction in growth delay is shown in Figure 5.3 to occur after each of these initial treatments, provided the second exposure is made no later than 24 hr after the first. In other words, the first exposure reduced the effectiveness of the second dose, indicating that indeed thermotolerance had developed. The kinetics after the 41°C pretreatment were somewhat different from those seen after 43°C (G.M. Hahn and I. Van Kersen, unpublished). Some level of protection was seen immediately upon completion of the 41°C exposure. The amount of protection depended upon the duration of the 41°C exposure. After 43°C pretreatment, several hours elapsed before the second dose was rendered less effective. This mirrored the experience *in vitro,* where 41°C was shown to be permissive for the development of tolerance, while 43°C was not. The relatively rapid disappearance (~24 hr) of much of the tolerance encountered is of interest.

Figure 5.3. Thermotolerance induced in RIF tumors. Cells derived from a radiation-induced fibrosarcoma (RIF) were implanted intradermally into the flanks of syngeneic C_3H mice. Tumors weighing approximately 100 mg were given conditioning doses of 41°C (15, 30, or 60 min). At times between 0 and 72 hr following the initial exposure, the tumors were given a test dose of 44°C (30 min). Mean tumor diameters (MTDs) were calculated daily from three-dimensional caliper measurements. In the figure, the time to double the MTD (in days) is plotted on the ordinate against the interval (in hours) between the two treatments. Shown also are MTD doubling times obtained from groups of mice whose tumors had received only the 41°C conditioning dose, or only the 44°C test dose. Exposure of tumors to 41°C for up to 60 min did very little; the MTD doubling time was 8–10 days, vs. 8–9 days for unheated controls.

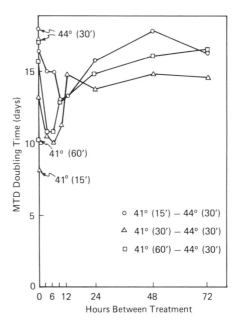

The 44°C exposure resulted in a doubling time of 16–18 days, an appreciable increase. Combined treatments led to intermediate doubling times, showing that the conditioning treatment introduced some thermal tolerance, even if the treatments followed each other without interval (0 hr point). Thermotolerance was maximum about 6 hr after completion of the test dose, and largely disappeared 24–48 hr later. Data from G. M. Hahn and I. Van Kersen (unpublished), with permission.

In tissue culture cells as well as in normal tissue, decay of tolerance proceeds more slowly than in this tumor. In several other studies, investigators did not find any evidence of thermotolerance in tumors (Overgaard and Overgaard, 1972; Suit *et al.,* 1977; Overgaard and Suit, 1979). Why such a discrepancy in results was seen is not known. Perhaps cells in only some tumors develop thermotolerance. If this were the case, it might have considerable clinical importance, because development of thermotolerance in normal tissue has been demonstrated in all studies designed to test for its occurrence. Obviously, if extra protection could be afforded specifically to normal tissue, thermotolerance could be utilized to increase the effectiveness of antitumor therapy.

In one instance an apparent discrepancy exists between tumor cure and cellular survival results. As shown in Section 5.2.2, a 50-min exposure at 43°C of the EMT6 tumor resulted in the cure of a rather astounding 80% of the tumor-bearing mice. The lesions, at time of treatment, weighed about 100 mg each and contained upwards of 10^{11} cells. Marmor *et al.*

(1977) utilized the ability of EMT6 cells to form colonies *in vitro* to determine the fraction of such cells surviving immediately following the heat treatment. At that time about 10% of the cells had retained their proliferative ability. Why did the remaining 10^{10} cells not commence to repopulate the tumor? Earlier results of Rockwell and Kallman (1973) provide a partial answer to this. They studied the X-ray response of the EMT6 tumor and demonstrated that at cell survival levels of 10^{-3}, tumor cures began to be observed. Presumably, because of the antigenicity of EMT6 cells, tumor-specific immune responses were able to deal with the remaining 10^8 cells. This still left unexplained the observation that after hyperthermia tumor cures were seen at a 100-fold higher level of cell survival. The most obvious hypothesis to invoke in order to try to explain this discrepancy appeared to be that hyperthermia reinforced the already potent antigenic response. A study designed to test this possibility (L. Nager, J. B. Marmor and G. M. Hahn, unpublished) was not consistent with this view. While, to be sure, animals cured of their tumor by hyperthermia became resistant to additional challenges with EMT6 cells, control groups of mice cured by either surgery or X irradiation were about equally resistant. Several other immune-related responses, e.g., macrophage cytotoxicity, chromium release from lymphocytes, etc., did not reveal any increased activity by cells from heat-treated animals when these were compared to cells from animals cured of EMT6 tumors by other modalities. These results were very consistent with an earlier study of Suit *et al.* (1977); neither of the two studies gave any support to the frequently made suggestion of a close connection between hyperthermia and immune response (Dickson, 1977; but also see Dickson and Calderwood, 1980, especially the discussion following this presentation).

To look for another explanation, Marmor *et al.* (1977) then followed the survival kinetics of cells in EMT6 tumors allowed to remain *in situ* for up to 48 hr after heating. Their results are shown in Figure 5.4, panel A. The major findings were that cell lysis (presumably of reproductively dead cells) occurred very rapidly, but more importantly, the number of clonogenic cells per tumor dropped by a factor of about 100 within the first 12 hr after treatment. After this very rapid cell killing, a plateau ensued. Cytotoxicity resumed after the first 24 hr, but at a much lower rate than that seen in the first 12-hr interval immediately following the treatment. An ultrastructural study of tumor sections obtained before and after heating of this tumor was carried out by Fajardo *et al.* (1980). In sections from heated tumors, early cellular damage was seen; particularly striking was the disintegration of plasma membranes within 6 hr of heating (Figure 5.5). But the most interesting suggestion made by the investigators was that vascular damage and ischemia resulting from such damage possibly led to the inhibition of blood flow and that this phenomenon was

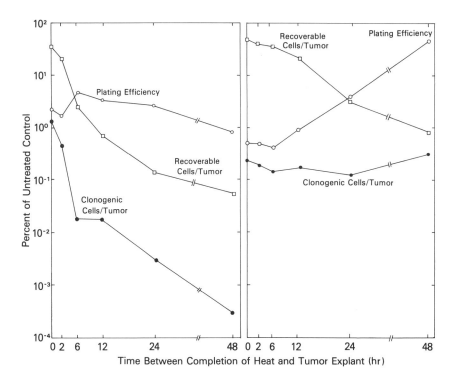

Figure 5.4. Cell survival kinetics following hyperthermic treatments of heat-sensitive (EMT6) and heat-resistant (RIF) tumors. Tumors were grown and treated according to the protocol described in Figure 5.2; heat exposure was 44°C (30 min). Control experiments showed that the exposure resulted in 100% cures of EMT6 and 0% cures of RIF lesions. Tumors were excised following hyperthermia at the times indicated on the abscissas. Single cell suspensions were prepared and the number of cells, as well as their survival "plating efficiency" (right ordinate), was determined. From these data the fraction of surviving cells per tumor, in reference to the number of viable cells in untreated tumors, was determined ("recoverable cells/tumor," left ordinate). Panel A shows results for EMT6, panel B for RIF turmors. Immediately following hyperthermia, approximately 10% of both EMT6 and RIF cells had retained their ability for colony formation. However, the survival of EMT6 cells declined rapidly in the next 12 hr; although plating efficiency actually increased, the number of countable cells per tumor declined drastically, so that the surviving fraction was reduced by a factor of 10^{-2} (panel A). No similar effect was seen with RIF tumors; surviving fraction fluctuated within statistical limits during 12–15 hr following completion of treatment and then started to increase, presumably as proliferation resumed (panel B). Data from Marmor *et al.*, (1977), with permission, and from G. M. Hahn and I. Van Kersen (unpublished), with permission.

the most likely candidate responsible for the rapid, initial cell killing observed within 12 hr after heating. Perhaps a combination of lack of sufficient nutrients and accumulation of metabolic products leading to low extracellular pH was responsible for the rapid cell inactivation. This suggestion is consistent with data obtained *in vitro:* cells placed in Hanks' Balanced Salt Solution at pH 6.4 after heating continued to be killed even at 37°C (Li *et al.*, 1980a). The slower rate of cell killing seen in the EMT6 tumor after 12 hr, when clinical evidence of ischemia had subsided, may very well reflect the tumor-specific immune response postulated by Rockwell and Kallman (1973) as being responsible for eliminating those EMT6 cells surviving X irradiation. Very similar results have been reported for the killing of cells after exposure of SCK tumors *in situ* (Song *et al.*, 1980). Blood flow measurements in heated tumors are also consistent with the views expressed in this paragraph. These are discussed in some detail in Chapter 6. Interestingly, cell survival kinetics in the heat-resistant, nonantigenic, RIF tumor show a different pattern (Figure 5.4, panel B). Cells from that tumor are also able to form colonies *in vitro*, and cell survival studies parallel to those described for EMT6 tumors were performed. While survival following a 60-min exposure at 43° was also about 10%, no subsequent reduction in the number of clonogenic cells per tumor could be demonstrated. The number of such cells remained constant for about 12–24 hr, and then started to increase, reflecting the resumption of proliferation. Thus, the difference between heat-curable and -incurable tumors may lie not so much in variations of cellular responses to heat (although these certainly could be important), but in variations of host responses, or in differences in tumor physiologies. A primary role may well be played by the maintenance of tumor vasculature.

5.2.3. Effects of Different Heating Modalities

Heating of murine tumors has been accomplished utilizing a variety of methods. Hence, a reasonable and important question to ask is the following: Are there antitumor effects associated with one or the other heating modality, effects that are not completely attributable to heat? In only one tumor system, the EMT6, have several heating techniques been compared to see if one or the other introduces any "nonthermal" effects, i.e., cell killing over and above that induced by an equivalent water-bath exposure. Marmor *et al.* (1977) compared cell survival in the EMT6 tumor immediately after radiofrequency or water-bath heating. Results as shown in Figure 5.6 demonstrate that there were no detectable differences in the fraction of cells surviving the treatment with radiofrequency (RF) or water bath if the temperature is used as the parameter against which cell killing (or survival) was measured. Similarly, Marmor *et al.* (1978b) showed that no significant differences existed between cell killing as induced by ultrasound when compared to the other two modalities. The same conclusions with respect to ultrasound and hot water heating were earlier reached by Lehmann and Krusen (1955). Although appreciable cell killing *in vitro* by ultrasound at hyperthermic temperatures was attributed by Li *et al.* (1977b) to nonthermal effects, this was seen only at sound intensities appreciably higher than those used in inducing hyperthermia. Finally, a comparison of cure rates in mice whose EMT6 tumors were treated with ultrasound or RF showed that these were very similar, provided the temperature used for comparison was the lowest temperature estimated to have occurred in the lesions (Hahn *et al.*, 1980). These results are illustrated in Table 5.1.

5.2.4. Modulation of Glucose Blood Levels

Cells *in vitro* are much more sensitive to heat if exposure is carried out at low pH (Chapter 2). The possibility of increasing the heat sensitivity of tumors by intentional acidification has been discussed in great detail and with great fervor by von Ardenne. His hypothesis is that excess glucose can shift cellular metabolism from oxidative to glycolytic pathways. This would result in the production of excess lactic acid, which in normal tissue might lower the pH from perhaps 7.4 to 7.1 or 7.2. In tumors, where the pH may already be lower at the beginning of glucose infusion, such a pH change would result in values of perhaps as low as 6.8, at least within some parts of the lesions. As has been discussed earlier and as shown by von Ardenne and others, lowering pH from 7.4 to 7.2 does little to increase heat sensitivity; below pH 7.0 a change of 0.2 pH units can cause a dramatic reduction in the survival of cells exposed to heat *in vitro*. But when pH changes are effected *in vitro*, say by the addition to the

TABLE 5.1
CURE RATES FOR EMT6 AND KHJJ TUMORS

Average temperature[a]	EMT6		KHJJ	
	Ultrasound[b]	RF[b]	Ultrasound[b]	RF[b]
43.0	0	50	17	30
43.5	27	85	15	45
44.0	30	100	20	60
44.5	60	100	30	N.M.[c]

[a]Duration of treatment: 30 min.
[b]RF-treated tumors have a relatively uniform temperature distribution, while the minimum tumor temperature in ultrasound-treated tumors is about 1° below the average temperature. Cure rates in percent.
[c]N.M.: Not measured.

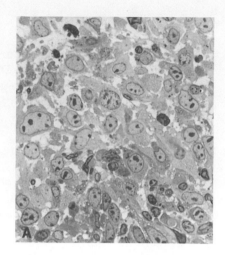

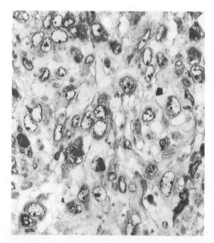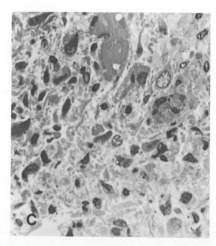

Figure 5.5. Histological changes in EMT6 tumors resulting from heating. EMT6 tumors implanted into the flanks of Balb/cKa mice were heated at 44°C for 30 min. Sections of untreated tumors, and tumors 15 min and 6 hr after heating were examined by light and transmission EM microscopy. Light microscopy: The untreated tumor shows cells having uniform, pale-gray chromatin, regular thin nuclear membranes and very prominent nucleoli (panel A). Fifteen minutes after heating (panel B) thickening of the nuclear envelope is observable, and cytoplasmic borders have lost their precision; some cells have developed vacuole-like clear areas of cytoplasm. At 6 hr (panel C), an obvious decrease in the number of tumor cells is observable; those remaining show marked karyopyknosis. Magnification: ×680. Electron microscopy in panel D on untreated EMT6 tumor cells is shown at 15,700 magnification. Chromatin is uniformly distributed, and the plasma membrane is sharply and continuously demarcated. Mitochondria are small and a few cristae are visible near the top of the picture. Only 15 min later (panel E, ×7800), peripheral aggregation of nuclear chromatin is visible. The cytoplasm appears "swollen" with irregular, electron-lucent areas, and the plasma membrane is no longer distinct. At 6 hrs (panel F, ×7800) the tumor cell is reduced to a small, dense, nuclear mass. The cytoplasm is fragmented, and the plasma membranes can no longer be identified. Data from Fajardo *et al.* (1980), with permission.

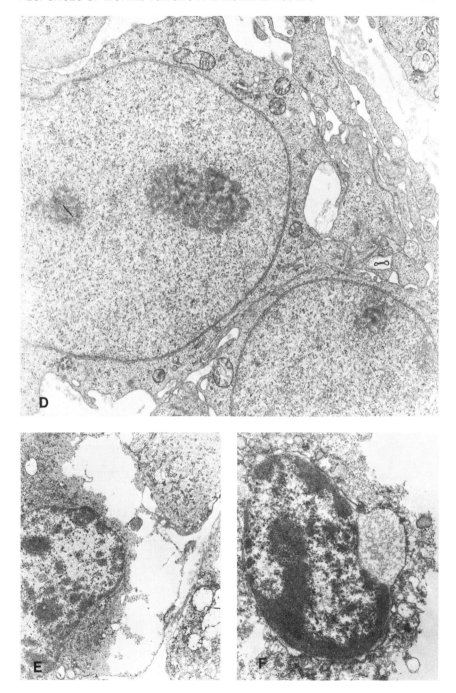

Figure 5.5. (continued)

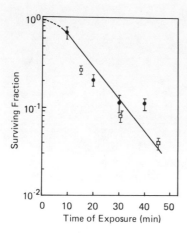

Figure 5.6. Effect of duration of 43.5°C exposure on cell survival in EMT6 tumors heated by either waterbath or RF fields. Tumors were held at 43.5°C for the indicated period of time, then excised, and cell survival was assayed immediately. In this, and other studies, cell killing appeared to be determined by the temperature–time profile and not by the mode of heating. ●: RF-heated tumors; □: water-bath-heated tumors. Marmor *et al.* (1977), with permission.

medium of small amounts of acid, there are no additional changes in the cellular environment. This is clearly not the case in tumors. Obviously, if long-term glucose infusions are used, the nutritional environment in the core of tumors would be modified appreciably. Primarily affected would be the glucose concentration itself, but also the availability of oxygen, for example, might be expected to increase as cells shift to anaerobic metabolism. Previously nutrient-deprived cells would now find themselves in a milieu rich in nutrients.

Since both chronic hypoxia and absence of glucose have been shown to increase greatly cellular sensitivity to heat, infusion of glucose might well accomplish the opposite of the desired effect. Any heat sensitization resulting from lower pH might be offset by increased resistance owing to the richer environment. Further, glucose infusion is known to induce fevers. Elevated body temperatures might well induce thermotolerance in cells, complicating treatment protocols. To my knowledge, there has been only one published study in which the effect of glucose infusion on tumor cure rate was evaluated. Dickson and Calderwood (1980) utilized heat treatments against the Yoshida sarcoma either with or without glucose infusion. In that one and very limited study, glucose infusion appeared to have no effect on tumor response to hyperthermic treatments. In the absence of additional data, comments regarding glucose infusions can only be classified as being on the level of speculation.

5.2.5. Factors Governing Variability of Tumor Responses

The high probability that the tumor temperature and blood flow distributions influence cure rates has already been mentioned. There are other aspects to the variability of tumor responses to hyperthermic treatment that I have not yet discussed. One of these is the possible relationship between heat resistance and the ability of the tumor to infiltrate surrounding normal tissue. One of the problems with many of the suggestions made in the literature about tumor eradication and tumor milieu is the implicit assumption that there is a strict delineation of tumor boundary. Frequently authors refer to one tumor environment as if pH changes, for example, suddenly increase in value as the tumor "boundary" is crossed. While this may be more or less true in some cases, in most it is not. Particularly in tumors able to infiltrate surrounding normal tissue, the tumor pH varies continuously from that observed near necrotic regions, to essentially that of normal tissue. It is fallacious to speak of one tumor environment for such tumors. In murine systems, it has been demonstrated that the curability of the tumor depends, among other things, on the site of implantation. Tumors which, if implanted subcutaneously, may be highly curable by hyperthermia alone, are rarely curable if implanted intramuscularly (E. W. Hahn et al., 1980). This point has also been discussed in the review by Overgaard (1978). He investigated possible correlations of tumor curability with the tissue of tumor origin, degree of tumor differentiation, growth characteristics, and with degree of tumor necrosis, but found none. There did appear to be an inverse relationship between invasiveness and cure rate. Very likely the relatively homogeneous microenvironment of cells in noninvasive tumors contributes to their curability. Suit (1975) suggests that there is a correlation between the X-ray dose required to sterilize a tumor and its curability by hyperthermia, and that both of these may be related to the degree of antigenicity of the tumor. Independent of whether it is immunogenicity or degree of infiltration or both that determine tumor response, in those tumors that are not curable by heat alone, the survival of relatively few cells, perhaps one in a thousand, determines regrowth of the tumor. In that case, combining hyperthermia with another modality capable of dealing with the cells surviving hyperthermia seems highly desirable if not essential. Finally, though this seems to be a relatively unimportant aspect, the variability of inherent sensitivities of the individual cells may contribute to heat resistance of tumors. Obviously, if a lesion contained a number of mutant, heat-resistant cells, these could survive treatment and later repopulate the tumor.

5.3. NORMAL TISSUE RESPONSES TO HEAT

The previous paragraphs have demonstrated rather clearly that at least some murine tumors can be eradicated simply by exposure to heat. Furthermore, it must have been true in these studies that normal tissue damage, within the immediate neighborhood of the region or elsewhere in the body, was not sufficiently severe to cause most of the animals to lose their lives. For example, in the study of Marmor *et al.* (1977) the death rate associated with the treatment of animals was about 13%. This rate was independent of the temperature of treatment (43 to 45°C) and very likely the deaths were associated with anesthesia. At autopsy, some though not all of the dead animals did show erythema and edema of the intestine underlying the tumor. Overheating may have resulted from the presence, during heating, of partially digested masses. Because these completely lack blood flow, they may have heated to temperatures over and above that of the surrounding tissue. Such masses may have been responsible for focal burns, leading to irreparable injuries. In later experiments, in which animals were starved overnight before being treated, the death rate was reduced, consistent with this hypothesis. Normal tissue damage was also seen in some survivors. Microscopic examination of various tissues from a series of animals sacrificed after treatment at 44°C showed small areas of focal necrosis in the liver, kidney, and intestinal tissue directly underlying the tumor (Marmor *et al.*, 1977).

Some level of normal tissue damage was therefore associated with the heating. Examination of the tumor area was carried out serially for a period of 30 days after completion of treatment. Shortly after treatment, animals developed black scabs overlying the tumor. This occurred in about 75% of the animals. These scabs disappeared within about a week, and although there was temporary epilation, hair started regrowing very quickly, and within two to three weeks, the former tumor area was no longer recognizable. The scab had been replaced by normal skin, and the hair had completely regrown. Microscopic examination of the tissue showed that two weeks after completion of heating, the only differences between untreated areas and those previously occupied by the tumor were a reduction in the thickness of the fat layer between skin and muscle, and a slight thickening of the skin. Thus, in the case of these heat-curable tumors, the complete eradication of the malignant lesion was not associated with the development of any appreciable level of normal tissue damage at the site of heating. Furthermore, the animals showed no functional deficiency, their eating habits were normal, and a month after the completion of treatment their weights and subsequent life spans were not statistically different from those of appropriate controls (G. M. Hahn and J. B. Marmor, unpublished).

Time–temperature heating profiles that cured animals of EMT6 tumors were ineffective against the heat-resistant RIF and KHT tumors. When an attempt was made to utilize a more severe heat dose, 45 min at 46°C, 30% of the animals died within a week after treatment (Faria and Hahn, 1982, in press). Several tumor cures were seen in the surviving animals, but obviously such treatment was associated with unacceptable levels of normal tissue damage. These results show the need to define what constitutes "acceptable" heat-induced damage, and to do so in a variety of tissues and organs. Then rational treatment plans for localized hyperthermia could be designed to maximally spare specific, heat-sensitive tissue. Currently we are far from having obtained such data.

5.3.1. Skin

Most of the tolerance results presented in the literature are on mouse skin. It is frequently suggested, or at least implied, that the response of skin to thermal insults is representative of all normal tissue responses. As was pointed out earlier, this is very unlikely to be the case. The normal temperature of the skin is several degrees below that of body core temperature. For example, in a mouse under anesthesia, the body core temperature is frequently between 31 and 32°C; the temperature of the skin is typically 28°C. Cells adapted to lower temperatures tend to become more sensitive to hyperthermic temperatures (Li and Hahn 1980b), and therefore skin responses likely reflect the heat sensitivity of adapted cells. I have also pointed out that if water-bath heating is employed, the skin is necessarily at a slightly higher temperature than is the tumor. In human treatments where water baths are not used the opposite is true, since it is relatively easy to cool the skin during the induction of hyperthermia by electromagnetic or ultrasound techniques. Thus, the response of the skin may be an excessively conservative predictor of tolerance of other tissues, and by itself may only have qualitative significance. This must be kept in mind when examining the data discussed in the following paragraphs, as well as in the later discussion on the effects that heat plus X irradiation have on normal tissue.

Perhaps the most intensive series of investigations of how heat damages skin (albeit not murine skin) were performed by Henriques and colleagues (Henriques, 1947; Moritz and Henriques, 1947). They were carried out toward the end of World War II under the auspices of the U.S. Army, and the goal was to define and quantitate a rather extreme form of hyperthermia, namely skin burning. Among other accomplishments, these investigators established a scoring system (hyperemia only; focal necrosis; complete epidermal necrosis) and determined the time–temperature relationships necessary to achieve a given level of damage. They examined the response of both porcine and human skin over the temperature range of 44 to 52°C, and demonstrated that in order to achieve a given effect with different time–temperature combinations each increase of one degree required a halving of the exposure time. Porcine and human skin behaved in a very similar manner. For example, complete epidermal necrosis occurred in the pig at 44°C after 420 min, while it took 360 min in the human;

at 45°C these numbers were reduced to 180 min for both, while at 47°C it required only 45 min in the pig and 30 min in the human. Henriques also performed an Arrhenius estimation of the activation energy associated with induction of necrosis and calculated a value of 150 kcal/mole. He concluded that proteins were the "targets" most likely at risk. These results are of course very similar to the values obtained by Pincus and Fischer (1931) for cessation of growth of tissue cultures exposed *in vitro* to elevated temperatures and the tumor data of Westermark (1927), and are not too different from the cell killing activation energies obtained by Westra and Dewey (1971).

Field *et al.* (1976) have looked at the rate of development of thermal injury in the ears of mice and plotted the percent of complete epidermal necrosis vs. time. It is clear that this damage is observable very rapidly (Figure 5.7). After an exposure of 45 min at 45.5°C, 100% of the animals developed this symptom 4 days after heating. Furthermore, because such necrosis can only be healed through the invasion of the affected area by cells from the surrounding tissue, recovery, if it appeared at all, was very slow. Hence, the percentage of animals in which such damage could be demonstrated remained at 100%, even if examination was carried out one or two weeks after treatment. For this reason, induction of necrosis is an inappropriate criterion when the repair rates of normal tissue damage are to be measured.

A different picture emerged if milder treatments were used. Also

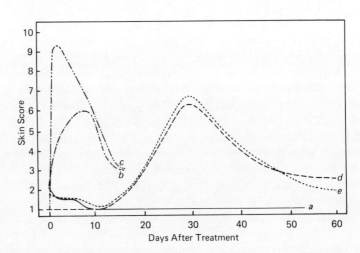

Figure 5.7. The time course of the skin reaction following various treatments. (a) Heat alone, 43°C for 1 hr (no reaction). (b) Heat alone, 44°C for 1 hr. (c) Heat alone, 45.5°C for 45 min. (d) X ray alone, 3000 rad. (e) X ray plus heat, 2000 rad followed immediately by 43°C for 1 hr. Dotted lines indicate deformed ears. Field *et al.* (1976), with permission.

shown in Figure 5.7 is a curve for the development of hyperemia in the absence of focal damage. Here the heating was 44°C for one hr. Again, the curve rose sharply, very closely mirroring that for focal necrosis, but if the animals were examined a week after treatment, no evidence of remaining damage was seen. Even if only 15 days were allowed to elapse between heat exposure and scoring, only 30% of the animals still retained any demonstrable effect of the treatment. This is a very short time for such marked repair to have occurred. After X irradiation for example, recovery takes place much more slowly, as is indicated in Figure 5.7. Repair occurs over periods of weeks, not days. Similar results were obtained by Law et al. (1978), who used a somewhat different scoring system to quantify damage induction and its subsequent repair in the ear of mice.

From these results the following conclusions can be drawn. The rate of induction of observable thermal damage is much more rapid than is the induction of such lesions by X irradiation. If heating is carried to the point where complete epidermal necrosis occurs, over a period of at least 3 weeks little if any recovery can be observed. On the other hand, if heating is limited so that the only manifestation of heat damage is hyperemia, both manifestation of damage and recovery are rapid; within 15 days after heating very little microscopic damage remains. Thus, recovery from damage is also more rapid after heating than after X irradiation. Currently no data exist on possible long-term effects of such heating; however, because the manifestation of local, heat-induced damage is so rapid, the probability of damage appearing at a later date is small.

The results quoted are consistent with the view that in mice, exposures of 1 hr in the range of 43 to 44°C cause no irreparable damage to skin. At higher temperatures, damage becomes important. Such temperature–time relationships are quite similar to those reported by Okumura and Reinhold (1978) for rat skin. But the murine data appear to be conservative estimates when compared to the porcine and human skin responses reported by Henriques (1947). For the skin of these two species, exposures to temperatures up to 45°C for 1 hr appear to cause no permanent damage. Henriques's results are reinforced by a recent study performed by Martinez et al. (1980). In that work, in which heat was induced by electromagnetic currents at approximately 1 MHz, neither skin nor fatty tissue of pigs showed serious ill effects below about 45°C (1-hr exposure) (Figure 5.8).

5.3.2. Cartilage

Quantitative data on hyperthermic damage to cartilage were obtained by Hahn et al. (1976) and by Field (1978). These two groups of investigators took advantage of the observation that damage to the tail of baby

rats or mice results in stunting of the growth of the tail during the animals'
subsequent development. For example, in the study of Field *et al.* (1976),
the tails of 7-day-old rats were immersed in heated water. Thermocouples
were used to monitor the internal temperature of the tails during heating.
After treatment, the animals were allowed to mature normally for 12
weeks. At that time growth was complete in normal and in treated cells.
Radiographs of the tail were obtained, and vertebrae were measured using
a traveling microscope. Vertebrae numbers 12, 13, and 14 in the treated
regions were compared with vertebrae 6, 7, and 8 in the untreated region
in order to obtain the percentage of stunting induced by the heat exposure.
Some of the tails became necrotic within a few days after heating. The
fraction of animals showing necrotic lesions was plotted against exposure

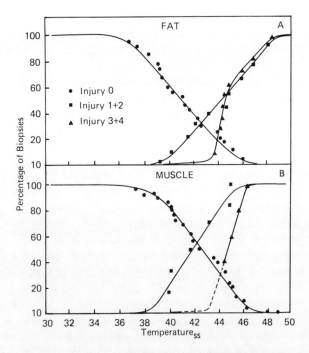

Figure 5.8. Heat sensitivity of porcine fat and muscle tissue. A scoring system based on
histologic observations was devised to quantify heat-induced damage to pig tissue. Biopsy
samples were obtained 30 days after heating to the indicated temperatures for 30 min with
a 13.65 MHz capacitively coupled radiofrequency system. Injury levels 1 and 2 were reversible; injury levels 3 and 4 involved necrosis and were irreversible. Panel A: Fat; panel
B: Muscle. In either tissue, heating for 30 min to temperatures up to 45°C appears safe;
above that temperature the rate of damage induction increases rapidly. Data from Martinez
et al. (1982), with permission.

time. Exposure of 43°C for 1 hr resulted in 10% stunting, but essentially no necrosis. The effect of heating on the induction of necrosis in baby rats is shown in Figure 5.9. The percentage of animals whose tail showed evidence of necrosis is plotted as the function of heating time for various temperatures.

Induction of necrosis was scored in normal tails and in tails that were clamped to prevent blood flow during heating. In the "oxic", i.e. un-clamped, case, 44°C for 1 hr resulted in approximately 50% of the rats' tails showing areas with necroses: reducing the heating time to 40 or 50 min prevented manifestation of such damage. Thus for the rat, 44°C for 1 hr seems to be the maximum heat dose for cartilage, if induction of necrosis is used as a criterion. This closely matches the time–temperature tolerance limits of skin. A different story emerged if blood flow was occluded during heating. Then even a 10 min exposure at 44°C induced 50% necrosis. Although the investigators suggested that hypoxia may be the primary reason for the difference in the responses of clamped and unclamped tails, very likely pH and nutritional effects were equally or more important.

5.3.3. Other Tissues

Gut may be a particularly heat-sensitive tissue, as indicated by the studies of Field *et al.* (1976) and Withers and Romsdahl (1977). There is also a suggestion that in mice a whole body exposure at 42°C for 1 hr introduces considerable structural changes in brain mitochandria. Gwozda

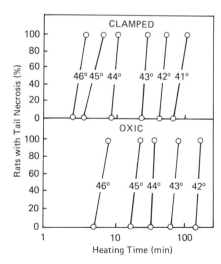

Figure 5.9. The effect of heat alone on baby rats' tails. Rats' tails were heated during in-fancy, and scoring of residual damage was performed in grown rats (see text). The per-centage of animals with tail necrosis is plot-ted as a function of heating time for various temperatures. Panel A: clamped; panel B: normal. Field *et al.* (1976), with permission.

et al. (1978) heated mice in an incubator. The temperature was monitored rectally. The changes observed were obliterated cristae at the lower temperature, and complete atrophy and the presence of cysts at the higher temperature, resulting either from the thermal exposure or from trauma secondary to the treatment. Effects from lack of adequate oxygen cannot be ruled out.

5.3.4. Discussion

The data, or rather the lack of additional results, clearly point out the need for more normal tissue studies before specific tissue tolerances can be discussed. Nevertheless, a few generalizations can be made. Tumor cure studies clearly demonstrate that certain animal tumors can be caused to regress completely and in some cases to be cured by heat–time profiles which, even in the absence of surface cooling, do not cause permanent skin damage. These relatively short-term heat exposures rarely result in any interference with the normal structure and function of tissue surrounding the treated tumor, implying that large portions of many tumors are more sensitive to heat than is normal tissue. Such conclusions will be strongly reinforced by the later discussion of the treatment of spontaneous tumors both in large animals and in humans.

5.4. RESPONSES OF TUMOR AND NORMAL TISSUE TO COMBINATIONS OF HEAT AND X RAY

5.4.1. Effects on Tumors

That heat does indeed sensitize tumors to the action of X rays has been demonstrated in many studies involving a variety of murine neoplasms. Beginning with an early work of Overgaard in 1935, investigators have demonstrated conclusively that when tumors are heated at the time of irradiation, or when heat is given shortly before or after irradiation, the X-ray dose required to sterilize a tumor is reduced sharply. Maximum dose reduction occurs for single doses. An example of the dose-modifying effect is shown in Figure 5.10. There I have used data from Robinson (1975) to demonstrate the reduction in X-ray dose required to sterilize 50% of transplantable mammary tumors (TCD_{50}) when the irradiation was administered during a 1-hr heat exposure. In these experiments the range of temperatures used varied from 38 to 44°C. A reduction in tumoricidal dose by a factor of 3 was seen if irradiation was carried out at the highest temperature. Intermediate temperatures resulted in a lesser, but still appreciable reduction in the TCD_{50}. Not only do these results show that heat very likely sensitized oxygenated tumor cells to X irradiation, but more importantly, the results demonstrate that the hypoxic cells, which this tumor is known to contain, must have been either sensitized preferentially by heat or killed outright. The most reasonable explanation of Robinson's data is that the highest heat–time profile used by him was by itself sufficient to kill most of the hypoxic cells, although preferential sensitization of these cells cannot be ruled out.

Hahn et al. (1974) have demonstrated that the addition of hyperermia to X irradiation results in increasing the cure rate not only if single doses are utilized but also if fractionated treatment regimens are employed. Unfortunately, the tumor used, the Ridgeway osteogenic sarcoma, is so radiation sensitive (TCD_{50} of less than 1000 rad), that it is not clear whether hyperthermia stimulated host responses against the tumor, if radiosensitization was involved, or if there was direct cell killing by hyperthermia. The same group also compared the interaction of sparsely and densely ionizing radiations and hyperthermia (Hahn et al., 1976). In that study, in which heating was effected by means of an infrared lamp, the temperature used was 42.5°C and the exposure period was 15 min.

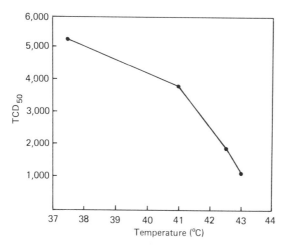

Figure 5.10. Dose-modifying effect of heat on a single X-ray dose. Transplantable mammary carcinomas in the legs of syngeneic mice were irradiated in the middle of a 60-min heat exposure at the temperature indicated on the abscissa. The X-ray dose required to cure 50% of the animals (TCD_{50}) was determined for each temperature and is shown on the ordinate. Drawn from data of Robinson (1975).

For this time–temperature profile little if any cell killing by heat itself was expected. Therefore, the investigators were examining specifically the ability of the heat exposure to sensitize cells to the two types of radiations studied. They showed that while the efficiency of X irradiation was enhanced by such a heat exposure, this was not the case for neutron irradiation, and concluded that "hyperthermia when used in combination with fast neutrons, and possibly other high-LET radiations, thus offers no advantage to local tumor control." Certainly as far as the sensitizing aspect of heat is concerned, these conclusions appear to be valid. Nevertheless, at higher temperatures and longer durations of heating, the cell killing effect of heat itself might appreciably modify cure rates. This may be particularly true for neutrons; although these represent an improvement over X-rays, even neutrons do not inactivate hypoxic cells as readily as they do cells in a well-oxygenated environment.

5.4.2. Effects on Normal Tissue: Therapeutic Gain Factors

Obviously, hyperthermia can increase the efficiency of ionizing radiations. What must now be examined is the effect of such treatments on normal tissue to obtain comparisons with effects on tumors. Several studies have attempted to do this. It has become accepted practice to define two parameters and use these for comparisons. The thermal enhancement ratio (TER) is the ratio of X-ray dose required in the absence of heat to the dose required in the presence of heat. Of course, a common endpoint must be designated, for example, the TCD_{50} or a specified level of damage for the particular normal tissue under examination. The second quantity of interest is the so-called therapeutic gain factor (TGF). This parameter is defined as the ratio of the TER for the tumor to the TER for the particular normal tissue. The larger the TGF the better. TGF values of less than 1 mean than the treatment results in increasing normal tissue damage to a greater extent than it affects the tumor. Considerable caution must be exercised if the TGF is to be truly meaningful. First of all, TERs for both tumor and normal tissue must be obtained over the same dose range. Secondly, the tumor TERs must be appropriate for the clinical setting. Very likely the TERs for single doses are much larger than those to be expected from fractionated courses of radiotherapy (Hahn *et al.*, 1974). Finally, and this is surely the most difficult part, the normal tissue TER should be obtained for the particular tissue that is treatment limiting. In almost all of the studies reported in the literature, this latter requirement, while not exactly ignored, is bypassed. Skin effects are much easier to measure than is damage to specific organs, and in most studies the investigators have used the response of that tissue for the comparison to tumor responses. The only exceptions are those studies involving cartilage and gut.

One of the most complete studies involving the examination of tumor and skin TERs (and resulting TGFs) is that of Hill and Denekamp (1979). Six types of transplantable mouse tumors were studied, differing with respect to the tissue of origin, growth rate, and degree of differentiation. Some of these variations were partially reflected in the lesions' radiation sensitivities. The tumors were of spontaneous origin, and were maintained in the mouse strain in which they initially occurred. Tumors were treated when they had mean diameters of 5–6.5 mm. Heating was in a water bath for a period of 60 min. In order to study the effect of sequencing of the two modalities, heating was applied at intervals between 0 and 24 hr before or after the X-ray dose. Tumor effects were assayed by determining the time required for the tumor to grow from 6.5 to 10 mm in diameter. The temperature chosen was 42.5°C, where little cell killing from heat alone was expected. Results obtained are tabulated in Table 5.2. Significant TERs were obtained for all tumors except for the very slowly growing RH carcinoma. TERs ranged in value from 1.8 to 1.1 and invariably were largest when the interval between heating and radiation was minimized. This last finding is consistent with that of Gillette and Ensley (1979) and consistent also with a wide range of *in vitro* data mentioned in Chapter 3. As the interval between heat and X-irradiation increased in either direction the TERs diminished, and usually by 24 hr little if any evidence of sensitization remained. Hill and Denekamp (1979) also obtained TERs for skin. An interesting fact emerged. If heat was given before X irradiation, the TGF hovered at or near 1, with a minimum value if the two treatments followed each other immediately (range 0.6 to 1.0). However, if the treatment sequence was reversed, X ray given first, as the interval between heating and X irradiation approached 6 hr, the TGF varied between values of 1.0 and 1.5, with no values below 1.0.

Hill and Denekamp compared their own data with the TERs obtained at various temperatures by a variety of other investigators and concluded that for heating and X irradiation immediately following each other, ''All of our tumor data fall within or below the range of TER values for normal tissues, indicating no therapeutic gain'' (Figure 5.11, panel A). Furthermore, data from Suit *et al.* (1977) as quoted by Hill and Denekamp also would imply that even at 43.5°C no therapeutic benefit would be obtained by combining hyperthermia and X irradiation.

The conclusion of Hill and Denekamp is very much at variance with that of Overgaard (1978), who collected similar data, as shown in Figure

TABLE 5.2 [a]
THE EFFECT OF HEAT AND X-RAY SEQUENCING ON TUMOR GROWTH

Tumor	Time interval (hours)	TER[b] Heat[c] after X ray	TER[b] Heat[c] before X ray	Volume doubling time, 6.5–8.2 mm	TGF[b] Heat[c] after X ray	TGF[b] Heat[c] before X ray
Squamous carcinoma D	0	1.5–1.7	1.6–1.8	2 days	0.8–0.9	0.9–1.0
	1	1.2–1.3	1.2–1.3		0.9–1.0	0.8–0.9
	2	1.4–1.8	1.5–1.9		1.1–1.5	1.1–1.4
	3	1.2–1.3	1.3–1.4		1.1–1.2	1.1–1.2
	6	1.0–1.2	1.4–1.5		1.0–1.2	1.2
	24	1.0–1.4	1.2–1.4		—	—
Carcinoma NT'	0	1.2–1.4	1.1–1.3	4.5 days	0.7–0.8	0.6–0.8
	1	1.3–1.5	1.2–1.4		1.0–1.2	0.9–1.0
	3	1.2–1.4	1.2–1.3		1.1–1.3	1.0–1.1
	6	1.2–1.5	1.2–1.3		1.2–1.5	1.0–1.1
	24	1.1–1.3	1.1–1.3		—	—
Slow sarcoma S	0	1.1–1.3	—	7.5 days	0.6–0.7	—
	1	1.2–1.4	—		0.1–1.1	—
	3	1.0–1.1	—		0.9–1.0	—
	6	1.0–1.1	—		1.0–1.1	—
Fast sarcoma F	0	1.2–1.4	—	1.8 days	0.7–0.8	—
	3	1.2–1.3	—		1.1–1.2	
MT2	0	1.5–1.7	—	2 days	0.8–0.9	—
Slow RH carcinoma	0	1.0	—	9 days	0.5	—

[a]Data from Hill and Denekamp, 1979, with permission.
[b]Thermal enhancement and therapeutic gain factors are relative to skin for the six mouse tumors.
[c]Heating: 42.5°C, 60 min, water bath; X ray: >2000 rad.

5.11, panel B. The tumor TERs shown by him imply a strong temperature dependence, with major increases at elevated temperatures. Obviously, there is a major discrepancy between the two sets of results. Several comments seem appropriate here to try to rationalize the discrepancy between these two compilations. First of all, most of the TERs for skin were obtained by hot water-bath heating. Skin, as has been pointed out several times, may be a particularly heat-sensitive tissue and in a water bath is invariably at a higher temperature than the tumor. Using skin as a typical normal tissue may then lead to pessimistic estimates of TGFs. This is consistent with the data shown by Overgaard. Almost all the skin data fall below his line for "normal tissue," i.e., are more sensitive, while all but one point of nonskin results are above that line. Secondly, the explanation put forth by Overgaard that at higher temperatures the results show not only sensitization but also direct cell killing by heat is surely correct. Were it not, cures in the absence of the X irradiation would have been impossible to obtain. If a tumor is extremely heat resistant, then cell killing is minor and the TER would tend to be constant over the temperature range. As I have pointed out in Chapter 2, this is in line with data showing that there is saturation of X-ray sensitization with respect to both temperature and duration of exposure. Of the data of Hill and Denekamp, only one point is at 43.5°C, and that was obtained with a fibrosarcoma that appears to be both heat and radiation resistant (Hill and Denekamp, 1979). In this connection it seems very unfortunate that no data exist at even higher tumor temperatures, since intratumor temperatures of 45°C and even higher seem consistent with clinical use.

Below temperatures of about 42 to 42.5°C, TGFs in the neighborhood of 1 seem to be the rule; it is only at higher temperatures, particularly above 43°C, that the combination of X irradiation and hyperthermia as used in these experiments leads to preferential tumor inactivation. Before drawing perhaps unnecessarily pessimistic conclusions from these experiments, the following considerations should be kept in mind. In all the studies described, no attempt was made to differentiate geometrically between the heating path and the portal for the X irradiation. Yet for many anatomical locations of tumors, utilization of a different path for heating than for X irradiation is not too difficult a proposition. If heat is delivered *via* ultrasound or electromagnetic techniques, one can think of heating along a line defined by the x-axis, with radiation directed along a line defined by the y-axis. (The tumor is assumed to be at the origin of such a coordinate system.) If the tumor is heated to a temperature that by itself kills few if any cells, i.e., 42.5°C, the only effect of heat would be to sensitize cells to X irradiation. Since overlap of the two modalities under the assumed conditions occurs only in or near the tumor, the effect of heat would be specific for that tissue volume. The only treatment-limiting tissue then would be structural normal tissue within the tumor volume. These considerations hold for any heating technique that leads to preferential heating of tumor volumes. Secondly, it has to be recognized that the studies so far have been done on a very limited number of tumors. When dealing with lesions that are extremely radioresistant, heating regimens may very well have benefits not considered in the studies described here. It has been demonstrated that some radioresistant tumors have an unusual capacity for repair of X-ray-induced, potentially lethal damage (Weichselbaum *et al.*, 1977). For such tumors, time–temperature profiles sufficiently potent to inhibit such recovery (Li *et al.*, 1978) would seem to offer considerable possibilities. For these tumors, an effective treatment would require that heating be carried out immediately after X irradiation.

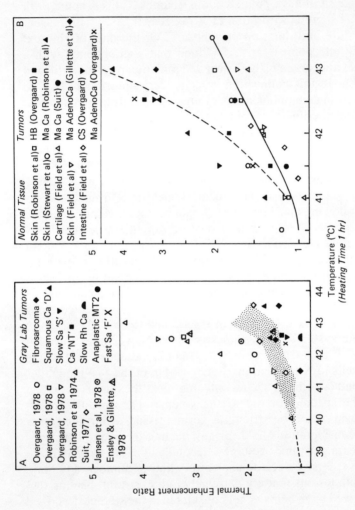

Figure 5.11. Thermal enhancement ratios for tumors and normal skin: two views of similar data. Tumor and normal tissue thermal enhancement ratios were compared by two groups: panel A, Hill and Denekamp (1979, with permission) and panel B, Overgaard (1977, with permission). In panel A, normal tissue responses are indicated by the shaded area, tumor responses by individual symbols. The solid symbols refer to data obtained by Hill and Denekamp utilizing water-bath heating. Their conclusion is that no advantage can be gained for heating and radiation if the two treatments are given in temporal proximity since normal tissue and tumor are affected in the same way. In panel B, the lower curve summarizes normal tissue responses, the upper curve tumor responses; Overgaard's conclusion is that at higher temperatures a considerable benefit may be derived from simultaneous treatments, as the lines for tumor and tissue responses diverge sharply.

Finally, the data mentioned so far have said very little about the possibility of using heat and X irradiation as independent modalities. This subject is discussed at some length in the review of Overgaard (1978). He advocates a treatment protocol in which heating and X irradiation are separated by 24 hr or more. The rationale here is that heat and X irradiation are individually optimum in effecting cell killing in different subpopulations of the cells making up the tumor. In particular, the most radioresistant cells are very likely those at low pH and in a milieu of nutritional deprivation, and therefore hypoxic. Such radioresistant cells would be expected to be very heat sensitive. Heat by itself, as was discussed in earlier sections, induces relatively little damage to normal tissue at temperature–time profiles that are capable of causing tumor regressions. These considerations make it reasonable to introduce an interval of sufficiently long duration between heat treatments and X irradiations in order to minimize any possible interactions between the two modalities. It is only these interactions that could be reflected as normal tissue sensitization. Two studies have been performed that strongly reinforce this concept. Overgaard (1977) studied the effects of sequence and time intervals of combined hyperthermia and radiation treatment of a mouse mammary adenocarcinoma. For that tumor, the TER was independent of the sequence used, even if treatment by radiation and heat were separated by as much as 24 hr. Since the TER for critical normal tissue is minimized by a long separation of heating and irradiation, a treatment schedule avoiding interactions should result in a large TGF.

Following this line of thought led Faria and Hahn (1982, in press) to compare the responses of the heat- and X-ray-resistant RIF tumor to a single-dose and a fractionated course of these modalities. The patterns of tumor volume changes following single doses of either X irradiation or heat were very different. Tumors treated with X irradiation regressed slowly; complete regressions were seen only after doses of 5000 rad and higher. Even larger doses were associated with progressively increasing tumor cure rates. The growth rate of regrowing, unsterilized tumors was appreciably lower than that of untreated controls, indicating an effect of the irradiation on the tumor bed. By contrast, RIF tumors heated 30 min at 44.5°C regressed promptly and completely but invariably regrew. The delay in regrowth was a function of the heating time. The growth rate of regrowing tumors was not affected by heating; growth curves of recurrences were parallel to those of unheated controls, implying an absence of tumor bed effect in areas exposed to hyperthermia alone.

When X-ray and heat doses were fractionated, additional differences were seen in the tumors' responses to the two modalities. Treatment consisted of X-ray fractions of 400 rad each given twice weekly (Mondays and Wednesdays) or heat doses of 30 min at 44.5°C, given once a week (Fridays). The assay used was tumor growth delay, measured as the time required for tumors to double in volume. For X rays, the delay increased with the number of fractions (up to eight); no cures were obtained, but the last fractions appeared as effective as the first in inducing additional growth delay. However, the tumor responded strongly to only the first two heat fractions, which induced a tumor growth delay equivalent to that induced by about 2000 rads of X rays. Additional heat doses were ineffective; four exposures resulted in a growth delay that was not very different from that seen following two heat fractions. Adding the two treatments was very effective: approximately 50% cures were obtained when two heat doses were added to six to seven X-ray doses.

What was particularly intriguing about this study was the finding that the heat doses did not affect skin scoring for a given X-ray dose; skin damage was similar in the animals receiving X ray only and in those receiving both treatments. It is dangerous to make too much of one set of experiments, and before drawing far-reaching conclusions verifications of these results by additional studies are highly desirable. Nevertheless, it appeared as though in this system heat either induced a type of damage in normal tissue that was not scorable by the technique utilized, or that the damage was scorable, but that the amount of additional damage induced at this time–temperature profile was insufficient to be measurable over and above the radiation damage. This latter possibility sounds almost too optimistic to be correct, but it is consistent with several findings. First of all, as I pointed out in the beginning of this chapter, heat treatments that routinely lead either to tumor cure or to substantial regressions of tumor volumes seem to cause no long-term normal tissue damage and very little short-term damage. Secondly, the fact that the tumor response shows very little additional growth delay once the effect of the initial heat treatments has been felt, suggests that a large number of tumor cells are essentially unaffected by the hyperthermic treatment. It is very likely that these latter cells are in an environment similar to that of normal tissue. They are either infiltrating tumor cells, cells at the very periphery of the tumor volume, or perhaps cells that are in close proximity to active blood vessels. If these cells are not affected by the hyperthermia treatment, it is not unreasonable to hypothesize that the normal tissue is equally little affected. In any case, it appeared that the hyperthermic treatment added the equivalent of 2400 rad to tumor damage, while adding little additional burden to the normal tissue. Needless to say, such a finding, if found to apply to tumors in general, would have far-reaching implications for radiotherapeutic practice.

A final word of caution about normal tissue effects. To date, few studies have been performed that examine the interactions of heat and X ray in tissue unusually sensitive to either modality individually. The importance of carrying out such studies is accentuated by the finding of Goffinet *et al.* (1977) that heat appreciably increases X-ray damage to the sensitive spinal cord.

5.5. RESPONSES OF TUMORS TO COMBINATIONS OF HEAT AND DRUGS

I have described several studies involving hyperthermia alone or hyperthermia and X irradiation, but there are very few investigations that examine the interactions of drugs and heat on murine tumors. This is a curious and unfortunate situation because the clinical application of combinations of heat and chemotherapy offers considerable promise. It is particularly curious that no study exists that examines the interaction of hyperthermia and various drugs on critical normal tissue. In the United States, this lack of data reflects in part prejudices currently existing in certain study sections of the National Cancer Institute. In rejecting one study in which it was proposed to examine a variety of drug–heat interactions in murine systems, the reviewers commented that such studies cannot "produce information on the basic physical–chemical interactions occurring within mammalian cells." Apparently it was felt that this is a *sine qua non* of research; empirical, phenomenological studies leading to possibilities of improved clinical applications are not deemed worthy. This unfortunate prejudice will certainly lead to complete domination of the hyperthermia field by radiotherapists who saw a clinical field develop successfully in the absence of an understanding of the interaction of X rays and cells on the biochemical level. Whether or not this is desirable is a matter of opinion. One thing is surely correct. If criteria such as those suggested by this study section had determined the development of radiotherapy, we would still be waiting for its beginning as a clinical modality for the treatment of tumors.

A recent review by Marmor (1979) describes the data on murine tumor studies available up to 1979. Since then there have only been one or two additional reports, and hence all I can do is to update her rather comprehensive review. I will also follow her organization. A few comments are in order about the type of studies that are likely to yield useful information. When performing tumor cure experiments, it is necessary to work with tumors that cannot be cured by heat alone; sensitive tumors such as the EMT6 cannot provide information with regard to cure rates of combined modalities (although such tumors can provide useful cell-killing data). It is also desirable to use tumors that at 37°C are at least somewhat responsive to the chemotherapeutic agent. If at that temperature the tumor does not respond at all, the absence of response in the presence of heat may not signify a lack of interaction. Such data may only show that even a synergistic interaction did not produce the effect at a measurable level. Finally, it is necessary to have a control group of mice in which the drug and heat are given with a temporal separation sufficiently long to preclude any interaction. This control provides information on additive effects. In the absence of such a control, reports of synergism must be treated with considerable skepticism. Because of the nonlinearity of tumor cure rates with either heat or drug dose, additive effects can easily be misinterpreted as appearing to show synergistic effects.

5.5.1. Alkylating Agents

The first report examining the interaction of an alkylating agent (mechlorethamine-N-oxide) and hyperthermia is that of Suzuki (1967). The combination of a 42°C local water bath with 5 mg/kg of the drug caused regression of Yoshida solid sarcomas in rats, whereas either of these treatments alone caused only the slowing of tumor growth. At higher doses of drug, 10 mg/kg, tumor regression occurred with and without heat. The addition of heat then caused no appreciable difference in the measurement of tumor regression. This is the only study that even mentions normal tissue damage. Local toxicity in terms of swelling and loss of heat was worse in the group that received the combined treatment. An alkylating agent, methylenedimethanesulfonate (MDMS), was used by Dickson and Suzanger (1974), also against the Yoshida sarcoma. No improvement in cure rates resulted from the combination of drug and heat. Tumors treated with heat and MDMS seemed to regress even more slowly than those treated with the drug alone. Using inhibition of glycolysis as the assay, Dickson and Suzanger (1976) found the treatments to be additive when the assay was performed 24 hr after the completion of hyperthermia. There is no way of knowing if inhibition of glycolysis is a meaningful assay for drug studies; not even its usefulness for hyperthermic inactivation is clearly established. This study was also insufficient in that curative doses of MDMS were used, and the drug and hyperthermia were not administered simultaneously; any effect resulting from the direct interaction of the two would not have been measured.

Yerushalmi and Hazan (1979) used the Lewis lung carcinoma implanted in the left hind leg of C3H/EB/BLF mice to examine the interaction of cyclophosphamide and hyperthermia. In a preliminary report, they showed that if the drug (150 mg/kg) and heat (tumor temperature approximately 42°C) were administered simultaneously, 10 out of 41 animals were cured of their tumors. If 30 min separated the two treatments, only 6 out of 46 animals were cured. Neither drug nor heat treatments by themselves resulted in any cures. The mean survival level of the animals not cured also reflected the increased efficiency of the combined treatment. It should be emphasized that in this last study heating was effected by blowing hot air over the lesion. Temperature elevations were local and no increase in body temperature of the treated animals was reported. Cyclophosphamide, in order to become cytotoxic, needs to be activated by the liver. The combination of cyclophosphamide and heat under conditions in which the liver is raised to elevated temperatures should await animal data on whether or not such treatments would affect the rate of activation of the drug.

5.5.2. Antitumor Antibiotics

Only three such antibiotics have been examined *in vivo:* adriamycin, bleomycin, and actinomycin D. Very different results have been found for them. The combination of adriamycin and 43°C hyperthermia for 30 min in treating BALB/c mice bearing EMT6 sarcomas was examined by Hahn *et al.* (1975). In this study, heating was localized to the tumor volume; cell cytotoxicity was examined in the dose range of 10 to 25 mg/kg. The combined cell killing by adriamycin and hyperthermia was clearly greater than that predicted on an additive basis. A study with the combination of adriamycin and heat against a mammary carcinoma in C3H × EBA/2F1 hybrids was carried out by Overgaard (1976); tumor cure was used as an assay. The dose used in that work, 25 mg/kg, was large and resulted in the death of 18 of 20 control animals that received the drug alone within 7 days after treatment. Both at 40.5 and 42.5°C the combination of adriamycin and heat gave a higher proportion of cures than did heat alone, although the numbers are not statistically significant. The very large number of animals that died from adriamycin and from the combination of the two treatments makes it difficult to draw meaningful conclusions from this study. Marmor *et al.* (1979) performed parallel studies of cell survival in EMT6 tumors and of the time for the tumor to double in C3H mice bearing KHT mammary carcinomas. Induction of hyperthermia was by radiofrequency currents, the temperature used was

43°C for 30 min, and heating was begun immediately after injection of the drug. As far as cell survival was concerned, a clear synergistic effect could be demonstrated only at doses of 10 mg/kg or greater. At 5 mg/kg, cell killing was not statistically different from that predicted on an additive basis. Neither at adriamycin doses of 2.5 mg/kg nor at 5 mg/kg did the addition of heat, given as described, result in increased MTD doubling times over those measured when the drug was given either 24 hr before or after heat. At these drug levels, there was no synergistic response either in terms of cell killing or in changes of MTD doubling times. At 10 mg/kg, a dose where the cell survival studies did show such an interaction, a large fraction of the animals died and the MTD doubling times were not considered meaningful.

Results for bleomycin at 15 mg/kg are shown in Figure 5.12. There is clear evidence of synergism in inducing growth delay. For example, when two treatments were given on alternate days, the growth delay was 20 days if bleomycin and heat (43°C, 30 min) were given simultaneously, but only 12 days if the treatments were given individually at 24-hr intervals. The 12-day growth delay is roughly what would be expected on the basis of additivity of individual heat and drug effects. When the study was repeated at lower temperatures, no synergism could be demonstrated, consistent with an *in vitro* finding of a marked threshold effect for this drug at about 43°C (Hahn *et al.*, 1975).

The only other study involving an antitumor antibiotic is that of Yerushalmi (1978), who studied the treatment of SV10 fibrosarcoma with actinomycin D and actinomycin D plus heat. A marked increase in median survival time was noted for the combined treatment compared to acti-

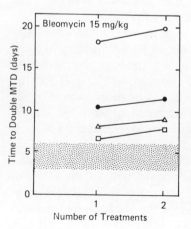

Figure 5.12. Mean tumor diameter doubling times for KHT tumors in C3H mice treated with combinations of heat and bleomycin. Points are median values for 7 to 15 animals. Shaded area: control range (mean ± 2 S.D.). □: 43°C for 30 min; △: bleomycin alone; ●: bleomycin and 43°C given 24 hr apart; ○: bleomycin and 43°C given simultaneously. Marmor *et al.* (1979), with permission.

nomycin D alone. Unfortunately, no control was done on the effect of heat alone, so one cannot tell if the effect was more (or less) than additive.

5.5.3. Nitrosoureas

The effect of BCNU and hyperthermia against EMT6 tumors was studied by Twentyman *et al.* (1978). Animals bearing either flank or leg tumors were treated with the drug at concentrations of 20 mg/kg immediately before being given a hyperthermic treatment by water bath. The average tumor temperature was 41.6°C, and the duration of treatment was 1 hr. Tumor regrowth studies showed that the effect of the combination treatment was superior to that of either treatment alone; cell survival assays, done in parallel, gave similar results. The study was done with only very few animals and therefore the conclusions that can be drawn from it are rather limited.

In a study in our laboratory, a variety of nitrosources were examined for their ability to retard the growth of KHT tumors or their cell-killing ability against EMT6 tumors (J. B. Marmor and G. M. Hahn, unpublished). Considerable potentiation of the *in vivo* cytotoxic effects of BCNU, chlorozotocin, and methyl-CCNU were seen at both 42 and 43°C; the effect was somewhat less significant at 41°C. Typical examples are shown in Figure 5.13 (panels A-C). These results clearly match the temperature responses found in Chinese hamster cells *in vitro* as discussed in Chapter 3.

5.5.4. Platinum Compounds

Enhancement of cytotoxicity *in vitro* for this agent, as described by Hahn (1978), is also matched *in vivo*. This is shown in Figure 5.13 (panel D). Here, results from Marmor *et al.* (1979) on the combined effect of this drug and hyperthermia on KHT tumor growth delay are shown. The results are very similar to those seen for bleomycin and for the nitrosoureas; increased growth delay if the drug and heat are given in close time proximity, and an additive effect only if a 12-hr interval is allowed to elapse between the two treatments.

5.5.5. Electron Affinic Compounds

There are by now several studies that demonstrate possible clinical benefits of drugs developed as radiation sensitizers specific for hypoxic cells in conjunction with hyperthermia. Bleehan *et al.* (1977) showed an interaction of the drug nitromidazole and hyperthermia against the EMT6

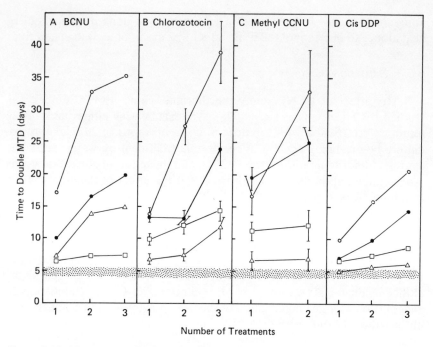

Figure 5.13. Mean tumor diameter doubling times for KHT tumors in C3H mice treated with combinations of heat and drugs as shown. Points: medians for 7 to 16 animals. Shaded area: control range (mean ± 2 S. D.). □: 43°C for 30 min; △: drug alone; ●: drug and heat treatment given 24 hr apart; ○: drug and heat treatment given simultaneously. A—BCNU, 10 mg/kg; B—chlorozotocin, 10 mg/kg; C—methyl-CCNU, 10 mg/kg; D—cis-DDP, 2 mg/ kg. Marmor *et al.* (1979), with permission, and J. B. Marmor and G. M. Hahn (unpublished).

tumor. Cell survival was used as an assay; no significant cell-killing effect of the drug was observed at 37°C, but it became markedly cytotoxic at 42.5°C. Similar results are found in another study, in which a tissue-culture-adapted line of a fibrosarcoma was studied (George *et al.*, 1977). An appreciable enhancement of the cytotoxic action of misonidazole, another electron affinic drug, against hypoxic tumor cells *in vivo* was observed when combined with 1 hr of heat at 40.5°C. This temperature, by itself, had no effect on cell survival. Another study examined the ability of the simultaneous administration of hyperthermia and nitromidazole to sensitize hypoxic tumor cells (L1210) to X irradiation (Hofer *et al.*, 1977). Cell survival was estimated by measuring the radioactivity of cells previously exposed to [^{125}I]iodo-deoxyuridine. Combined administration of hyperthermia and nitromidazole produced potentiation of radiation damage in hypoxic L1210 populations, with the dose-modifying factor as high as 4.2. Under optimal conditions, hypoxic L1210 cells subjected simultaneously to the drug and to heat became more radiosensitive than untreated, fully oxygenated L1210 cells. Two other cell lines (BP8 murine sarcoma and Ehrlich ascite cells) behaved in a somewhat similar manner when exposed to the two modalities *in vivo*. Finally, in one study the combination of all three treatments—hyperthermia, misonidazole, and radiation—was studied to determine local tumor control in a mammary carcinoma growing in C3H mice (Stone, 1978). Dose modifying factors of 3.8 and 5.03 to single dose TCD_{50} were found when the tumors were immersed in 42.5 and 43°C water baths. The dose of misonidazole used to achieve such tremendous modifying factors was 1 mg/kg, given 30 min before irradiation.

5.5.6. Lidocaine

The final study that will be described here involved the use of the local anesthetic lidocaine infused into CA755 mammary adenocarcinomas in order to try to accentuate hyperthermic effects (Yatvin *et al.*, 1979). This experiment appears to be the only known attempt *in vivo* to use what I have called a hyperthermic sensitizer. Lidocaine and several other local anesthetics, as well as other agents, such as short-chained aliphatic alcohols, act as temperature modifiers. They do this at concentrations that are not necessarily cytotoxic at 37°C. Young BDF1 mice grafted with mammary adenocarcinoma CA755 had lidocaine injected into three areas of the tumor (total dose 2 mg/mouse) within 5 min before heat treatments in a water bath. Control groups were similarly infused with .05 ml of isotonic saline. A 3 × 3 block design of treatment regimens with three temperatures (room temperature, 42°C, and 43.5°C), and three injection options (no injection, saline injection, and lidocaine injection) were used. Results are shown in Table 5.3. There was considerable interaction between the anesthetic agent and hyperthermia. At 43.5°C, survival times were increased threefold over the control, and 4 out of 20 animals treated, still alive at day 60, were presumed to be cured. It was only in the groups given both drug and heat treatments that any cures were obtained; animals in all other groups died of their tumors.

This interesting study opens an entirely new field for investigation. There are, however, some cautions. As has been discussed earlier, lidocaine acts to shift temperature. What is needed, in order to make the results obtained by Yatvin *et al.* more compelling, is a study in which the amount of temperature shift induced by the amount of lidocaine is determined, and an appropriate control is carried out at the higher temperature.

TABLE 5.3
SURVIVAL OF MICE AFTER TREATMENT WITH HEAT
OR HEAT PLUS LIDOCAINE[a]

		Survival (days) after injection[c]	
Heating[b]	None	Saline	Lidocaine
None	12.8 ± 0.90 (25)	12.7 ± 0.70 (17)	14.6 ± 1.21 (17)
42.0°C	12.6 ± 1.36 (10)	16.5 ± 1.61 (10)	13.6 ± 0.89 (10)
43.5°C	18.5 ± 0.88 (31)	19.4 ± 1.08 (30)	>37.3 ± 6.21 (31)

[a]Data from Yatvin et al., 1979, with permission.
[b]For 1 hour.
[c]Values are means ± standard errors; number of animals is shown in parentheses. Analysis of variance indicates that the increase in survival when lidocaine is present during heating at 43.5°C for 1 hr is significantly different (P < .05) from the results for the other eight treatments. Heat alone at 43.5°C significantly prolonged survival. The figure for lidocaine plus 43.5°C is minimal, as it included four animals that were still alive.

The alcohol data of Li and Hahn (1978) would suggest a temperature shift of about one degree. Thus, an appropriate control would have been a group of animals exposed at 44.5°C (43.5°C of the experiment plus one degree shift to compensate for the lidocaine). It would then be desirable to have a demonstration that the presence of lidocaine induces greater tumor effects than the accompanying normal tissue effects of the 44.5°C exposure. In the absence of this control, the possibility remains that lidocaine plus heat yields the same effects as treatment at an appropriately increased temperature. Nevertheless, the development of techniques to sensitize tumors to heat, particularly with agents that at normal temperatures do not show cytotoxicity, is an area of considerable promise.

5.6. DO TUMOR CELLS DIE IN THE SAME MANNER IN VIVO AS THEY DO IN VITRO?

The answer to this question seems to be yes and no. In Table 5.4, which is an adaptation and update from a similar compilation by Overgaard (1977), I have listed several characteristics of tumor cell death in vivo and in vitro. Clearly there is considerable similarity in many aspects of cell death. The heat sensitivity of cells per se does not seem to be too different under the two conditions. Effects of the environment may be most important. This is demonstrated by the cells' sensitization in vitro by chronic hypoxia, lack of glucose, and low pH, features also encountered in the core of some tumors. Cells are sensitized to X irradiation and to many

TABLE 5.4
HEAT DEATH OF CELLS[a]

	In vitro	*In vivo*
Selectivity for malignant cells	Malignant cells may be slightly more sensitive.	Selective destruction of all cells from some tumors, but only some cells from other tumors.
Heat sensitivity	Function of cell type and environment. Survival after 1 hr at 44°C (pH 7.4): 10^{-1} (typical value).	Some, but certainly not all, tumors exquisitively sensitive to heat. 1 hr at 43°C produces many tumor cures. However, cell survival as measured immediately after treatment may be comparable to *in vitro* survival.
Histopathology	Only minor immediate damage to most cells; no clear indication of primary lesion. Expression of death may take several days.	In one tumor, lysosomal damage appears to lead to cell destruction. In another, the initial lesion appears in the cytoplasmic membrane. Expression of cell death rapid (1–6 hr).
Effect of cellular environment	Chronic hypoxia, lack of glucose and other nutrients, as well as low pH interact to make cells heat sensitive.	In some tumors, core more sensitive than periphery. Reduced blood flow during and after heating may increase cell killing.
Cell cycle effects	Late S and M phase cells, and some plateau phase cells more heat sensitive.	Not known, though mitotic cells appear to be very sensitive.
Development of thermotolerance	Found in all cell systems examined; rate of development is a function of initial treatment temperature and duration, and perhaps of environment during incubation.	Demonstrated only in one or two tumor systems, though found in all normal tissue examined to date.
Recovery from sublethal damage	Probably, though difficult to demonstrate because of development of thermotolerance.	No evidence for recovery, though difficult to measure.
Heat increases X-ray cytotoxicity	Yes	Yes
Heat modifies drug cytotoxicity	Depending upon drug, may increase, not affect, or reduce cytotoxicity.	Increased cytotoxicity in some cases or lack of interaction in others has been demonstrated.

[a]Source: Overgaard, 1977, with permission.

chemotherapeutic agents, whether *in vitro* or *in vivo*. There are, however, some major differences, which seem to relate primarily to events occurring after the cessation of the hyperthermic treatment. In particular, for several tumors if cells are allowed to remain *in situ* after heating, there occurs an additional cell killing that proceeds fairly rapidly over 6 hr. This was demonstrated clearly for the EMT6 tumor (Hahn *et al.*, 1978a) and has been discussed in Section 5.2.2. This may reflect the behavior of cells *in vitro*. For example, (Li *et al.*, 1980a) have shown that if cells heated in buffer are forced to remain in a nutrient-deprived state after heating, their survival is reduced. Similarly, low pH after heating can lead to additional cell killing.

It does not seem likely, however, that the massive cell death of EMT6 cells *in situ* can be ascribed to minor variations in pH or nutritional status of the cells, as these conditions exist before heating. *In vivo* we must look to host responses to the tumor, or to host–tumor interactions that could accentuate cell death and eventually lead to tumor cures even after relatively mild hyperthermia time–temperature combinations. The two major areas to be examined are the various immune responses the body can mount against the tumor and the role of regional blood flow.

5.6.1. The Role of Immune Responses

A thorough examination of the interaction of immune processes and hyperthermia is well beyond the scope of what I am attempting to do here. I will restrict myself to an attempt to survey the existing literature to see if data can be found that would definitely implicate a unique, hyperthermia-stimulated immune response as being responsible for some of the tumor cures obtained after only very mild heat exposures. It is appropriate to recall that 100% of animals bearing EMT6 tumors were cured after 30-min exposures of the tumor to 44°C. This heat dose reduced cell survival *in vitro* by, at most, a factor of 10. There is no question that animals cured of tumors by hyperthermia are able to mount a response specifically against that tumor, and that this response is over and above that of animals that had never been exposed to that tumor. However, if the comparison of the ability to reject tumor cells is made among animals cured by hyperthermia, cured by irradiation, or cured by surgery, to date no significant differences have been demonstrated (C. Nager, J. B. Marmor and G. M. Hahn, unpublished; Suit *et al.*, 1978). Experiments performed to evaluate immunocompetence included determination of the number of cells required to initiate new tumors in cured mice, chromium release experiments involving cytotoxic lymphocytes obtained from cured animals, and a comparison of the ability of "armed" macrophages to inhibit growth of EMT6 cells *in vitro*. In all these experiments, no unique property could be ascribed to the heat treatments. A review by Szmigielski and Janiak (1978) details many of the immune responses affected by hyperthermic treatment. However, none of the data specifically allow one to isolate mechanisms responsible for the tumor cures. In fact, Harris and Meneses (1978) showed that protein synthesis, which is necessary for cell-mediated immune cytolysis, was markedly depressed in T-lymphocytes by heating to 43°C. Heated lymphocytes were less able to mount an attack against P-815 neoplastic cells than were unheated cells. The workers looked at the total cell killing effected and found it to be additive; cell death induced by heat alone plus cell death induced by the lymphocytes was equivalent to the total cell death measured, without any evidence for synergism. Another possibility is that heating increased the antigenicity of tumor cells. There is indeed one report suggesting this (Mondovi *et al.*, 1972), but this finding has not been duplicated by others (Suit *et al.*, 1978). In any case, the data of Mondovi refer to heating of cells *in vitro*, and no equivalent of such a putative increased antigenicity has been demonstrated *in vivo*.

This is not to suggest that immune responses are not involved in the sterilization of tumors by hyperthermia. There is no doubt that manipulations of immune responses can have considerable effects on the progression of cancer treatment in experimental animals and probably also in man. One need only mention the work of Coley with streptococcal bacterial toxins, particularly as demonstrated in the analysis of long-term survival of the patients treated by him as carried out by his daughter Helen Nauts (Fowler and Nauts, 1964). Additionally, the work of Okamoto *et al.*, (1966) and Kurokawa *et al.*, (1972) indicate that the use of specific purified streptococcal bacteria can influence the progress of malignant diseases in man. Many of the data results have been reviewed by Huth (1977). He presents an interesting historical review of the entire subject and additionally reproduced *in vitro* some of the more pertinent results of Okamoto *et al.* and of Kurokawa *et al.* But it is not at all clear that the use of microbial substances in cancer therapy is necessarily related to hyperthermia. This is brought out in a recent review of the human data by Nauts (1975). Many of Coley's patients who responded favorably to treatment developed fevers limited to perhaps 40 to 41°C, and there was no clear correlation between the effectiveness of the treatment and the highest temperature of the patients' fevers. After looking at the data relating to hyperthermia and the immune response, I conclude that while there are many hints that suggest an association between hyperthermia and immune responses, no firm data exist that prove any connection.

5.6.2. Effect of Hyperthermia on Spread and Growth of Metastases

Before widespread clinical applications of hyperthermia can be recommended, the possibility that increased temperatures affect the formation or progression of metastases needs careful study. Beneficial effects of the treatment of primary tumors resulting in the reduction in size or disappearance of secondary tumors have been reported (Dickson, 1977). These experiments clearly involve antigenic, transplanted tumors, and the relevance of such data to the human situation is not certain. Of considerably greater possible importance are data that suggest that heat may increase the rate of metastatic spread.

The earliest studies that seem to suggest that this problem is one of concern are those of Suzuki (1967) and Muckle and Dickson (1973). Both groups noted that in spite of some effects of the combination of drugs and heat against primary tumors, there was no survival advantage resulting from the treatments. Dickson and Ellis (1976) heated rats bearing Yoshida sarcomas for 1 hr. The local tumor temperature rose to 42°C, but the water baths employed for the heating induced whole-body temperatures of 41.5°C. This treatment was fatal to 151 out of 167 animals. The life span of the survivors was much reduced when it was compared to that of unheated controls (16 ± 2.5 vs. 26 ± 3.1 days); the animals died of widespread disease. In a later study, Dickson and Muckle treated rabbits bearing VX-2 carcinomas with either local or whole body heating. Localized heating was found to be more effective in achieving tumor cures. However, in animals in which cure was not achieved, there appeared to be an increased spread and growth of metastases. Even with "local" heating it is very likely that the core body temperature was also raised. Walker et al. (1978) also suggested such an adverse effect from localized heating. However, that study involving murine tumors was based on retrospective controls, and the control animals were not handled in the same way as were the heated mice. Therefore results from that study cannot be evaluated.

The influence exerted by either whole-body or localized heating on 3L Lewis carcinomas was studied by Yerushalmi (1976). Mice bearing tumors in their left hind legs were subjected to heating with streams of hot air; whole-body heating was achieved by additionally placing the animals in an insulated cylinder during the hot air exposure (30 min). Tumor temperatures ranging between 41 and 43°C were obtained, with somewhat lower values for whole-body heating. The 3L tumor metastasized to the lungs with very high efficiency in untreated animals. The mice treated with whole-body hyperthermia developed lung disease before the controls, while those treated only locally maintained healthy lungs for a longer period.

Two other studies also indicate that localized heating does not increase the rate of metastatic spread or growth. Schechter *et al.* (1978) used a carcinoma implanted into the hind legs of Wistar rats. This cancer metastasizes from that site to the retroperitoneal lymph nodes in 100% of tumor-bearing animals. Heating the tumors to 42.3°C for 90 min inhibited the growth of both primary and preexisting metastases; inadequate heating did not result in increased growth of metastasis or of the primary tumor.

In a somewhat similar study, Marmor *et al.* (1979) investigated the treatment of KHT tumors with localized hyperthermia (43°C, 30 min) or hyperthermia and drugs (adriamycin, bleomycin, BCNU, and/or cis-platinum). This tumor was implanted in the flanks of C3H mice. From that site it metastasizes to the lungs with 100% regularity. Marmor *et al.* developed a scoring system that permitted a quantitative estimation of the severity of the metastatic lesion at the time of sacrifice of the mice. In lungs excised 23–25 days after either hyperthermia or sham treatments, the average metatasis score in heated animals was 3.4 ± 0.14, while in controls it was 3.7 ± 0.13 (out of a possible maximum of 4). Scores of lungs of animals exposed to combinations of drugs and heat were uniformly lower than either those of controls or of animals exposed to heat alone.

Finally, the effect of heat and heat plus X ray on the production of disseminated disease was studied by Hahn *et al.* (1979). Dunn osteogenic sarcoma was implanted in the footpads of syngeneic mice. Localized treatment of 40.5 or 42.5°C (15 min) with or without the addition of three or four fractions of 200 rad did not increase metastatic spread of the disease.

In sum, these results indicate that whole-body heating of mice very likely does increase the rate of spread of metastases. There are no data on the effects of whole-body heating on the rate of growth of individual metastatic lesions. Caution is therefore in order where such treatments of localized human cancers are considered.

The experimental evidence favors the view that localized heating does not affect metastatic spread. The results that show disappearance of metastases after the successful treatment of primary lesions probably reflect the antigenicity of the transplanted tumors and likely do not apply to the treatment of spontaneous tumors. As to possible deleterious effects, the properly controlled studies show no increases of metastatic lesions following localized heating. The one possible exception, that of Dickson and

Ellis (1976), probably reflects the effects of the high level of whole-body heating encountered rather than the slight additional increase in tumor temperature.

5.7. SUMMARY

Studies on mice with transplantable tumors have demonstrated that some tumors can be cured by hyperthermic exposures that involve only a modest amount of cell killing; other tumors are considerably more heat resistant. Cell death induced directly by the heating process does not necessarily reflect tumor cure results. Tumor antigenicity and heat-induced modifications of tumor blood flow appear to be important factors that influence tumor curability. The uniformity of temperature distributions may further affect cure rates.

Ultrastructural studies show that cells heated *in vivo* show rapid disintegration of lysosomal and plasma membranes, though whether or not these events are secondary to heat death resulting from other lesions is not known. Attempts to sensitize tumor cells by hyperacidification with glucose infusions have not as yet produced any positive results. In the absence of appropriate experimental data to the contrary, the possibility that such infusions may result in increased cellular resistance brought about by an improvement in the nutrient environment cannot be dismissed.

Thermotolerance develops in some, though perhaps not all, murine tumors. It also develops in all the normal tissues that have been examined. While the onset of tolerance in tumors and in normal tissue follows similar kinetics, in at least one tumor system the decay of tolerance is more rapid.

Normal tissue damage from heating may be an all-or-nothing phenomenon in the sense that tissue necrosis is irreparable (at least over a 30-day period) while most other damage is repaired rapidly. Skin may be a particularly heat-sensitive tissue, and heating with hot water baths may introduce damage of a nonthermal nature.

Heating in conjunction with X irradiation clearly increases antitumor effects; TERs of 1.5–1.6 or higher have been observed. The TERs are maximum if heating and X irradiation are simultaneous; potentiation is reduced if a time interval is introduced between the two treatments. However, depending upon the tumor system, the TERs may still be appreciable even if heating follows X irradiation by several hours, up to 24 hr in one study. Fractionation treatments reduce the TERs. Normal tissue effects are potentiated similarly, so that for combined treatments with simultaneous exposures, those volumes of normal tissue that are at the same temperature as the tumor will be affected equally. However, if the treatments are separated, particularly if heat follows X irradiation by several hours, there may be a tumor-specific potentiation. In one murine tumor system, separating the fractionated radiotherapy from weekly heatings indicated that two 30 min treatments at 44.5°C are the equivalent of approximately 2000 rad against the tumor, without affecting the skin in a measurable way.

Combinations of drug and heat also increase antitumor effects. Of particular efficacy against KHT and RIF tumors is the simultaneous application of localized heat and nitrosoureas, bleomycin, or cis-platinum.

While there is considerable evidence that in mice whole-body heating increases the spread of metastatic disease, the available data do not support the suggestion that localized hyperthermia causes a similar effect.

6

Technical Aspects of Hyperthermia

6.1. INTRODUCTION

Any attempt to cover, in one chapter, the physiology and physics of heating tumors, as well as the means of measuring tumor and normal tissue temperatures, is a difficult undertaking. It would not be unreasonable to write several treatises on these subjects. For example, the two major competing physical techniques that apply to localized heating, electromagnetics and ultrasound, each merit thorough expositions. To do so would require two textbooks, and I would hardly be competent to be the author of either. Therefore, to stay within space (and my own) limitations, I am going to be very selective in the choice of topics to be covered. As a guide to determining appropriate subject matter, I am taking what might be described as a consumer's viewpoint. I don't mean the ultimate consumer, the patient, who rarely is in a position to choose the treatment, but I am thinking of the physician. His or her questions relate not so much to specific aspects of the design of various systems, but to the machines' capabilities and limitations, i.e., to their utility in a clinical setting. In Table 6.1 I have summarized much of the information available regarding advantages and disadvantages of various heating modalities.

A topic of importance is that of biological hazards associated with each mode of heating. These include not only possible damages to the patient who is subjected to high intensities of energy flow, but also possible adverse effects on the operators of the equipment, although the latter are likely to be exposed only to leakage levels. After all, no one wants to duplicate the situation encountered by many early radiologists, who used ionizing radiations without adequate safeguards because the carcinogenic aspects of such radiations were then not known. Unfortunately, the possible biological hazards of neither microwaves nor of ultrasound have been explored in the detail warranted by the wide use of these modalities in medicine and elsewhere.

TABLE 6.1
COMPARISON OF HEATING TECHNIQUES[a]

Heating technique	Advantages	Disadvantages	Possible applications
Ultrasound Single transducer	Simplicity; fatty tissue not preferentially heated; does not interfere with temperature measurements.	Relatively poor depth–dose distribution for unfocused system; focused transducer has little flexibility; maximum dimensions determined by crystal availability (currently 5-cm diameter); differential heating of bone.	Near-surface tumors; skin lesions; some head and neck tumors.
Ultrasound Multiple transducers	Fatty tissue not preferentially heated; does not interfere with temperature measurements; depth dose distribution 10–15 cm with focusing; isocentric system feasible; precise localization possible; can be combined with echoing for alignment.	Air–tissue interfaces cause reflections; inability to heat lung; bones may present difficulties; possibility of pain at higher power levels; volume to be heated is limited by size and number of transducers.	Soft-tissue tumors, bladder, liver, head and neck lesions, bone; brain (?).
Radiofrequency[b] Capacitive coupling	Applicators (invasive or noninvasive) can be tailored to individual requirements; multiple applicators may permit some depth–dose optimization; surface of applicators easily cooled to permit skin protection.	Skin and fatty tissues are high-absorption tissues; fatty tissue is dose limiting, even with maximum cooling; heating pattern difficult to measure and hard to predict; metal temperature probe distorts field and gives false readings.	Chest, upper abdomen, pelvis, extremities; brain (?).

TECHNICAL ASPECTS OF HYPERTHERMIA 181

Method	Advantages	Disadvantages	Applications
Radiofrequency Inductive coupling	Simple equipment; maximum heating is in tissue with very little heating of skin or fatty tissue; no direct skin applicator(s) required; large volumes can be heated.	Heating not easily localized; preferential heating of tumors depends on low blood flow—hence not useful for well-vascularized tumors; metal temperature probe distorts field and gives false readings.	Liver and some abdominal tumors, large lesions in extremities; brain (?).
Microwave heating	Fatty tissue not preferentially heated; large volumes readily heated; technology far advanced; multiple applicator systems feasible; specialized insertable applicators for local heating feasible.	Limited penetration using a single applicator even at optimum frequencies; localized heating possible at higher frequency (e.g., 2.45 GHz) but depth distribution poor; shielding of room may be necessary; possible adverse biological effects; metal temperature probe distorts field and gives false readings.	Large near-surface lesions (e.g., chest wall, large lesions in extremities, mycosis fungoides); with special applicators: bladder, prostate, colon, cervix.

"Source: G.M. Hahn et al., 1980, with permission.
b0.5–100 MHz

The physiologic aspects of hyperthermia, particularly the great importance of blood flow rates before, during, and after heating, would really require careful exposition, but because of the lack of adequate data, this subject can only be discussed in more or less general terms. However, one topic is based on firm data. The measured values of blood flow in many unheated tumors tend to be lower than those in normal tissue; when this evidence is combined with our knowledge about the very limited amount of heat-conduction in tumors, it points conclusively towards the advantage for localized heating *via* continuous energy deposition. When using either electromagnetic or ultrasound techniques to accomplish this, the equilibrium temperature in many tumors, or at least in parts of the tumors, can be expected to be higher than that of surrounding normal tissue, even though the rate of energy deposition in the two tissues may be similar.

Thermometry is covered in survey fashion. The presently available thermocouples and thermistors all have more or less similar properties (though thermistors with high-resistance leads do offer some advantages) and there is little reason to choose one over the other, except availability of units and size of the probes. Several optical probes that neither disturb nor are disturbed by electromagnetic fields will soon become available, but at the time of writing of this book, no satisfactory unit can be purchased "off the shelf." Noninvasive thermometry, the ultimate goal, is possible in theory. However, it appears that many years will elapse before devices capable of adequate accuracy and spatial resolution will be available for clinical use.

6.2. LOCALIZED HEATING

6.2.1. System Requirements

Tumor eradication by heat alone very likely would require equipment that has the ability to raise the temperature of all malignant cells through a temperature–time profile that would insure that the probability that any one such cell survives can be made arbitrarily small. An ideal hyperthermia system would have to accomplish this. Further, it would need the capability of measuring tumor and surrounding normal tissue temperatures in such a way that constant monitoring would be possible. Additionally, the pattern of energy transmission and deposition used must insure that damage to normal tissue does not exceed "maximum acceptable thermal damage." This term is as imprecise as "maximum acceptable normal tissue damage," the equivalent term currently used in radiation therapy.

Hyperthermia is such a new modality that in the absence of long-term survivors, one cannot even assess the dangers of possible late effects, or to state if, in the absence of acute damage, these constitute a realistic concern.

It is perhaps useful to point out some things *not* included in my requirements for an ideal system. I don't suggest that a uniform tumor temperature is a necessity. In some situations it may not even be desirable. Nor have I said that all tumor temperatures must exceed that of normal tissue. If it can be demonstrated (and there is good indication that it can) that some tumors are more sensitive to heat than are normal tissue, or that normal tissue can be protected by intentionally produced thermo-tolerance, then such a requirement is unnecessary. Furthermore, it is not difficult to conceive of a system that utilizes an appropriate temporal variation of energy flow. For such a device, high levels of instantaneous heat may occur in some normal tissue (perhaps skin and fat), but the weighted average temperature could still be maintained sufficiently low so that the basic maxim of "no excessive thermal damage" is not violated. However, the nonlinear relationship between damage induction and time at different temperatures must be kept in mind when determining what constitutes the appropriate weighting to establish the correct average temperature.

Very likely most early hyperthermic systems will operate with fixed geometries, so that during the "on" time, energy flow will be constant. Under these conditions, and neglecting the favorable possibility of the higher heat resistance of normal tissue, the vague term "maximum thermal damage" can be translated to a concrete limitation on absorbed power. Experimental results show that it takes somewhere near 30 mW/g to maintain animal or human tissue at a temperature of 43 to 44°C, this temperature can be maintained in most dog, pig, and human tissue for at least 1 hr. without doing measurable normal tissue damage. For this reason, an acceptable restriction to be placed on hyperthermia systems might be the following: Except during the initial heating periods, in no part of the body, except the designated tumor volume, may absorbed power levels exceed 30 mW/g of tissue. Even this requirement may be somewhat too severe: if surface cooling is used, higher absorbed power values are tolerable in the cooled part of the skin and immediately adjacent fatty tissue.

The ideal hyperthermia system is not likely to make its appearance very soon, if ever. In its absence, the most realistic approach, it seems to me, is not to rely on heat exclusively, but to combine hyperthermia with other modalities, particularly with radiation therapy. I have already pointed out the biological reasons that suggest that these two modalities are complementary. It seems equally clear that equipment considerations reinforce this view. If combination treatments are used, it is not necessary to attempt to eliminate by heat each and every cancer cell. Advantage can then be taken of the physiology of many tumors, which permits preferential heating of at least parts of the lesion. Those cells in volumes heated less effectively and therefore surviving hyperthermia could be dealt with by X irradiation or possibly by chemotherapy.

6.2.2. Blood Flow in Normal Tissue and in Tumors

Heat transfer within the body occurs *via* conduction and convection, although at the body's surface, radiation and heat loss by evaporation of liquids are also of importance. The relative amounts of heat transferred depend on the thermal properties of the tissue and on the rate of blood flow, since it is the latter that is responsible for essentially all convective transfer. One tissue that may be an exception to this statement is the lung, where air flow probably contributes significantly. Blood flow rates in normal tissue vary tremendously, having a maximum value of 450 ml/100g/min in the kidneys to a low of perhaps 2 ml/100g/min in some fatty tissue. Table 6.2 lists values for some normal tissues and available data for tumors. If a temperature gradient is established in the body, for each degree of temperature difference blood can transfer between 2 and 400 cal/100g/min of heat, depending upon the location of the temperature gradient. By contrast, the amount of heat transferred by conduction is usually much lower. For a specific case, a sphere of 100 g of tissue surrounded by a layer of equal tissue at a lower temperature, conduction accounts for about 4 cal/100g/min/°C of heat transfer in brain and about 1 cal/100g/min/°C in fat. Typical values of conductive transfer are about 25% of those for convective transfer. In other words, in many tissues, blood flow accounts for about 80% of total heat transfer. These values are in the absence of vasoconstriction or vasodilation; obviously under conditions where blood flow rates are modified by external means or in response to thermal stress, these values can change appreciably.

The data in Table 6.2 indicate that net blood flow in many tumors should be lower than that in most normal tissue, though the wide range of blood flow values for tumors also indicates that this is certainly not true for all tumors. Since blood flow, as just discussed, is responsible for most of the removal of heat, these results definitely show that an optimum way of heating many isolated solid tumors is *via* continuous creation of heat, both in cancerous and in normal tissue. This can be accomplished by the absorption of energy from the passage through tissue of electromagnetic waves, electric currents, or ultrasound pressure waves. In each

TABLE 6.2
BLOOD FLOW RATES OF SOME NORMAL AND
MALIGNANT HUMAN TISSUES

Tissue	Blood flow rate (ml/100g tissue/min)	Source
Kidney	350–550	Rowell, 1974.
Liver	50–100	
Skin	10	
Muscle—resting	2–20	
—active	>100	
Fatty tissue	2–5	
Brain	50	
Tumors		
Corpus uteri (various)	10–40	Nystrom *et al.* (1969).
Lymphangiomas	10	Touloukian *et al.* (1971).
Gliomas	33–92	Cronquist *et al.* (1966).
Brain (metastatic and primary)	25–55	Capon (1970).
Brain (metastatic carcinomas)	<<50	Oleson and Paulson (1971).
Primary tumors	30–50	Oleson and Paulson (1971).
Brain (various)	~50	Damir *et al.* (1972).
Differentiated carcinomas	22.8 ± 14.9	Mäntylä *et al.* (1976).
Lymphomas	34 ± 21	Mäntylä *et al.* (1976).
Anaplastic carcinomas	15.4 ± 11.4	Mäntylä *et al.* (1976).

case, the amount of energy absorbed per unit volume of tissue depends both upon characteristics of the tissue and upon the spatial distribution of the energy flow. Additionally, the homeostatic process of vasodilation may accentuate the differences between the equilibrium temperatures of tumors and of normal tissue.

One important word of caution about what I have said in the previous paragraphs: While some tumors are well-defined, encapsulated entities, this is not the case for the vast majority of human cancers. Malignant growths frequently infiltrate surrounding tissue to the point where distinction between tumor and normal tissue is difficult, if not impossible. Such tumors may or may not have a rather well-defined core, but at their periphery they gradually blend into the normal tissue surroundings. In such cases, the description of blood flow rates by one number is not very meaningful. This is illustrated by the results of Mäntylä *et al.* (1976). These investigators used the xenon clearance technique to estimate blood flow in a variety of human neoplasms. ^{133}Xe was injected into one location in the tumor, and the rate of disappearance of activity was monitored at the site of injection. From these data, blood flow values were inferred (Figure 6.1). A very striking finding was the range of blood flow values found within tumors of one histology. I suspect that this finding relates only partially to actual tumor-to-tumor variations; much of the difference in measured blood flow rates might well be attributed to the particular site of injection. For example, if that site happened to coincide with a necrotic focus, a very low clearance rate would have been measured, even though blood flow rates in other parts of the tumor may have been much higher. In this sense, the data of Mäntylä *et al.* probably can be used to estimate the range of blood flow rates within individual tumors. These vary by at least one order of magnitude.

Similar considerations apply to tumor pH and to concentrations of oxygen, glucose, and other nutrients. Again, very likely these are not uniform. Therefore, the inference that is frequently made in the literature that there exists one well-defined "tumor milieu" that differs from that of normal cells, is really very misleading. It is much more realistic to think of a range of tumor microenvironments. Some of these are characterized by low pH, poor nutrients, etc. But others closely resemble those of normal tissue. Furthermore, conditions in any specific part of the tumor do not remain static. Motion by the patient, breathing, temperature variations, and anesthesia can all be expected to modify dynamically the cellular environment in any particular location within the tumor. On the other hand, assigning a uniform environment to normal tissue may be a reasonably accurate approximation of the true state of affairs.

6.2.2.1. Hyperthermic Modification of Blood Flow

An ultrastructural study by Fajardo *et al.* (1980) strongly implied that edema and reduction of blood flow secondary to ischemia were involved in the cell killing observed in heated EMT6 tumors within 24 hr following the cessation of hyperthermia. Going well beyond this speculation, several groups of investigators have actually measured blood flow rates as well as tissue permeability both during and after hyperthermia.

Song (1978) implanted Walter 256 carcinomas into the right thighs of inbred ST rats. Heating at 43°C for 1 hr was accomplished by hot water baths, and both vascular volume and vascular permeability were measured. After the completion of hyperthermia, the rate of blood flow in the tumor had remained unchanged, but that of the surrounding tissue had

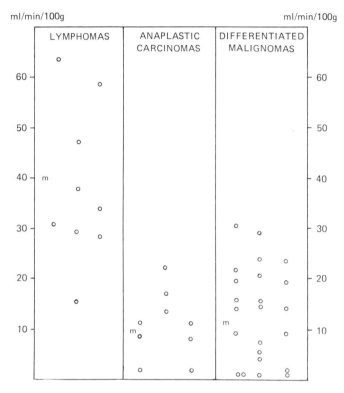

Figure 6.1 Blood flow values in different human tumor groups. Superficial tumors were injected with xenon and the clearance rate of the radioactive gas was monitored by gamma-counting. This rate was then converted to blood flow. Note the wide range of blood flow values within each tumor group. From Mäntylä *et al.* (1976), with permission.

increased between 160 and 360% over rates measured before heating. Appreciable changes of vascular volume, at least as far as the tumor is concerned, are in contrast to the results of Reinhold *et al.* (1978), Eddy (1980), Bicher (1980), and Hughes *et al.* (1979). All these workers found that hyperthermia actually reduced the blood flow rates in rodent tumors. Reinhold *et al.* used an ingenious system, the "sandwich tumor." The cancer, a Rhabdomyo sarcoma, grew in sheetlike fashion 100 to 200 μm thick between a mica plate and a glass cover slip. This entire assembly was on the back of a live rat (strain WHE/RJ). The microstructure of the tumor could be observed visually before, during, and after treatment. During 42.5°C exposure, blood circulation within the central part of the tumor was impeded progressively with increasing exposure time. At the end of a 3-hr treatment, circulation had ceased in the center of the tumor and the onset of necrosis was observed. Toward the tumor's periphery circulation was maintained, and the tumor retained its viability. A visual demonstration of this effect is shown in Figure 6.2, which consists of photomicrographs from Reinhold's work. These show vascularity of the tumor before, and 60 min and 180 min after the initiation of exposure to 42.5°C. The effects of heat on the vasculature are unmistakable.

Bicher et al. (1980) measured blood flow, oxygen tension, and pH values in adenocarcinomas growing in C3H mice. Implanted microelectrodes were used for measurements. These workers found that in the tumors, blood flow increased as the temperature rose from 35 to 41°C; but at higher temperatures it was reduced dramatically. In parallel, oxygen tension rose in the tumors during periods of increased blood flow. Heating also affected pH, which dropped from an average value of 6.8 to 6.4 after one hour of heating at 43°C. A detailed study showed that at the initiation of heating, pH values ranged from about 6.2 to 7.0. This range was reduced to 5.8 to 6.4 after heating (Figure 6.3, panel A). Each of eight points was examined individually over the heating period. A microelectrode left in situ measured changes in pH (Figure 6.3, panel B). To some extent the change in pH may have resulted from electrode-induced modifications of vasculature and perhaps from cellular destruction. However, the careful use of microelectrodes and the multiplicity of data showing similar results make this unlikely.

Another study that suggests major heat-induced reductions of tumor blood flow is that of Eddy (1980), who exposed a squamous cell carcinoma growing in the cheek pouch of hamsters to hyperthermia (41, 43, 45°C; 30 min). His results, shown in Table 6.3, also indicate major changes in blood flow rates, depending upon the temperature of the hyperthermic exposure.

Finally, Hughes et al. (1979) reported that blood flow in scalp nodules of rats was completely inhibited by 1 hr of hyperthermia at 43°C. The authors used a novel technique of proton irradiation to induce activation of ^{15}O in the nodules, and then they measured the decay of radioactivity as a measure of blood flow.

These results show that hyperthermia can accomplish modifications of tumor microenvironments, and that these may well enhance the selective antitumor effects of heat therapy.

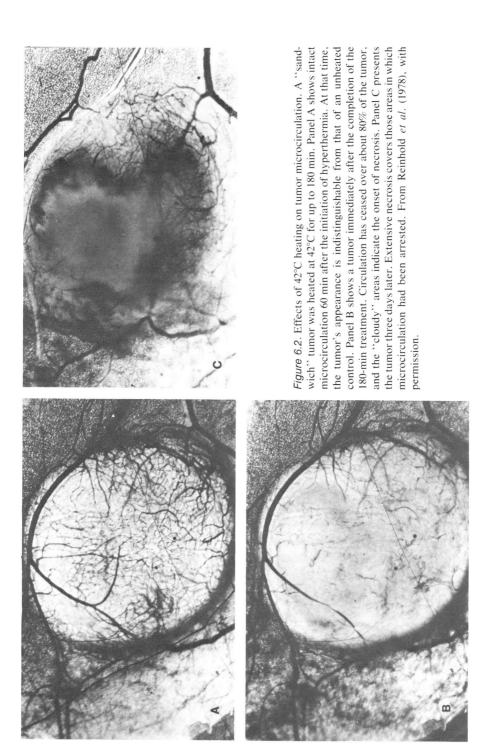

Figure 6.2. Effects of 42°C heating on tumor microcirculation. A "sandwich" tumor was heated at 42°C for up to 180 min. Panel A shows intact microcirculation 60 min after the initiation of hyperthermia. At that time, the tumor's appearance is indistinguishable from that of an unheated control. Panel B shows a tumor immediately after the completion of the 180-min treatment. Circulation has ceased over about 80% of the tumor, and the "cloudy" areas indicate the onset of necrosis. Panel C presents the tumor three days later. Extensive necrosis covers those areas in which microcirculation had been arrested. From Reinhold *et al.* (1978), with permission.

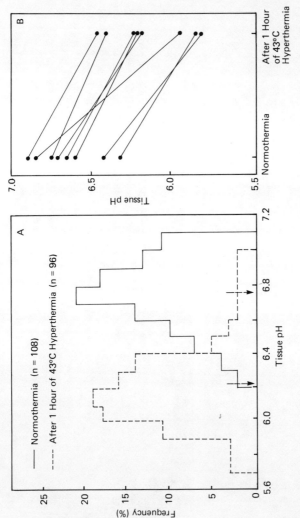

Figure 6.3. Tissue pH in unheated and heated lesions. Mammary tumors implanted into syngeneic C3H mice were heated with 2.54 GHz microwaves for 1 hr at 43°C. Microelectrodes were used to make pH determinations before and after heating. Panel A shows a comparison of pH values measured before and after microwave exposure. The mean pH was 6.75 in unheated tumors, and dropped to 6.2 in heated tumors (arrows). Panel B demonstrates pH changes in eight selected sites. In this experiment, the microelectrodes were left in place during heating, and values before and after were recorded. From Bicher *et al.* (1980), with permission.

TABLE 6.3
TIME COURSE OF EVENTS DURING 30-MIN HYPERTHERMIA[a]

	41°C	43°C[b]	45°C[b]
Reduced vascular caliber and filling	3–5 min	1–2 min	1–2 min
Return of vessel caliber to preheating levels	15 min		
Return of vessel caliber to greater than preheating levels		15 min Mild to moderate	6 min in some tumors Mild
Stasis in tumor vessels	10–15 min Very few	10–15 min →Mild[b]	5–6 min →Severe
Diapedesis and/or petechiae	10–15 min Very few	10–15 min →Mild	5–6 min →Marked

RETURN TO 34°C, OBSERVED FOR 10 MIN

	41°C	43°C[b]	45°C[b]
Dilatation of vascular network	2–3 min Moderate	No change	No change, total stasis
Histopathologic changes in vasculature at 24 hr postheating	No significant alteration	Hyperemia, few thrombosed vessels, continued petechiae, some loss of endothe- lial cells	Nonfunctional vessels packed with red cells, some loss of endothelial cells, thrombosis

[a]Source: Eddy, 1980, with permission.
[b]→ = progressive during the remainder of the heating period.

6.2.3. Methods of Local Heating

6.2.3.1. Microwaves

6.2.3.1.a. Single Applicator. Perhaps because of the availability of appropriate equipment for diathermy as well as for many nonmedical uses, most of the equipment used for clinical hyperthermia utilizes microwaves. While this is not unexpected, what is very surprising is that so much of the work is done at 2.45 GHz, a frequency already recognized in the 1950's by Schwan and Piersal (1954; 1955) as being unsuitable for heating to depths exceeding 1 or 2 cm. The problem is that absorption occurs as the electromagnetic wave enters tissue, and at 2.45 GHz absorption defeats attempts to heat to adequate depths. While on a submicroscopic level molecular mechanisms are involved, on a macroscopic scale the values of conductivity (σ) and dielectric constants (ϵ) are the parameters that permit calculation of fractional power reduction as the wave passes through tissue. Both σ and ϵ are frequency dependent. The molecules that determine the values are primarily, though not exclusively, those of free water. However, the values of σ are also affected by the orientation of the electric field with respect to tissue and possibly by charge distributions at cellular interfaces.

Both an increased negative charge distribution on cellular membranes as well as an increased content of free water has been reported to be associated with malignant tissue. Both of these effects are said to be in a direction to increase energy absorption, particularly in the frequency range of 400 MHz or lower; some experimental data exist to support this view (Joines *et al.*, 1980).

In muscle, the maximum ratio of absorption by malignant vs. normal tissue is claimed to be 1.5 : 1, a remarkably high value if found to apply to human tumors (Joines *et al.*, 1980). However, this is of scant help if the amount of energy that reaches the tissue is not sufficient to achieve adequate heating. To present an idea on the rate of energy dissipation in fat and in muscle, the microwave power absorption patterns for four frequencies are shown in Figure 6.4. The calculated values shown are based on plane wave geometry and assume normal incidence of the wave on tissue. Looking first at 2.45 GHz, two features are evident. In fat, a peak of absorption occurs at a distance of 1 cm from the fat–muscle

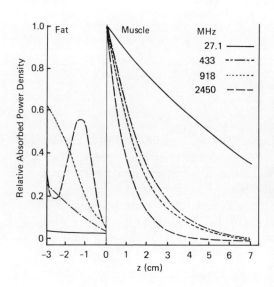

Figure 6.4. Relative absorbed power density patterns in fat and muscle tissue exposed to a plane wave source. The peak of absorption in fat at 2.450 GHz results from the addition of incident and reflected waves; even at 918 MHz considerable energy is absorbed in a 3-cm fat layer. Deep penetration in muscle is only achievable at low frequencies (i.e., 27 MHz). From Johnson and Guy (1972), with permission.

interface (toward the skin). This peak results from a standing wave pattern established by the reflection occurring at this interface. Because of the limited capacity of fatty tissue for energy dissipation, this results in an undesirable, sometimes unacceptable local increase in temperature. As the transmitted part of the wave enters muscle, absorption per unit path length increases appreciably, so that in that tissue the penetration of any appreciable amount of energy is limited to 1 or 2 cm.

Going to lower frequencies improves the situation. At 918 MHz the reflection coefficient at the fat–muscle interface is reduced and, because of the longer wavelength, the peak of the standing wave pattern is not observed until about 3–4 cm from the interface. Except in highly obese individuals, this is outside the volume of interest for clinical applications. This situation is improved even more at 433 MHz, where absorption and heating in fatty tissue becomes relatively unimportant. However, there is little improvement in absorption in muscle: going from 2.45 GHz to 918 MHz improves the penetration distance to 2–2.5 cm, but going to 433 MHz gains only a few additional millimeters. Clearly, 2.45 GHz is an unsatisfactory frequency to use; 918 MHz is superior, and the major advantage to be gained by going to 433 MHz, leaving aside any possibility of increased absorption specifically in malignant tissue, is the improved absorption pattern in fat. Figure 6.4 also shows re'sults at 27.1 MHz. Here improvement is quite appreciable indeed; absorption in fat is almost negligible, and in muscle, penetration of 7–8 cm is obtainable.

A number of tumors, because of their location, do lend themselves to heating with microwaves at 918 or 433 MHz. Specially designed antennas can be placed in close proximity to tumors of the cervix, rectum, oral cavity, and esophagus. Lesions in such locations can be heated with relatively simple techniques, although for most geometries the temperature distributions achieved will be far from uniform. Specific devices have been constructed (Taylor, 1978; Mendecki *et al.,* 1977; Wang, 1980) and used in the clinic (D. S. Li *et al.,* 1982). However, equipment design is complicated at low frequencies. Treatment applicators become excessively large and radiation patterns are difficult to control.

6.2.3.1.b. Multiple Applicators. So far I have only mentioned single applicators. The design of multiple applicators operating either independently or phased to optimize radiation patterns is certainly possible, though the amount of benefit derived from such arrays is not as large as one might expect. At 27 MHz, where, as was shown in Figure 6.4, penetration is favorable, the wavelength is so large that very likely little can be gained by vectorial addition of fields from multiple applicators in order to achieve selective heating of well-defined volumes. At higher frequencies, where the advantages increase, attenuation of individual beams again becomes important. A system using twelve radiators operating in a cylindrical geometry for regional body heating has been described by Holt (1977). This unit operates at 434 MHz. An idea of heat distributions that can be obtained with one, two, or three applicators from this device is shown in Figure 6.5, taken from the work by Paliwal *et al.* (1980). To obtain these results, phantoms consisting of material having electrical characteristics very similar to that of muscle were exposed to 200 W of microwave power (per antenna) for up to 15 min. Readings with implanted thermocouples were made after the power was turned off. Although the authors suggest that their data show that hyperthermia of tumors can be achieved to a depth of 10 cm, this claim is rather questionable. During 10–15 min of heating, considerable conduction of heat may have taken place. In a static phantom, heat conduction would manifest itself as a temperature increase even in those volumes where little or no deposition of energy occurs. However, in the presence of blood flow, cooling by the circulating blood would neutralize effects from conduction almost completely. For the geometry employed by those workers, conduction could certainly have influenced the temperature distribution obtained. These results therefore cannot be used to determine maximum heating distances. In order to provide evidence for local deposition of energy, data on specific absorption ratios (called SARs in the literature) must be provided.

The data of Figure 6.5 do show rather clearly that even with multiple microwave applicators, maximum temperatures occur near the surface of the phantom. Only in panel D is there any suggestion that preferential heating may have occurred in a specific area inside the phantom volume. Even in the geometric arrangement of that figure, with three microwave horns apparently pointed at one position within the phantom, only a small volume about 5 cm below the "skin" was heated to a temperature 0.5 to 1° above that of its surroundings.

Unfortunately, neither the work of Holt nor that of Paliwal *et al.* describes details of the equipment, not even to the point of informing the reader whether the signals emitted from the individual antennas were coherent or incoherent; most likely, judging from the shapes of the isotherms, the outputs were incoherent. Such signals avoid problems of destructive and constructive interference. On the other hand, they preclude the type of signal addition possible for coherent systems, i.e., one in which phase relationships between individual emitters is either maintained or changed in a specified manner. With a coherent-phased array operating in the frequency range of 400 MHz, it should be possible, at least in principle, to heat preferentially specific, small ($\sim$100–500 cm^3) volumes of tissue at depths of several centimeters below the phantom surface. Whether or not in heterogeneous tissue this can also be done predictably and reliably remains to be seen. Heating of larger volumes

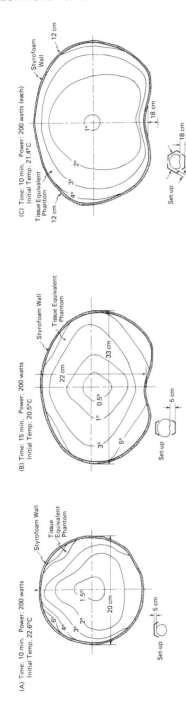

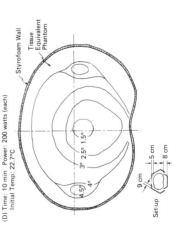

Figure 6.5. Temperature distributions measured in "abdominal" phantoms exposed to 433 MHz microwaves. Phantoms were subjected to microwave heating with one to three applicators (arranged as indicated in the small diagrams) for either 10 or 15 min. The isotherms shown are departures from ambient temperatures. The data combine effects from specific absorption as well as from possible conduction; therefore they do not exactly reflect energy deposition. From Paliwal *et al.* (1980), with permission.

may also present problems, because the constructive phase addition relationships can only be maintained for distances that are at most one quarter of the wavelength as measured in the tissue.

6.2.3.2. Resistive Heating

The basic problem of any hyperthermic methodology employing lower frequency (<50 MHz) electromagnetic techniques is to achieve sufficient penetration of the heating currents without heating excessively outside the tumor volume. At least conceptually, the easiest way to achieve this is to implant two or more electrodes at the periphery of the tumor to be heated (Doss, 1974) and then to pass currents between these. Heating takes place *via* the ohmic losses occurring in the lesion. The technique is relatively simple, does not require sophisticated equipment, and can result in very favorable temperature distributions. Since heating is entirely local, no concerns exist about skin temperatures or indeed about temperatures outside the volume of interest. Very low frequencies (<1 MHz) can be used, so that equipment problems and temperature measurement difficulties are minimized. At these low frequencies the capacitive impedance becomes large; hence isolation of the probes is readily achievable. The overriding disadvantage, for all but the most superficial lesions, is the need for invasive placement of electrodes. In the case of the combination of hyperthermia with brachytherapy, this disadvantage disappears, since in any case the implantation of radioactive sources requires invasive procedures. It is possible to utilize the same structures for heating and for radioactive loading (e.g., Cetas *et al.*, 1980). Figure 6.6 shows an example of such a device used for the treatment of tumors of the cervix. It has been modified from the usual implant device, so that the loading needles also serve as heating electrodes.

Electrodes need not necessarily be placed inside the body for resistive heating; in some situations adequate heating currents can be induced in tumors by placing electrodes outside the body. Commercial units that employ watercooled electrodes to do this are already available. The usual problem exists: to deliver adequate power to deep-seated structures, excessive surface heating may be required. This situation is shown schematically in Figure 6.7. Several body tissues, i.e., skin, fatty tissue, and muscle, act as elements in series with the generator. The ohmic heat generated in any volume of tissue is proportional to the local resistivity times the square of the current flow in that volume. Thus, any tissue that has high resistivity and that must be traversed by the flow of current will generate considerable heat. Unless this heat is carried off by appropriate

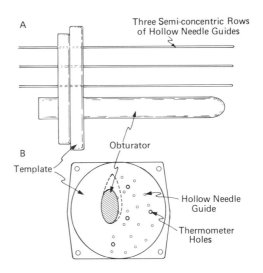

Figure 6.6. Interstitial applicator for combined hyperthermia and brachytherapy. A Syed-type applicator (A) was designed to treat a smooth-muscle tumor of the vagina. The device consisted of a hollow copper obturator ($2 \times 3 \times 11$ cm^3) and 19 hollow needles, which were spaced as shown in B. One side of an RF generator was connected to the outer semicircle of copper needles. Radiation was given following heating (43°C, 30 min) by loading ^{192}Ir into the hollow guides. From Cetas *et al.* (1980), with permission.

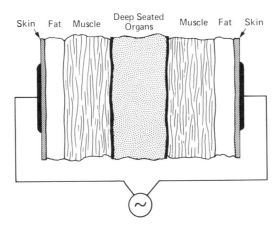

Figure 6.7. Schematic of two-electrode capacitive heating. A radio frequency current is impressed between the two electrodes. In order to reach deep-seated lesions, this current must pass through skin, fatty tissue, and muscle. Heating in any of these tissues is determined by local resistivity. This is high in fatty tissue, and high temperatures there are frequently treatment limiting. From G. M. Hahn *et al.* (1980), with permission.

blood flow, such tissue will rise to higher temperatures than its surroundings. Some typical conductivities (i.e., resistivity^{-1}) are shown in Figure 6.8 for the frequency range 1–100 MHz. Of importance is the low value shown by fatty tissue. As is suggested by Figure 6.7, in order for currents to penetrate deeply they must pass through a layer of fat. The data of Table 6.2 indicate that fatty tissue is not particularly well vascularized; blood flow rates are low. Therefore, the high temperatures reached in fatty tissue frequently limit the usefulness of heating with external electrodes. To some extent, cooling the electrodes can ameliorate this situation. However, the heat conductivity of fat is low, and for this reason external cooling is beneficial only down to a few millimeters below the dermal layer. Even in situations in which fatty tissue is not treatment limiting, the heating of deep-seated tumors cannot be assured. Electrical and physiological characteristics of the tumors become important. Only if enough current enters the tumor and/or enough heat is retained, will adequate temperatures be reached.

Very similar considerations apply for electrodes not touching the skin. These can be employed at frequencies where so-called capacitive heating becomes appreciable (>20 MHz). Because of the poor coupling

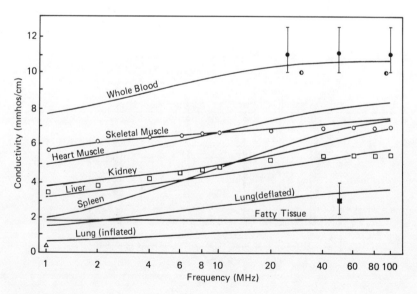

Figure 6.8. Electrical conductivities of pig tissue as measured in live animals. Magnitudes and phase angles of reflection coefficients were measured with an impedance bridge, and conductivities and dielectric constants were calculated. Shown here are the conductivities in the frequency range of interest for capacitive RF heating. From G. M. Hahn *et al.* (1980), with permission.

efficiency frequently associated with such systems, the power requirements to achieve a 30 mW/mg absorbed power level have to be considerable. While systems employing contact electrodes require a power density at the electrodes typically of 0.5–1 W/cm², capacitively coupled systems
frequently need two or three times this density. Furthermore, the energy
reflected by the body is scattered in the treatment area and may be a
health hazard both to the patient and to others. However, capacitively
coupled systems with nontouching electrodes are simple to construct and
patient set-up time is short, perhaps balancing these adverse features.

In neither the directly nor the capacitively coupled mode can the
distribution of current flow or of the resulting temperature be predicted
with accuracy. This is illustrated in Figure 6.9, which shows the temperature distribution measured in the breast of a patient suffering from recurring carcinoma of the breast. She had her tumor heated with a capacitively coupled system operating at 27 MHz. The electrodes were placed
as sketched in the figure. The highly uneven temperature distribution
probably reflects several factors including vascular variations within the
tumor, possibly local variations in conductivities within the tissue, and
the uneven current distribution induced by the electrodes.

One might think that multiple external electrodes, perhaps activated
two at a time, in a "cross-fire" mode (i.e., by opposed pairs of electrodes),
would greatly improve the situation. This may indeed be true in some
cases; in most, the presence of extra electrodes so modifies current flow
that deep penetration (and heating) is not improved and, unless the extra
capacity introduced by additional electrodes is minimized, may even be
reduced.

Instead of causing a flow of electric currents by utilizing electric fields,
time-varying magnetic fields can also serve to generate local currents by
magnetic induction. Maxwell's equations, which describe the behavior of
electromagnetic systems, show that in conductive media eddy currents
are introduced whose magnitude is proportional to local conductivity and
to the instantaneous rate of change of the magnetic field. Systems employing this technique have been used both for physiotherapy and for
heating tumors.

Von Ardenne (1978) describes a unit operating at 27.12 MHz. The
device, called "CHT selectotherm," employs two coils each of about 10
cm in diameter, which are placed at opposing sides of the body to be
treated. The coils are continuously moved in a raster motion in a plane
parallel to the body. This is done in order to improve the homogeneity
of energy deposition. The presence of two coils rather than a single coil
reduces the rate of fall-off of the magnetic field from the skin. Because
of the considerable power requirement to achieve the desired magnitude
of the magnetic field (about 1000 W), the coils are cooled continuously.

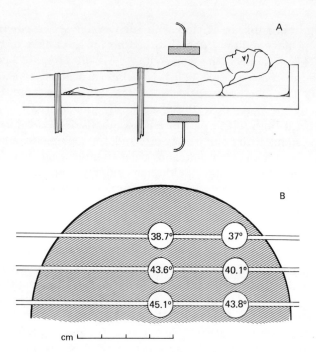

Figure 6.9. Temperature inhomogeneity during RF heating. A patient with a massive recurring carcinoma of the breast was treated with RF (27 MHz). The geometry of the capacitively coupled electrodes is shown in panel A. Panel B shows the temperatures measured during short-term interruptions of the heating. These results are not atypical for tumor distributions during heating with noncontact electrodes. Unpublished data of J. Dutreix and J. M. Cosset (Inst. Gustave Roussy, Villejuif, France).

Measured results in a homogeneous phantom (matched to "tissue" for electrical characteristics) show that even under optimum conditions, the fall-off in temperature is appreciable. For a phantom thickness of only 12 cm, the center of the phantom rises to a temperature differential of only 50% of that expected at the phantom's surface (Von Ardenne, 1978).

A very different approach has been taken by Storm *et al.* (1979). These workers have constructed what appears to be essentially a large, "one turn" coil made of a sheet of conducting material, forming a section of a right circular cylinder. The diameter of the cylinder is sufficiently large so that a patient can be placed inside the unit (Figure 6.10). The axial dimension of the cylinder can be made to fit the volume to be heated. The device, called a "Magnetrode," sets up magnetic fields throughout the body, although a substantial reduction of current flow toward the center of the unit is inevitable. Eddy currents are generated; in homogeneous phantoms these would be expected to be maximum at the surface

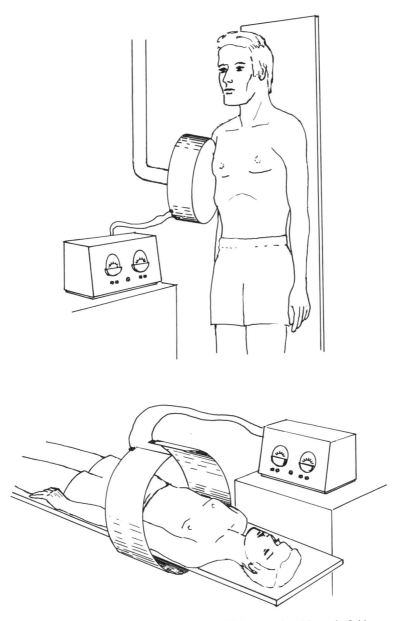

Figure 6.10. Schematics for inductive heating at RF frequencies. Magnetic fields are set up in tissue by the currents flowing in the coils. The magnetic fields oscillate at the radio frequency, and thereby induce eddy currents. These in turn cause local heating. Panel A: Usual diathermy geometry. Panel B: Single-turn coil with patient at center. Both geometric arrangements favor the heating of surface tissue. Illustration from G. M. Hahn *et al.* (1980), with permission.

of the phantoms. In patients it is claimed that superior temperature distributions are obtained. Unfortunately, no details of the measured energy distributions (or temperature distributions in homogeneous phantoms) are provided by the authors, nor, apparently, can they be obtained from the manufacturer. In a unit that is sold commercially for "investigative" hyperthermia of patients, such data should readily be available.

The inductive units described are very limited in their ability to deposit energy in specific tissue volumes. A tumor temperature superior to that of normal tissue can be achieved only under favorable physiological conditions. Only those tumors showing a greatly impaired ability to exchange heat with surrounding tissue can be expected to rise to temperatures sufficiently elevated for adequate treatment. While such units are useful as interim solutions, they seem to offer only limited long-term prospects. Just as radiotherapists have demanded more and more precision of their accelerators in order to deposit ionizing radiations in precisely controlled volumes, very likely in the future practitioners of hyperthermia will demand precisely predictable patterns of deposition of thermal energy.

6.2.3.3. Ultrasound

One method of localizing the deposition of energy in a more or less precise manner is through the use of ultrasound. The passage of a pressure wave through an inelastic medium results in transfer of energy, just as does the passage of an electromagnetic wave through resistive tissue. Of course the molecular mechanisms involved are very different. Why then should the use of ultrasound offer an easier way of localizing energy than do electromagnetic techniques? The reason lies in the absorption vs. frequency (or wavelength) characteristics of the two modalities. In order to establish a well-defined beam of energy, the linear dimensions of the transducer (or applicator) must be the equivalent of several wavelengths in tissue. As is illustrated in Figure 6.4, the absorption in muscle of microwaves at frequencies of about 1 GHz is so rapid, that without excessive surface heating penetration of energy in useful amounts is limited to a depth of about 1–2 cm. At 1 GHz, the wavelength of an electromagnetic wave in an aqueous medium is about 5 cm; at 400 MHz it is 12.5 cm. Obviously, to achieve an appreciable amount of "beam shaping" a large aperture would be required, one much larger than the body dimensions that are available for placement of the applicator. Absorption graphs for ultrasound in the frequency range of 0.2 to 5 MHz are shown in Figure 6.11. Even in muscle, where absorption is higher than in fatty tissue, good penetration is achievable below about 1 MHz. At that frequency, the wavelength of ultrasound in tissue is only 0.15 cm, so that beam shaping is readily achievable.

A block diagram of a simple, unfocused ultrasound system is shown in Figure 6.12 (Hahn and Pounds, 1976). The function generator develops a continuous signal at or near the resonance frequency of the piezoelectric crystal. The signal is appropriately amplified and applied to the transducer, where it is converted to ultrasound energy (typical conversion efficiency is 50%). The sound is then transmitted through a layer of degassed water and passes through a deformable membrane and into the tissue to be heated. Degassing of the water is necessary to prevent cavitation, i.e., the formation of small air bubbles that resonate, absorb energy, and prevent transmission of the signal. The water "cuff" serves two purposes: it cools the skin and introduces a path between the transducer and the tissue so that the severe variations in sound intensity that develop in the "near field" of the transducer (Figure 6.13) occur in the water and not in the tissue, where they might cause undesirable hot (or cold) spots. The

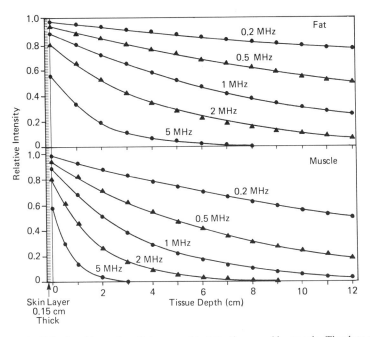

Figure 6.11. Calculated intensity of ultrasound in fatty tissue and in muscle. The data shown are calculated on the basis of a plane wave incident on tissue covered with a 0.15-cm layer of skin. On the abscissa is the penetration into tissue; on the ordinate is the relative intensity of the wave at the indicated frequency.

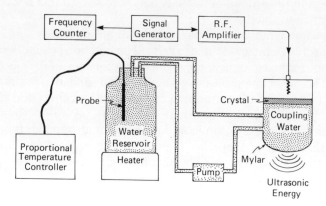

Figure 6.12. Block diagram of a simple ultrasound system. The tumor to be heated is in contact with the flexible mylar (or latex) membrane. The water "cuff" introduces a path between the transducer and the skin, so that near-field hot (and cold) spots (see Figure 6.13) do not occur in the tissue to be heated. The temperature of the water, which is continuously degassed during treatment, can be adjusted to protect the skin from overheating. Both focused and unfocused transducers can be used. Adapted from Hahn and Pounds (1976), with permission.

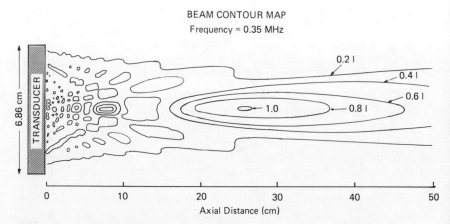

Figure 6.13. Ultrasound intensity distribution near an unfocused transducer. The figure shown assumes a uniform, in-phase output across the face of the transducer. The "near field" is characterized by rapid changes in sound intensities. In the "far field" such changes disappear and the formation of a well-defined beam becomes apparent. Numbers show isointensity contours. D. Pounds and T. Anderson (unpublished).

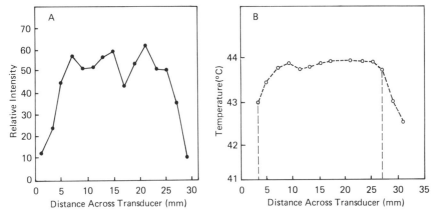

Figure 6.14. Spatial intensity variation in the output of a 3-MHz transducer and the resulting temperature distribution in the muscle of a dog. In panel A, the distribution of sound output 1 cm from the membrane was measured in a water bath. In panel B, a thermistor was implanted in the muscle of a dog 1 cm from the membrane, and the transducer slowly moved across the skin overlying the muscle. From G. M. Hahn *et al.* (1980), with permission.

actual distribution of energy, measured in a water bath 1 cm from the membrane on a line perpendicular to the axis of the transducer, is shown in panel A of Figure 6.14. Panel B of that figure shows the measured heat distribution in a muscle of a dog, also at a distance of 1 cm from the transducer membrane. Obviously the fluctuations of incident energy seen in the water bath are not reflected as temperature variations *in vivo*. Presumably, scattering of energy and heat conduction and convection efficiently mask these. These results should not be interpreted as suggesting that ultrasound magically induced uniform temperature distributions. Tissue inhomogeneities can cause reflections that can modify energy and temperature distributions. At 2 MHz or less, the only serious reflections are those caused by bone and by air–tissue interfaces. Considerable care must be taken to minimize these, because the standing waves resulting from interference patterns or even the power addition of incident and reflected waves can cause considerable local burning. There are some simple methods that can be employed to reduce the danger from reflections. For example, by avoiding normal incidence of sound on large, bony surfaces, reflections into the transmitted beam can be reduced; this can frequently be accomplished by a simple change in the orientation of the transducer. For some air–tissue interfaces, reflections can almost be eliminated by replacing the air with liquid; for example, during the heating of tumors in extremities, the treated limb can be placed in a water bath. Frequency or phase modulation, pulsing of signals, or continuous physical motion of the transducer can all be used to minimize the deleterious effects of standing wave formation.

As far as depth of penetration is concerned, the use of even such unfocused ultrasound beams offers some, albeit limited, advantages over electromagnetic techniques. Heating to depths of 3–4 cm is readily accomplished. For deep penetration, the basic problem remains: tissue at or near the skin is exposed to a higher energy density than deeper tissue and therefore rises to maximum temperature. Surface cooling can only protect the skin and tissue a few millimeters below the skin. To heat to greater depth, two techniques are available: focusing of single beams or superimposition of several beams utilizing different entry portals. These techniques can be combined: several focused beams can be superimposed, or one single focused beam can be moved continuously to simulate the behavior of multiple beams.

Two systems have been designed, built, and tested that employ either multiple or dynamic ultrasound beams. One of these, developed jointly by Stanford University and Hewlett-Packard Corporation, employs six transducers operating at about 300 KHz. These are mounted in an isocentric fashion on a spherical surface (Figure 6.15). The tumor volume is placed at the isocenter, and the path length between the tumor and the transducer is adjusted by means of a very flexible membrane whose position can be changed by varying the pressure of the degassed water between it and the transducers. The maximum distance between the membrane and the center of the overlap volume is about 15 cm so that tumors can be heated to that depth without inducing excessive skin (or other

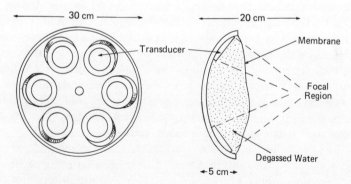

Figure 6.15. Schematic of a six-transducer isospherical system. The unit operates at 300 kHz; each transducer has a maximum acoustic power output of 50 W. The transducers are mounted on a spherical surface so that the acoustic output patterns overlap at the center of the sphere. (D. Pounds, G. M. Hahn, and T. Anderson, unpublished).

tissue) temperatures. The maximum volume of tumor that can be heated is an ellipsoid with axes of about 5 and 6 cm. A series of isotherms measured in the muscle of a live pig are shown in Figure 6.16. The temperature of the circulating liquid can be adjusted so that the water can either cool or heat the tissue in touch with the membrane. The decision on whether to cool or to heat depends on the configuration of the volume to be treated, particularly on the closeness of the tumor to the skin.

A second unit developed at the Massachusetts Institute of Technology (Lele, 1979) utilizes focused transducers at frequencies from 0.6 to 2.7 MHz. They are mounted on a precision, computer-controlled unit that effects translation of the transducer(s), so that a more or less arbitrary volume of tissue can be heated. Frequency, sound intensity, and the trajectory and velocity of the transducers are under computer control to attempt to match them to the dimensions, location, and heat diffusivity of the particular tumor. Inputs to the computer of the depth and size of the tumor are either entered manually or they are inferred from pulsed, low-power signals and temperature measurements that are obtained from sensors embedded in 30-gauge needles. Additional thermocouples are retracted in 0.5 mm steps through the region of interest. Both the thermocouple motion and the data acquisition system are under computer

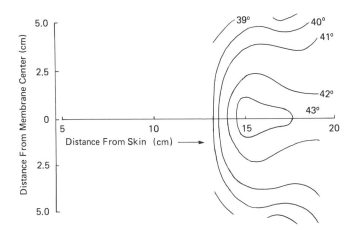

Figure 6.16. Temperature distributions induced in muscle of a live pig by the isospherical ultrasound system. The unit described in Figure 6.15 was used to heat muscle tissue of an anesthetized pig. The sound was coupled from the water-filled membrane to the skin of the animal with a commercial ultrasound jelly. Temperature measurements were made by multiple thermocouples implanted in an area centered around a point 15 cm from the membrane. The isotherms shown are estimates based on data from multiple heatings. Hahn et al. (1981) with permission.

control, and a temperature display is provided. Such a unit can, in principle at least, avoid temperature variations introduced by reflections from bone or air cavities, since the dwell time of the transducer(s) can be varied to achieve desirable patterns of energy deposition.

6.2.3.4. Other Techniques

There are no other techniques available that allow heating of deep-seated lesions. Absorption characteristics of tissue at optical frequencies are such that heating at depths of more than 1 or 2 cm is precluded, even if lasers are utilized to optimize energy distribution. However, simple techniques, such as infrared irradiation, can be used to good effect for specific near-surface lesions. For example, small tumor nodules located in bony structures, e.g., scalp or shoulder, are readily heated with infrared lamps. Infrared might also be of use to heat large surface areas with multiple lesions as are seen for example in patients suffering from micosis fungoidis. However, infrared lamps or other optical heating, as well as conductive systems, have only very limited appeal and do not warrant detailed discussion.

6.3. REGIONAL HEATING

6.3.1. Perfusion of Extracorporeally Heated Blood

The use of heated blood in isolation perfusion of regional volumes results in the more or less uniform heating of the perfused volumes. These usually are an arm or leg (Cavaliere *et al.*, 1967; Stehlin *et al.*, 1975; Cavaliere, 1976). The technique is conceptually very simple. Typical is the description provided by Cavaliere *et al.* (1980) for the heating of hind limbs of dogs. The iliac vessels are exposed and cannulated. They are then connected to a heart–lung machine, a tourniquet is applied, and perfusion is carried out using blood that has been warmed with a heat exchanger and oxygenated through a disk-oxygenator before it is introduced into the leg *via* the arterial line. Problems encountered include a high level of hemolysis and "sludging" of the blood to be heated, requiring dilution of the blood with isotonic saline solution. The rate of heating is about 0.25°/min, and this rate is maintained from 36 to about 42°C. However, in humans, where much larger volumes need to be heated, the rate of heating may be slower and local departures from linearity are to be expected. Human limbs require thermal isolation to prevent excessive heat loss, and rubber blankets may be used to achieve this. While a variety of other relatively minor physiological problems have been encountered, all relating to impairment of circulation, these have been overcome, so that today hyperthermic perfusions are routinely carried out in several treatment centers. It appears to be the treatment of choice when regional hyperthermia is combined with regional chemotherapy (Stehlin *et al.*, 1975). Then the drug can be added to the blood during the heating procedure.

6.3.2. Other Techniques

Techniques usually thought of as applying to localized heating can also be used for regional heating. In fact, microwave hyperthermia such as described by Holt (1977) or inductive heating as practiced by Storm *et al.* (1979) is really a form of regional treatment. For example, in the "Magnetrode," all that is required to make the system truly regional is an increased length of the cylindrical "coil" and an appropriate increase in the power available. Advantages over the perfusion method are not inconsiderable; no invasive procedures are necessary, heating is more rapid, and complications resulting from impairment of vascular function should be minimized. The primary disadvantage is that heating may well be nonuniform, since as discussed earlier, control over the spatial deposition of energy is limited.

6.4. WHOLE-BODY HEATING

Obviously, whole-body heating is an extreme form of regional hyperthermia, and indeed those techniques used for regional heating are also usable for whole-body heating. However, other methods are also available, and historically the development of whole-body hyperthermia has been very different from that of regional heating. Simple considerations show that approximately 400 W of net input power are needed to raise the temperature of a man of approximately 70 kg from 37 to 41.8°C (Law and Pettigrew, 1980). As long as loss of an appreciable amount of heat is prevented, any mechanism for adding this amount of energy to the body results in the appropriate increase in temperature. Of particular importance is heat loss resulting from sweating. At a maximum rate of evaporation, heat losses of an equivalent of 1100 W can occur. Heat loss also occurs in the lungs, but quantitatively this is of less importance (approximately 10 W). Finally, radiative losses are not inconsiderable. The magnitude of such losses depends on the environment, the ambient temperature, and body temperature. Radiation losses of 50 W are typical in a normal, clothed individual, but can rise substantially in surroundings favoring emission.

An early technique for whole body hyperthermia has been described by Suryanarayan (1966):

> "After premedication with 50 mgm. of Pethidine (I.M.) the patient is made to lie in a porcelain bath tub naked, the whole body and the extremities immersed in warm water, 100°F (37.7°C). The head and the face up to the neck are enclosed in a polythene bag in which warm air is circulated during therapy. Provision is also made to cool the carotid arteries by means of iced water which is circulated through an inner tube of a car tyre. This tube can be wound round the neck and head in case of any necessity to cool the head. This adaptation has been found very useful when the body temperature rises beyond 42°C to 44°C (107.6°F to 111.2°F)."

6.4.1. "Pettigrew" Technique

Henderson and Pettigrew, in 1971, described a technique for effective induction of hyperthermia. This pioneering method involves placing the subject in a sealed covering of polyethylene and then immersing him (or her) in a bath of melted paraffin at a nominal temperature of about 50°C. Paraffin has a melting point of 46°C; its latent heat of fusion is appreciable (129 cal/g), although its heat capacity is relatively low (2.6 cal/g/°C in the liquid state). As the relatively cold body is immersed in the liquid wax, solidification occurs at the cold surfaces and heat is transferred to the body. Vasodilation occurs rapidly so that blood flow cools the skin as core temperature begins to rise. As the thickness of the solid layer of wax begins to increase, heat flow into the body is reduced until the desired equilibrium temperature of about 41.8°C is reached. Behavior of the skin and core temperature, as well as the change with time of the thickness of the solid wax layer, are shown in Figure 6.17.

The wax technique has now been used by several treatment centers; at Edinburgh alone, Pettigrew and his associates have heated over 125 patients with a total of over 400 heating sessions. No unusual problems have been encountered, and the technique appears to be safe and reliable. The rate of heating is approximately 4°C/hr.

6.4.2. "Blanket" Technique

Another, simpler technique is to surround the patient with an insulator ("blanket") and then raise his temperature by a combination of the accumulation of metabolic heat and active external heating. Several such approaches have been described (Bull *et al.*, 1979; Larkin, 1979; Barlogie *et al.*, 1980). Heating of the "blankets" can utilize electric currents (Larkin; Barlogie) or circulating water (Bull). In these techniques, the heating rate is also about 4°C/hr; the maximum rate is dictated by skin tolerance. This technique has also been shown to be safe and reliable.

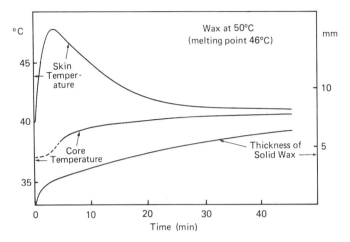

Figure 6.17. Theoretical skin and core temperatures during whole-body heating employing a paraffin wax bath. Initially the wax is at 46°C in its molten state. Skin temperature and wax temperature therefore coincide. As heat is transferred into the body, raising the core temperature, the wax solidifies and forms an insulating layer. The thickness of the layer increases with time as shown in the lowest line, and skin temperature drops. Thermal equilibrium is reached slowly; heating of core (and skin) to a final 41.8°C takes about 80 minutes. From Law and Pettigrew (1980), with permission.

6.4.3. Heating Cabinet

A very different approach was described by Pomp (1978). A cabinet was constructed with a transparent plastic top as shown in Figure 6.18. The patient is placed in the cabinet with his head outside the heating chamber. The air inside the enclosure is elevated to temperatures between 53 and 60°C. Additional heat can be provided with a coil located below the patient, and in some units, by a 468-MHz microwave unit capable of producing 200 W of radiated energy. No data are provided on the rate of heat induction, but rates appreciably exceeding those of the previous two techniques are to be expected, since heating occurs not only at the skin, but also in tissue to a depth of 1–2 cm below the skin.

6.4.4. Perfusion with Extracorporeally Heated Blood

At least three groups have described an extension of the technique of regional perfusion to whole body hyperthermia (Frazier, 1979; Parks *et al.*, 1979; Cavaliere *et al.*, 1980).

The technique developed by Parks *et al.* has been described in considerable detail. It involves the use of a high-flow arteriovenous shunt, which is anastomosed to the common femoral artery and vein. This is

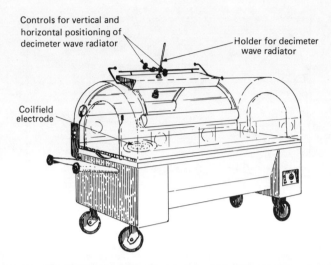

Controls for vertical and
horizontal positioning of
decimeter wave radiator

Holder for decimeter
wave radiator

Coilfield
electrode

Figure 6.18. Siemens ("Pomp") cabinet for whole body heating. Both hot air and 468 MHz microwaves are used to elevate core temperature. From Pomp (1978), with permission.

done several days before the hyperthermic treatment in order to allow enough time for adequate healing of the shunt wound. Hyperthermia is carried out under anesthesia. A part of the shunt is exteriorized and connected to a heat exchanger and temperature regulating device. The sensor for the thermoregulator is a thermistor inserted *via* a catheter into the patient's bladder. Temperatures reached were 41.5°C, a temperature that was reached "in as little as 22 minutes," implying a heating rate of about 12°/hr. Frazier (1979), in a discussion of the work of Parks *et al.*, also reports that heating rates as high as 12°/hr can be accomplished with this technique.

6.4.5. Discussion of Whole-Body Heating Techniques

In comparing the various heating techniques utilized for whole-body hyperthermia, it becomes obvious that to date no consensus for a desirable protocol has been achieved. While it seems generally accepted that 42°C is the upper limit for long-term exposures, Frazier (1979) suggests short-term "pulsed" therapy, that is, treatments lasting no more than 15–30 min, going up to 43.2°C, with intermediate times at 41°C. No data on optimum rates of induction of hyperthermia exists, nor is it clear that the variable temperature technique suggested by Frazier has either theoretical or practical advantages over uniform temperature treatments.

If heating and cooling rates can be shown to have important therapeutic consequences, extracorporeal circulation of blood at the appropriate temperature may indeed be very useful. If not, the surgical procedure required for the placement of the arteriovenous shunt may place an unnecessary burden on what is usually already a very sick patient. One conclusion can be reached with certainty: whole body hyperthermia could benefit immensely from the development of an appropriate small-animal model. Such a model would permit rapid answers to be obtained for these important questions. As an example, while I could speculate about the possible need for rapid induction of high temperatures to bypass development of thermotolerance, only appropriate animal studies can provide data for rational decisions.

6.5. POSSIBLE ADVERSE ASPECTS OF HEATING

Most cancer treatment techniques have associated with them special dangers to both patient and treatment personnel. Ionizing radiations are the best known (and certainly the most publicized) example. The carcinogenic properties of X rays are certainly appreciated widely. But most anticancer drugs are hardly innocuous. These agents are usually highly mutagenic and carcinogenic, a fact that is much less appreciated, certainly by the general public, but frequently even by hospital personnel. It is ironic to see in one area of many institutions the great care taken to protect both patients and technicians from unnecessary exposure to X rays, while around the corner equally dangerous drugs are handled without even minimal care. Frequently, personnel handle them without gloves and do not use a fume hood for preparing drug dilutions. Obviously the problem is largely one of ignorance. In the case of hyperthermia, a similar situation may be developing. In spite of the hundreds of papers dealing with various clinical aspects of treatment, the subject of possible adverse effects is essentially ignored. There are really two different aspects to consider: the possible dangers of elevated temperatures *per se,* and the dangers associated with the particular modes of induction.

6.5.1. Dangers Associated with High Temperatures

The four areas of concern here are: burns, carcinogenesis, teratogenic properties of heat, and induction of cataracts. Burns will be discussed in the next chapter under normal tissue damage. Carcinogenic properties of heat have not been examined *in vivo;* the limited data obtained *in vitro* have been mentioned in Section 4.3. There the paradox was brought out that although mutation rates increase at temperatures of 43°C, no con-

comitant increase in transformation rates has been seen. Possible teratogenic problems must be considered. Exposure of pregnant females from
many species to temperature–time profiles not exceeding those used in
anticancer treatments has been shown to result in a variety of malfor-
mations in the newborns. Tooth defects (Kreshover and Clough, 1953),
hernias (Edwards, 1967), vertebrate abnormalities (Lecyk, 1966), etc.,
have been observed in animals ranging from rodents to primates. In these
studies, many workers noted that exposures of pregnant females to elevated temperatures were also correlated with high rates of abortions,
stillbirths, and postnatal deaths. In humans, too, the suggestion exists
that high temperatures may be teratogenic. Women exposed to hyperthermia during pregnancy have given birth to children with malformation
rates apparently exceeding those of control populations (Miller *et al.*,
1978; Smith *et al.*, 1978). In these retrospective human studies, the hyperthermic exposure resulted either from viral and bacterial infections or
from sauna bathing. Presumably in all of these situations it was exposure
of the fetus to the high temperature that caused the subsequent malformation. This clearly suggests that localized hyperthermia treatments during pregnancy should be designed to minimize the exposure of the fetus
and that regional or whole body heating of pregnant women be undertaken
only in cases of absolute necessity.

The induction of cataracts was, for a long time, suspected of being
a specific consequence of microwave exposure (Zaret, 1964; Aurell and
Tengroth, 1973). However, the studies of Kramer *et al.* (1976) tend to
show that the formation of cataracts even after exposure to low-level
microwaves results from localized hyperthermia induced by the microwaves. The eye lens is not vascularized and therefore can rise to unsus-
pectedly high temperatures in any electromagnetic environment. This is
a problem that clearly needs to be considered when treating head and
neck lesions with electromagnetic techniques, or when using ultrasound
in areas adjacent to the eye. It ia also a matter to keep in mind with respect
to protection of attending personnel.

6.5.2. Dangers Associated with Methods of Induction of Hyperthermia

6.5.2.1. Electromagnetic Techniques

There exists an enormous amount of literature that suggests that
electromagnetic radiation at levels of 10 mW/cm^2 or even lower can cause
a variety of adverse effects in humans. The literature is amorphous, appearing in many journals that span several disciplines. Much of the work
has been done in Eastern countries, and a controversy exists between

experts in Eastern and Western countries as to the "safe" background levels of electromagnetic radiation. Eastern standards are several orders of magnitude more stringent than the 10 mW/cm² level accepted in the United States and Western Europe.

The adverse effects claimed to be associated with low levels of electromagnetic radiation include: chromosomal aberrations, effects on the reproductive systems of both males and females, adverse effects on pregnant animals, and a syndrome of general malaise, said to be associated with chronic exposure to electromagnetic fields. Anyone interested in this topic will find several records of recent symposia of interest (Cleary, 1970; Czerski *et al.*, 1975; Johnson and Shore, 1975). While none of the reports unequivocally show danger at leakage levels, they do indicate a great area of uncertainty and therefore suggest caution. In the clinic, the use of Faraday cages to surround treatment areas would almost surely obviate any need for anxiety on the part of personnel. The danger posed by electromagnetic fields to patients is so minimal in comparison to the dangers posed by their malignancy as to not warrant discussion, except of course in the case of gross negligence.

6.5.2.2. Ultrasound

There is little if any danger to operating personnel associated with the clinical use of ultrasound. The reason for this is found in the almost complete impedance mismatch that an air–tissue interface represents to the passage of a sound wave. Therefore, leakage of sound energy is essentially zero. Patient danger associated with ultrasound exposure is probably also not great, though very little work has been done at the intensities required for induction of hyperthermia. Liebeskind *et al.* (1979) describe chromosomal aberrations introduced in tissue culture at diagnostic ultrasound power levels; this implies that if similar findings could be obtained *in vivo*, ultrasound would have a carcinogenic potential. No such results *in vivo* have been presented to date, and therefore little can be said about this subject except that this is an area that should be studied in detail, not only because of the possible dangers during hyperthermia induction, but primarily because of the exponentially growing use of the "safe" ultrasound to replace X rays in diagnostic procedures.

6.6. MEASUREMENT OF TEMPERATURES

During whole-body or regional hyperthermia, temperature measurements present no great difficulties. Measurement devices can be placed in several body cavities, or hypodermic needles can be used to insert one or even several sensors into limbs. Temperature distributions are relatively uniform, so that detailed temperature mapping is not required. The methods of temperature induction (except in the case of the heating cabinet) do not involve electric currents or electromagnetic irradiation; therefore, the process of heating does not interfere with measurement.

Very different considerations arise when localized heating is considered. Nonuniform temperature distributions are the objective of localized heating: high temperature in the tumor, lower in the normal tissue. Clearly, to ascertain actual temperature distribution becomes very important. Not only is it desirable to monitor critical normal tissues, but it is imperative to obtain temperature distributions within tumors. To underscore this, I have pointed out already that it is the lowest, not the highest or average tumor temperature that tends to determine tumor response to hyperthermic treatment. Therefore the knowledge of the existence or absence of "cold spots" within a tumor is likely to be important and may influence treatment strategy. To obtain meaningful temperature distributions, even for tumors accessible from the body surface, is not easy. The use of electromagnetic heating techniques, furthermore, entails serious problems because of the interactions of electric fields with the measurement apparatus. The optic approaches to thermometry, currently under development and discussed later in this section, may facilitate the physicist's task in this respect. Multiple sensors implanted within a single needle may also help.

To obtain temperature distributions in most deep-seated lesions, however, almost surely will require the development of noninvasive temperature measurement techniques. While these are theoretically possible, no system exists today that is sufficiently far advanced in development to permit even estimates of performance limitations. Without question, the current inability of instruments to measure temperature distributions noninvasively represents a serious limitation to the development of standardized hyperthermic treatment techniques. In fact a very good case can be made for the proposition that evaluation of the limits of the potential of hyperthermia as an anticancer agent cannot be made until noninvasive temperature measurement techniques become available.

6.6.1. Invasive Techniques

6.6.1.1. Thermistors and Thermocouples

Leaving aside devices such as mercury or alcohol thermometers, which are much too large for most clinical applications, the most widely used sensors for clinical temperature measurements are thermistors and thermocouples. Thermistors are semiconducting elements (e.g., a combination of palladium, silicon, and chromium) whose resistance varies greatly with temperature. The change in resistance over small temperature differences is reasonably linear, although for precise measurements ($\pm$ 0.05°) calibration of individual thermistors is required. This is not a serious problem for medical applications where such precision is not required. Operation of the "thermometer" is achieved by measuring the resistance of the element, as for example, in one arm of a Wheatstone bridge. Thermistors are very sensitive and have short time constants, so that in the absence of external electric fields rapid and accurate temperature measurements are possible. The thermistor elements are usually bonded in hypodermic needles and the bonding material may act as a local heat sink. This can be a problem of considerable importance when measuring temperature in an ultrasonic field and must be tested before such elements are used indiscriminately. Minimum dimensions of thermistor elements are of the order of 0.5 mm.

Thermocouples are constructed from two different metals. When a temperature difference exists between the two, a voltage difference is set up and from this a current can be generated whose magnitude is proportional to the temperature difference. A variety of metals are employed, depending upon the temperature range of interest; for biological applications, copper–constantan or chromal–constantan is frequently used. Thermocouples can be reduced in size to 0.1 mm diameter. Their accuracy is better than $\pm$ 0.1°, and both their time constants and their sensitivities are perfectly acceptable for hyperthermic measurements. Multiple thermocouple sensors (at least up to three) can be placed in one needle, and these can give readouts at three points of a tumor. Such units are currently commercially available.

Both thermistors and thermocouples are subject to interference by an electromagnetic field, and the hypodermic needles in which they are encased modify the field configurations. This is responsible for two types of errors: false temperature readings introduced by signals generated on the sensor itself and on the cabling associated with the sensor, and raising of the local temperature in a small volume around the metallic components resulting from a concentration of electric fields around the sensor. Safeguards such as appropriate filtering, shielding, using high-resistance leads, minimizing the magnitude of metal objects in the field, and orienting leads or needles as much as possible at right angles to electric fields can reduce the error introduced by these factors considerably. But, even under the best of circumstances, at frequencies of 10 MHz or higher, errors of the order of 1 to 2° or more can be expected if measurements are made in the presence of strong external fields. At lower frequencies, insulation of the part of the sensor exposed to external fields can be used to good effect.

Whenever possible, for example while treating experimental animals, the magnitude of error introduced by the presence of the sensor during heating should be investigated. The procedure to do this is simple. First a temperature reading is done with the sensor in place during heating. Usually interference with the system's electronics manifests itself as erratic readings; values change rapidly without obvious reasons for doing so. If this is found to be the case, both the electronics box itself and the input lead(s) must be carefully shielded, or readings must be undertaken only with the heating device turned off. To check for local heating resulting from the concentration of electric fields around the metal, the usual procedure is to heat to the desired temperature, shut off the heating unit and then construct a temperature vs. time curve, such as is shown in Figure 6.19. If heating was uniform throughout the curve, this decay curve is characterized by a single exponential (curve a). If a small volume in the immediate neighborhood of the sensor had reach higher temperatures, the

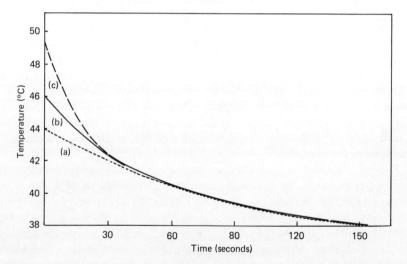

Figure 6.19. Correction for artifacts introduced by the presence of the metallic sensor: Temperature decay curves during RF (or microwave) heating. After the electromagnetic source is turned off, the time–temperature curve indicates the presence (or absence) of local heating resulting from field distortions introduced by the metallic sensor. Line a: The decay curve is characterized by a single exponential, indicating no hot spots of differing temperatures. Lines b and c show expected temperature fall-off if excessive heating in the immediate neighborhood of the probe had occurred. However the macroscopic (tumor) temperature in all three situations was 44°C.

temperature in the immediate area of the sensor would decay rapidly and the resulting curve would show two components of temperature decay, such as in curves b and c. From such measurements, estimates of the magnitude of the error and of the true average temperature can be made.

The practical problems of interactions between electric fields and either thermistors or thermocouples can be so severe that many investigators choose not to have any sensors in the field during the times that the heating devices are turned on. The usual method adopted is to insert one or more plastic catheters into the treatment volume, and then periodically to turn off the heating unit, rapidly insert the measuring device into the catheter, and then perform the temperature determination. While this procedure is somewhat cumbersome, it does bypass the interaction difficulties just discussed.

6.6.1.2. Optical Temperature Measurement Techniques

Replacing metallic sensors with nonmetallic ones would obviously greatly facilitate the measurement problems during induction and maintenance of hyperthermia by electromagnetic techniques. Several attempts at constructing optic temperature sensors have been made. In general, the approach is to attach a temperature-sensitive optical material to two or more lengths of optical fibers or bundles of fibers, one for an input and the other for an output signal. Usually a comparison of the two signals yields the required temperature data; this comparison is carried out in an appropriate opticoelectrical instrument package, that many times also contains the display and/or recording unit. The optical components are nonconductive and as such are neither affected by the alternating electromagnetic fields, nor do they distort them.

6.6.1.2.a. Liquid Crystal Sensors. Some cholesteric crystals show a rather remarkable temperature dependence of their reflective properties. This is most strikingly shown by the change in the color of these materials with even minor temperature changes. A sensor using such crystals was developed more or less specifically for hyperthermic applications by Rozell *et al.* (1974). This unit, available commercially, combines three different types of crystals to obtain a temperature range of 35 to 50°C with a sensitivity of about ± 0.2°. The device measures the amount of light generated by a red-light-emitting diode and that reflected from the crystal back to a phototransistor.

In clinical applications, the device has not proven very satisfactory. The dimensions are large for insertion with hypodermic needles (minimum diameter >1 mm); the materials are not very stable, and hysteresis effects make frequent calibrations necessary. The major positive aspect of the liquid crystal probe has been the demonstration that an optic temperature sensor can be built, and that it can operate within an electromagnetic environment.

6.6.1.2.b. Birefringent Crystals. Birefringent crystals are anisotropic in the sense that their indices of refraction are different for light polarized in two different planes. For some materials this difference is a sensitive function of temperature. Cetas (1975) has taken advantage of the favorable temperature characteristics of lithium tantalate to construct a thermometer that uses the differential phase shift introduced by a thin (0.1-mm thick) plate of this material to determine temperature changes. Signals from a light-emitting diode are passed through optic fibers to a mirror coated with a polarizer and a layer of lithium tantalate. The reflected light is then retransmitted to the opticoelectronic package for analysis. The phase change introduced by the birefringent properties of the crystal is seen as a change in magnitude of the signal at the output of the polarizer after reflection. The device has a potential sensitivity of $\pm$ 0.1°, its maximum dimension can be held to less than 1 mm, and its useful operating range can be adjusted to be in the range of 20 to 50°C. Because the temperature measurement is related to the amplitude of the signal at the end of the output fiber optics, variations in input intensity, as well as light scattering in the transmission path, must be monitored. This is accomplished by including a reference signal that does not pass through the lithium tantalate, but encounters all other environments seen by the signal beam.

6.6.1.2.c. Devices Depending on Light Absorption. Many materials exist that show temperature-dependent absorption characteristics for signals at specific frequencies. The most useful class of materials for temperature sensing may be those semiconductors that show greatly increased absorption when the incoming signal has energies just sufficient to raise an electron from the valence to the conduction band. In gallium arsenide, this difference is highly temperature dependent. Christensen (1979) has used this property of the semiconductor as well as the availability of light-emitting diodes made from this material to construct a temperature sensor useful for hyperthermic applications. Maximum dimensions can be kept below 1 mm, and a sensitivity of better than $\pm$ 0.2° has been demonstrated. Again, because the measurement of temperature depends upon the magnitude of the reflected signal, monitoring of source energy and optical path scattering is necessary to achieve maximum accuracy and sensitivity.

6.6.1.2.d. Phosphor Sensors. Another group of optical temperature sensors utilizes materials, actually uniquely phosphors, that once excited, return to their ground states in a temperature-dependent manner (Wickersheim and Alves, 1979). At lower temperatures luminescent processes dominate, but at higher temperatures nonradiative relaxation processes become important. Thus, the fluorescence of some phosphors rapidly "decays" as the temperature range is reached where luminescence loses its dominance. Some phosphors have the property that these temperatures are in the physiological range, and a temperature-dependent luminescent signal can be obtained. By combining two phosphors that "quench" at appreciably different temperatures and also fluoresce at different wavelengths, it is possible to derive, by appropriate separation, filtering, and individual detection, two signals: one temperature independent and one temperature dependent. Taking the ratio of the two produces a single measurement whose magnitude is an indication of temperature, and is independent of fluctuations of input signal amplitude and of light path scattering. Thus the need for control signals is obviated (Wickersheim and Alves, 1979). The ultimate accuracy of such a device far exceeds hyperthermia requirements; dimensions of fractions of a millimeter are theoretically possible, though certainly will not be obtained for some time. (Current units have minimum dimensions of about 1 mm).

6.6.1.2.e. Discussion. Of the optical instruments discussed, only the liquid crystal is readily available. Unfortunately, it is the least useful. Very likely by the time this volume is published, at least one or two of the other devices will also be purchasable. On paper at least, the performance of all three should be adequate. Only routine use of the devices will be able to provide data on their relative advantages and disadvantages. It is certain, however, that within another year or so reliable and accurate measurement of temperature will be possible even in an environment of alternating electromagnetic fields and currents.

6.6.2. Noninvasive Techniques

The need for detailed temperature mapping in tumors and normal tissue almost surely precludes the routine use of invasive techniques. The number of thermocouples (or thermistors, or other invasive devices) that can realistically be inserted into a patient's tumor is obviously very limited and certainly not sufficient to allow enough heat measurements to be obtained. Therefore, heat measurements can only be performed at an extremely limited number of positions. To obtain real tumor temperature mappings, noninvasive measurement techniques are required. Unfortunately, these techniques, except for thermography, are not available now and very likely will not become available for another five years if then.

6.6.2.1. Thermography

This passive technique depends upon the radiative parameters of skin and the immediately underlying tissue. In principle, the power radiated per unit volume of tissue (or any other material) is proportional to the fourth power of the absolute temperature; however, the net power received by an instrument at temperature T_1 from a surface at T_2 is proportional to $T_2 - T_1$. provided this difference is small compared to the absolute temperature. By scanning a surface optically, usually at infrared frequencies, and measuring T for each area examined, it is possible to construct a thermal map of the surface under consideration. However, because of the absorption properties of tissue, this temperature distribution is almost exclusively an indication of the events occurring within a few millimeters of the skin. That does not mean that deep-seated thermal sources may not also be noticed with thermography. However, when this happens the effect is not owing to diffusion or of direct measurement of emitted infrared radiation, but of blood flow from the deep-seated source carrying heat to the skin. The infrared camera "sees" only the actual subcutaneous (or cutaneous) temperature.

Infrared cameras certainly have their use in clinical hyperthermia. There they can give an indication of subcutaneous heat distributions and draw attention to potential hot or cold spots. Some users find these devices very helpful indeed (T. C. Cetas, private communication). However, they are no aid in obtaining real temperature distributions in depth. Chen *et al.* (1977) have suggested a method of transient tomographic thermography that could provide temperature (or blood flow) data to a depth of 2 cm with spatial resolutions of the order of 0.5 cm. A simulation carried out by M. M. Chen and P. Pantazatos was used to "reconstruct" an assumed blood flow distribution. Presumably, a transient temperature distribution could have been "reconstructed" similarly (although it could not easily have been separated from blood flow changes if these had occurred concurrently). Whether or not such techniques can ever be made sufficiently sophisticated so that useful temperature distributions can be obtained at depths below a few millimeters remains to be seen.

6.6.2.2. Microwave Radiometry

Significant quantities of radiation are given off by "black bodies" not only in the infrared region but also in the microwave and somewhat lower frequency regions. While maximum radiation occurs at infrared frequencies, radiation in the GHz and lower region is readily detectable. Because of the absorption characteristics of mammalian tissue, the energy reaching the skin from points 1 cm or more below the skin is actually larger at GHz frequencies than that from an emitter of equal intensity at infrared frequencies. Furthermore, the microwave emmision, because of its larger wavelength, is less subject to scatter than it is that at infrared wavelengths. This allows at least some degree of spatial resolution. Microwave radiometers, i.e., antennas that passively intercept the signals emitted from various points in the body, are readily constructed (e.g. Myers *et al.*, 1979). Because, in the microwave region, the absorption characteristics of tissue change very rapidly with frequency, two radiometers tuned to different frequencies will receive signals from somewhat different emitters, even though they may be "looking" at the same surface area of tissue. Because of the reduced absorption by the intervening tissue, signals measured at lower frequency will be weighted somewhat more toward parts of the volume away from the surface. If measurements at a series of frequencies were obtained, it seems that these, coupled with the knowledge of tissue absorption characteristics, could be used to "reconstruct" a temperature-depth profile. I have seen no serious examination of such a project, but it would seem worthwhile at least to undertake a feasibility study.

6.6.2.3. Ultrasound Velocity

Changes with temperature in the mechanical properties of the propagating media result in changes of ultrasound velocity. Such velocity differences are measurable and can be used to determine induced temperature changes, at least in homogeneous media. The magnitude of the velocity change is quite sufficient so that at sound frequencies of about 1 MHz temperature changes of $\pm$ 0.2° can be observed. Small changes in velocity are measured by determining the phase change of the affected signal. This change is directly proportional to velocity change and can be measured by the usual methods of detecting phase modulation. Highly sensitive methods of measuring phase differences of electrical signals are well known to sonar and radar engineers and need no discussion here. Thus there is no doubt that noninvasive measurements of uniform temperature changes in homogeneous media can be obtained *via* ultrasound techniques.

Can this method be applied to heterogeneous media undergoing nonuniform temperature changes? Obviously phase changes can still be measured. These now no longer relate to velocity in a simple way, but represent the sum of local velocity changes, integrated over the path length of the particular "ray" of sound from its origin to the point of measurement. If the velocity dependence on temperature of each element of path length is known (theoretically or by measurement) and enough measurements are performed on phase changes of individual sound rays, a tomographic reconstruction of the velocity (and therefore temperature) distribution is theoretically possible. Such a reconstruction could result in a two- (or three-) dimensional mapping of induced temperature shifts. Several groups are attempting to develop both the hardware and software required to utilize ultrasound velocity measurements for this purpose (Bowen *et al.*, 1975; Johnson *et al.*, 1975; Sachs and Tanney, 1977). However, because of the difficulty of the problem, it may be many years before practical instruments of this type will be available.

6.7. SUMMARY

Localized heating presents levels of technical difficulty not associated with regional or whole-body heating. On the other hand, only localized heating offers the possibility of using high (>42°C) temperatures as well as geometric isolation of the heated volume.

The "ideal" system for localized heating should have the capability of raising the temperature of every malignant cell to a lethal level without introducing unacceptable levels of damage in normal tissue. For systems designed to work as adjuvants to radiotherapy, such unrealistically high requirements can be relaxed appreciably.

Blood flow rates in normal and malignant tissue greatly influence heat distributions. Under normal physiological conditions, heat transfer is about 80% via blood flow and 20% via conduction, although these figures depend upon the tissue in question and upon the magnitude of the heated volume. Blood flow rates in normal and malignant tissue overlap, although on the average, tumors probably have somewhat lower rates. Blood flow rates within tumors of one histology can vary appreciably, and blood flow rates are probably very heterogeneous even within the same tumor.

Hyperthermia increases blood flow rates in normal tissue but either does not affect rates in tumors or reduces them. Some studies even report complete inhibition of blood flow in some tumors following heating at 43°C for 1 hr. Not only blood flow rates but also pH is affected by hyperthermia. Particularly exposures of tumors to temperatures above 43°C cause substantial acidification of tumor tissue.

Heating with microwaves using single applicators is made difficult by absorption characteristics of tissue. At 2.45 GHz, penetration in muscle is limited to about 1 cm, and reflection from muscle–fat interfaces can cause excessive heating in the fatty tissue. At lower frequencies both problems are ameliorated. At 400 MHz, reflection is no longer troublesome, and penetration in muscle is increased to a depth of 2–2.5 cm. Specialized applicators for heating lesions in and around human cavities have been constructed and have useful potential. Use of multiple applicators might improve heating patterns.

The implanting of electrodes, wherever feasible, offers a simple way of heating specific tumor volumes with currents in the frequency range of 0.5–27 MHz. This approach is particularly attractive in conjunction with implants of radioactive sources, where much of the same equipment can be used to effect heating and to serve as containers for the radioactive materials. Noninvasive, capacitively coupled electrodes can also be used for heating some tumors, though excessive heating in fatty tissue frequently becomes treatment limiting. Inductively coupled systems are not limited by heating in fatty tissue. However, these suffer from the difficulty of precise delivery of energy.

The use of multiple electrodes offers some possibility of improving patterns of energy deposition; however, the impedance modifications introduced by the presence of the additional electrodes so modifies current flow that the improvements are frequently limited or even nonexistent.

Precise deposition of energy is possible with focused ultrasound systems. Multiple transducers or movable single transducers can be utilized to optimize heating patterns. Except in situations where air–tissue interfaces or bony obstructions make ultrasound penetration impossible, this technique probably offers the best opportunity for precise localized heating.

Regional heating, particularly of the extremities, is most frequently accomplished by perfusion of extracorporeally heated blood. Systems employing heat exchangers and disk-oxygenators in conjunction with heart–lung machines are described in the literature. Regional heating by microwaves or inductively coupled radiofrequency currents is also quite feasible.

All the techniques for regional heating can, in principle, be extended to whole-body heating. Additionally, the "wax technique" of Pettigrew is widely used. Care must be taken in all whole-body heating techniques to limit heat losses, particularly *via* evaporation and radiation.

Temperature measurements today involve primarily thermistors and thermocouples, usually embedded in hypodermic needles. These devices, although accurate and having time constants with only a few seconds, interact with electromagnetic fields. Temperature measurements in such fields are technically difficult and should only be undertaken by experienced physicists or engineers. Temperature measurements in ultrasonic fields are much easier, although care must also be taken particularly when using thermistors, since the plastic used to bond these in place is frequently an absorber of sound energy.

Several systems that do not interact with electromagnetic fields are currently under development and should be commercially available at the time of publication of this book. Noninvasive techniques of temperature measurement are also under development, but their realization is probably years away.

7

Effects of Hyperthermia against Spontaneous Cancers

7.1. INTRODUCTION

The previous chapters have developed the biological and physical data that suggest the use of hyperthermia as a treatment modality against cancer. In this chapter I'll present a spectrum of results that show the responses to heat of spontaneous tumors in animals and in man. These are generally in line with the expectations raised by the cellular and murine data. A word of caution: it is essential that the results shown, particularly those relating to human tumors, be regarded in the proper context. To date no controlled clinical trials have taken place; thus, all the results reported are preliminary in nature. Equally importantly, the reported response rates must not be looked upon as reflecting the limits of hyperthermic usefulness. Patients treated were usually suffering from far-advanced disease. In the best protocols, the temperature–time profiles employed as well as fractionation schedules and timing of heat applications when given in conjunction with X-ray therapy, were based on cellular or mouse data. At worst, they were random guesses. Superimposed on the limitation implied by the range of biological uncertainties is the current lack of adequate heating and temperature monitoring equipment.

Based on these considerations, I see the major value of the data presented here as a demonstration that hyperthermia is a safe technique involving (at current treatment levels) a minimum of normal tissue complications and that many though certainly not all tumors respond and sometimes respond quickly to treatment. The clinical details of treatment are changing so rapidly that their detailed exposition is hardly warranted now; by the time this book is published, different procedures and schedules and probably equipment may well be in use.

7.2. HISTORICAL BACKGROUND

Reports on attempts to treat malignancies by elevating body temperature go back many years (Busch, 1866; Fehleisen, 1883). Some of the impetus for the attempts to treat cancers with heat derives from well-documented occurrences of "spontaneous" remissions in patients who had episodes of high fevers while suffering from malignant disease. An excellent review of this subject is that of Selawry *et al.* (1957). This study showed that out of 450 spontaneous remissions of histologically proven malignancies, at least 150 were demonstrably associated with the development of acute fevers that resulted from concurrent diseases such as malaria or typhus. A somewhat similar observation was made by Huth (1957), who noticed that one third of spontaneous remissions of lymphomas in children were also associated with high fever. While most of the lymphoma remissions were of short duration, several "cures" of carcinomas and sarcomas have been described. Therefore it is not at all surprising that many physicians attempted to treat patients suffering from malignancies by elevating their body temperatures. This was achieved *via* intentional infections with bacterial agents or by injections of chemical pyrogens. The most prominent of these studies has been discussed earlier. Coley (1893; 1894; 1911) developed a bacterial toxin which, when injected into patients, induced fevers ranging from 38 to 42°C. Quite impressive results were obtained by him against osteosarcomas and soft tissue sarcomas (Coley-Nauts *et al.,* 1946). Other effects not necessarily related to the induction of hyperthermia, perhaps stimulation of immune responses, may have been involved. Nevertheless, these results surely provided sufficiently encouraging data so that one would have expected that the use of heat in the treatment of human cancers would have undergone a continuous development. However, this was not the case. For half a century after Coley's work, perhaps because of the advent of the new magic method of curing cancer, the X rays of Roentgen, reports of heat treatments almost disappeared from the literature.

7.3. CANCERS IN OUT-BRED ANIMAL POPULATIONS

Based on his results obtained from heating transplantable tumors in mice, Crile (1963) treated thirty spontaneous cancers in dogs. The malignancies included nine osteogenic sarcomas, six cancers of the breast, five lymphosarcomas, three mast cell tumors, three adenocarcinomas, and four "miscellaneous" carcinomas. Considerable variation of the heat sensitivity of these tumors was found. Mast cell tumors were very sensitive and disappeared after immersion of the affected part in a hot waterbath at 48°C for 75 min. Lymphomas were also heat sensitive, even within the temperature range useful for systemic hyperthermia (<42°C). Many of the animals treated systemically died 8–18 hr after treatment, perhaps because they had had such extensive involvement of mesenteric and mediastinal nodes. Crile attributed these deaths to sudden and excessive destruction of massive amounts of tumor tissue. Only in mast cell tumors, in the lymphomas, and in one or two carcinomas did heat alone appear to destroy the local tumor completely. As far as the lymphomas were concerned, there was essentially no follow-up, so by destruction of tumor presumably only an immediate rapid regression is implied. In other cases, the tumors, usually infiltrating carcinomas or osteogenic sarcomas, regressed, but were not controlled.

Two additional later studies were those of Miller *et al.* (1977) and Marmor *et al.* (1978b). The findings of Marmor *et al.* are illustrated in Table 7.1. Ultrasound was used to induce hyperthermia. Both complete and partial remissions were obtained by heat treatments that ranged from 43 to 45°C. A course of treatment was arbitrarily defined as six treatments, each session lasting between 30 and 45 min, and given twice a week in order to minimize the possible effects of thermotolerance. Thermocouples were always implanted in order to monitor temperatures during treatment. Most of the animals involved had been treated previously, unsuccessfully, by surgery or by radiation therapy or by both. These animals were then referred by members of the Veterinarian Association of the San Francisco

TABLE 7.1
TREATMENT OF SPONTANEOUS TUMORS IN DOGS AND CATS WITH
ULTRASOUND[a]

Pathology	Courses	Animals	Complete regression	Partial regression	No effect
Squamous cell carcinoma	8	7	3	4	1
Fibrosarcoma	5	5	0	1	4
Perianal adenocarcinoma	3	3	0	1	2
Mastocytoma	2	1	0	2	0
Osteogenic sarcoma	1	1	0	0	1
Mammary carcinoma	1	1	0	0	1
Liposarcoma	1	1	0	0	1
Hemangiosarcoma	1	1	0	1	0
Total	22	20	3	9	10
Percent (all courses)			14	41	45

[a]From Marmor *et al.*, 1978b with permission.

Peninsula to Stanford for treatment with hyperthermia. The histologies of tumors treated are also shown in Table 7.1. These histologies more or less reflect the range of canine and feline tumors before rapid generalization of the disease as seen in veterinary practice.

Obviously, hyperthermia was capable of eliciting many positive responses against these spontaneous tumors. What about normal tissue damage? Table 7.2 shows the complications encountered by Marmor *et al.* They were limited to small superficial burns that occurred at the site of implantation of the thermocouple. It is remarkable that so few complications were found. One caveat: the follow-up on most of these animals lasted only a few months. Thus, long-term deleterious effects would not have been observed in the study. But acute effects were essentially absent. Results very similar to the ones described by Marmor *et al.* were also found by Miller *et al.* This group also commented on the lack of normal tissue damage.

Very recently, M. Dewhirst and associates (personal communication) have started a program of combined X ray and heat and also heat alone to treat spontaneous tumors in dogs and cats. As of this writing, 30 animals had been treated with RF-induced hyperthermia. Temperatures were sampled at seven points in the tumor. This is illustrated in Figure 7.1, which shows the placement of seven thermistors in a giant-cell tumor located on the dorsal surface of the foot, and the temperature recorded during treatment by each sensor. Temperatures within the tumor varied by almost 5°; furthermore, the changes in temperature during treatment varied from location to location. For example, in the center of the tumor the temperature rose to a maximum of 45°C at 8 min after initiation of hyperthermia, and then remained at that level throughout the session. A thermistor located in the central part of the tumor measured a rapid increase in tumor temperature to 44°C almost immediately upon the start of heating; by 8 min the temperature dropped to just below 42°C.

Several interesting observations were made with respect to tumor responses. The correlation between the lowest tumor temperature and the probability of regression was high; other tumor temperatures (highest, average, etc.) were not good prognostic indicators. Large tumors (>10 cm³) responded almost as well to the combined treatment as did smaller tumors (complete response rate 77% and 63%, respectively), quite in contrast to tumors treated with radiation only. In the latter, the complete response rates were 55% and 13%, respectively. (Larger tumors also responded relatively well to heat alone; ³/₁₁ showed complete regressions vs. ⅕ for smaller tumors. These numbers are so small that no conclusion can be drawn). These well-conceived and carefully executed studies should yield data of direct applicability to human treatments.

TABLE 7.2
TOXICITY OF ULTRASOUND

Tumor	Site	Treatment resulting in burn	Peak tumor temperature (°C)	Frequency (MHz)	Toxicity	Duration (weeks)	Healing
Squamous cell	Nose	4th	45	2.970	Superficial burn—small	2	Good
Hemangiosarcoma	Flank	1st	46	0.708	Superficial burn—small	<2	Good
Fibrosarcoma	Neck	2nd	46	5.000	Superficial burn—small	2	Good
Osteogenic sarcoma	Maxilla	2nd	46	5.000	Superficial burn—small	1	Good
Squamous cell	Eyelid[b]	2nd	>46	2.970	Superficial burn—small	3	Good
Squamous cell	Maxilla	2nd	49	0.910	Superficial and deep burn	1½	Good

[a]From Marmor et al., 1978b, with permission.
[b]Heating done over styrofoam contact lens.

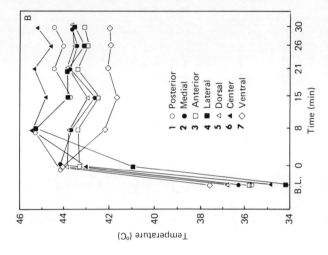

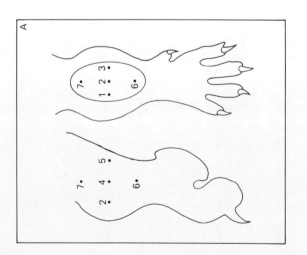

Figure 7.1. Heat distributions during treatment of a feline giant cell tumor. Panel A shows the placement of seven thermistors, panel B the temperature recorded by each of these sensors. Heating was by direct-coupled RF (1 MHz). Both spatial and temporal heterogeneities of up to several degrees are clearly observable. These results are not too different from temperature distributions measured during the treatment of human malignancies. Data from M. Dewhirst (personal communication).

The studies just described all involved localized heating of tumors. To my knowledge, no studies have been published involving treatments of tumor-bearing animals by regional or whole-body hyperthermia, although some of these are in progress (D. Kapp, personal communication). This is indeed a great pity. As I pointed out several times earlier, small animals simply are not a useful model for either whole-body or regional hyperthermia. Two reasons for this are: (1) Rodents tend to be too heat sensitive, so that temperature–time profiles that can easily be used with patients are lethal to both mice and rats. (2) Relating to regional perfusion, the geometry of small animals cannot be scaled appropriately, and technical problems dominate because of the small veins and arteries of these animals. To test specific aspects of whole-body hyperthermia, it would seem that out-bred dogs with spontaneous neoplasms constitute a very reasonable experimental model.

7.4. HUMAN CANCERS: HEAT ALONE

7.4.1. Whole-Body Heating

Based both on the anecdotal results of the early treatments and on the view that malignant cells are more heat sensitive than are normal cells, several groups of investigators have treated patients with advanced malignancies by raising their body temperatures to 41 to 42°C. Certainly such an approach is very attractive. Once a cancer has generalized, localized or regional treatments can only offer palliation by treatment of particularly bothersome tumors. Conceptually at least, a regimen of fractionated whole-body hyperthermia might eliminate enough malignant cells so that a cure might be achieved. It should be clearly understood that whole-body heating can only succeed if the tumor cells involved are more heat sensitive not only than their normal counterparts, but also more subject to destruction by heat than the most sensitive normal population in general. Furthermore, the treatments required to kill the malignant cells must not be so severe as to interfere with necessary physiological function. These are severe restrictions. The data that I presented in Chapter 2 suggest that at least as far as murine cells are concerned, many tumor cells are fully as heat resistant as normal cells. Thus, cures of cancers with whole-body hyperthermia as the sole modality appear unlikely. This is not to imply that other antitumor responses may not be observed. But these might well be based on the modification of cellular responses by tumor microenvironments rather than on intrinsic cell sensibilities.

Whole-body hyperthermia has been practiced now by many groups

(Henderson and Pettigrew, 1971; Pettigrew, 1975; Larkin *et al.*, 1976; 1977; Blair and Levin, 1978; Euler-Rolle *et al.*, 1978; Fabricius *et al.*, 1978; Bull *et al.*, 1979; Parks *et al.*, 1979). The techniques used for inducing whole-body hyperthermia have been described in the last chapter. Although the various methods differ with respect to difficulties and practical problems associated with heating, there seem to be only small differences in the results obtained. Larkin (1979) treated a total of 92 patients over a 4½-year period with total-body hyperthermia either alone or in combination with other modalities. Body temperature was gradually raised, usually over two hr, to 42°C. Fluid replacement was used, averaging 12 ml/kg per hr, and over this time urine output averaged a total of 100 ml/ hr. During treatment, vital signs, core temperature, electrocardiogram, and urine output were carefully monitored. The patients were under anesthesia induced by barbiturates.

A total of 205 treatments were completed. Good tolerance of the treatment was indicated by serial analysis of hematological, metabolic, and organ-function parameters. An interesting finding was that pulse rates increased from a mean of 90 before treatment to an average of 160 during treatment. The range of pulse rates measured varied from 100 to 207. A mild metabolic acidosis usually developed, but this required no therapy; potassium replacement was used to prevent hypokalemia. Other imbalances in the concentrations of divalent ions were observed, and these led to some focal muscle irritability. In diabetics, hyperglycemia was seen and usually required insulin therapy. Mild elevations in the concentration of liver enzymes were observed, but they returned to base levels 96 hr after the completion of therapy. No lung or kidney damage was seen.

The patients had ninety-three different tumors in sixteen different primary sites. In almost all cases the investigators stated that there was a large tumor burden that disease was progressing in spite of various other therapies. Most patients had a measurable lesion or a biochemical marker available for objective evaluation. The overall response rate, which includes some patients who were given radiation and chemotherapy concomitantly, was 43%, with an additional 15% achieving "good 'subjective palliation." Complete regressions were seen in only four patients.

No deaths occurred during treatment; however, six patients suffered complications that were eventually fatal. Larkin suggests that these can be avoided by the proper selection of patients and appropriate monitoring of life-support measures. Unavoidable side effects of the procedure included fatigue, diarrhea, anorexia, and a circumoral herpes.

Parks *et al.* (1979) treated approximately 60 patients with extracorporeally heated blood utilizing an arteriovenous shunt. One third of these patients received only hyperthermia, one third received hyperthermia and

250 mg/m² cyclophosphamide, and one third received hyperthermia, 250 mg/m² cyclophosphamide, and 50 mg of BCNU for each treatment. Eleven patients were treated with 42°C for six forty-five with 41.5°C for six hr, and four with 41.5°C for nine hr, at 2 to 7-day intervals. Hyperthermia increased the urinary excretion of potassium, sodium, and organic phosphates, as well as creatinine, 200% to 600%, elevated the metabolic rate 150% to 200%, and shifted the respiratory quotients. Neurological abnormalities occurred in some of the patients treated at the beginning of the study, but were eliminated later by maintaining serum phosphate levels. Of 36 patients at risk for two or more months, antitumor effects were evident by clinical X-ray or histological findings in 25 (69%). However, whether or not these responses can be translated to increased life spans remains to be seen.

At the National Institute of Cancer, Bull *et al.* (1979) reported on a Phase I clinical trial of whole-body hyperthermia. A trial utilizing heat alone was begun as a step preliminary to combining systemic hyperthermia with chemotherapy. Neither rectal nor esophageal temperature was allowed to exceed 42°C with an average temperature plateau of 41.8°C. Patients were heavily sedated but required no respiratory assistance. Monitoring was carried out by four professionals and involved esophageal, rectal, and skin thermistor probes, block electrocardiogram leads, and arterial and venous pressure measurements. For the first treatment, the patient's cardiovascular status was monitored, using a Swan–Ganz pulmonary arterial catheter.

For the first series of patients, who were exposed to heat alone, the most acute physiological stress observed in actual treatment was a large change in cardiovascular function. Baseline cardiac rate increased from 70 to 160 beats per min, duplicating the findings of Larkin. Systemic arteriopulmonary pressures decreased somewhat, but the cardiac index increased from 3.3 to 7.2 liters per min. Despite the major cardiac stress, there was no evidence of cardiac damage in any patient as reflected in data on the levels of glutamic–oxidoacetic acid transaminases, serum glutamic–pyruvic acid transaminases, and LDH and CPK isoenzymes, as well as in serioelectrocardiograms. The patients were maintained with 0.6–1 liter/hr of fluid replacement, and no changes were observed in electrolyte or renal functions. However, sharp drops in serum phosphate and magnesium levels were documented in all patients. Patients experienced severe fatigue for several days following the procedure. Seven of fourteen experienced mild nausea; four had mild diarrhea for 24 hr. Some patients developed fever of up to 40°C after cooling, 12–36 hr after the completion of therapy. Four patients unexpectedly developed symptoms of peripheral neuropathy following the exposure to heat. Two of these had had a previous exposure to vinka alkaloids, and this finding may be akin to the "recall" phenomenon observed in irradiated patients treated with actinomycin D or adriamycin. Antitumor responses were seen in some of the patients, but the response rate was only about 20% at best. All of these three groups of authors comment on the high cardiac activity of patients undergoing hyperthermia.

Euler-Rolle *et al.* (1978) show that the administration of beta-receptor inhibitors can reduce cardiac problems. These workers treated twenty-nine patients bearing tumors of different types. Thirty-six courses of whole-body hyperthermia supplemented with the administration of some drugs were combined with hyperglycemia. The thermal dose was 42°C for a period of 120 min. In fifteen cases beta-receptors were blocked with pindolol. Blocking beta-receptors was found to prevent the occurrence of extremely high heart rates, kept the systolic blood pressure relatively constant, reduced the incidence of serious arrhythmias, and "prevented acute heart failure." The implication of this is that acute heart failure was found in the other groups, but in fact only one such case occurred.

An examination of all the data from the groups that have utilized whole-body hyperthermia and hyperthermia in conjunction with chemotherapy shows that, depending on the criteria used and the temperatures reached in treatment, objective response rates between 10% and 50% or even higher can be obtained. The better results generally involve combinations of drugs and heat. Complete regressions are very rare, probably less than 5%. Durations of responses tend to be short, a few months at most. Retreatment is possible, although the early data of Pettigrew (1975) tended to show that retreatment was less efficacious. Further than that, the data are hard to evaluate. Most practitioners did not stick to well-defined protocols, and the addition of chemotherapy and radiotherapy even further complicated the analysis of the findings. Most medical complications resulting from whole-body hyperthermia are potentially severe but manageable, although clearly monitoring of vital functions is a necessity. Douglass *et al.* (1981) point to one danger: three patients that had previous spinal cord irradiation developed serious transverse myelitis after whole-body hyperthermia. Careful selection of patients can aid in minimizing complication problems.

7.4.2. Regional Heating

Very much the same conditions apply to regional heating as to whole-body heating; treatment success depends upon thermosensitivity of the malignant cell population and is limited by the response of normal cells and by physiological complications. Because the volume of treatment is limited, these problems are less severe: fewer normal cell populations are affected and the danger of causing physiological disorders is reduced.

Regional perfusion with externally heated blood was first started at the Regina Elena Institute in Rome (Cavaliere et al., 1967; 1980; Moricca et al., 1977), and that group has maintained an active program over the years. Tumors of the extremities, particularly osteogenic sarcomas, melanomas, and soft-tissue sarcomas, were treated. In early studies, tourniquets were used in an attempt to isolate the treatment volume. This practice was abandoned when it was found that nerve damage and severe reduction of limb mobility resulted from the compression maintained during the several hours of treatment time. In later work, perfusion rates and pressure were maintained at levels sufficiently high to insure that heat loss via the normal circulation did not represent a problem. Typical survival results are shown in Table 7.3 for stage III melanomas. These patients were treated with hyperthermia and then had their affected limbs amputated. The number of patients is small (forty) and no controls not involving hyperthermia (e.g., chemotherapy and amputation) are presented. Nevertheless, the results are interesting and encouraging. In most other studies the prognosis for patients having regionally metastic melanoma is considerably poorer. Results for osteogenic sarcomas were somewhat similar; 60% of the patients survived 5 years. Less favorable results were found for soft-tissue sarcomas. Cavalieri et al. are convinced that

TABLE 7.3
SURVIVAL OF PATIENTS WITH MELANOMA
(STAGES IIIA, IIIB, IIIAB)[a]

| Year | Percent survival | |
	HP[b] only (18 patients)	HP[b] plus chemotherapy (20 patients)
1	90	95
2	84	70
3	60	45
4	50	45
5	50	45
6	50	45
7	50	45
8	50	45
9	50	45
10	50	45

[a]From Cavaliere et al., 1980, with permission.
[b]HP: hyperthermic perfusion

enhanced immune reactions are associated with regional heating because "the heated cells act as an antigenic source to immunize the host against recurrences and metastases." No data exist to buttress this optimistic view.

7.4.3. Heating of Isolated Lesions

There are very few studies in the literature that attempt to quantify the effect of hyperthermia (without adjuvant treatments) against tumors. Of those studies that have been reported, some can best be described as anecdotal. For example, LeVeen *et al.* (1976) reported on their experience treating twenty-one patients with a capacitively coupled radiofrequency system operating at 13.65 MHz. Unfortunately, very few details of the treatment were provided, nor were temperature distributions obtained. This situation mirrors an earlier one found in the literature of Horvath (1944). This investigator used ultrasound to heat superficial human tumors. He observed that insonified tumors had reduced growth rates, and noted some tumor regressions. All effects seen were short term. No temperature estimates were obtained (small thermocouples and thermistors were of course not then available); in fact Horvath did not explicitly attribute his findings to hyperthermic effects.

Recently, three studies describing the use of ultrasound for heating superficial human lesions have been published. An unfocused system was used at Stanford and at the M.D. Anderson Tumor Institute (Corry *et al.*, 1980b). The Stanford system utilized an ultrasound transducer with a uniform power output over a 4-cm circular field. The system operated between 2 and 3 MHz and was used to treat forty patients. The results are shown in Table 7.4. The temperature obtained ranged between 43 and 45°C. Treatment sessions lasted between 30 and 45 min and were repeated twice a week during a three-week course, for a total of six treatments. Very similar results were obtained by the M.D. Anderson group, who who utilized a similar system. Their results are shown in Table 7.5. This group utilized higher temperatures, with some lesions heated up to 50°C. Durations of the remissions, grouped according to temperature exposure, are show in Table 7.6. Side effects were minimal. They are listed in Table 7.7. Pain was observed in twelve patients; ten of those had their tumor located directly over bone. Superficial burns were seen at the site of thermocouple puncture, and these healed very rapidly. Tumor ulceration was primarily an augmentation of already existing ulcerations. None of the side effects required medical intervention, and no long-term deleterious effects were seen over the follow-up periods involved. However, they were short, and any potential long-term effects would have been

TABLE 7.4

OBJECTIVE TUMOR RESPONSES FOLLOWING LOCALIZED ULTRASOUND
HYPERTHERMIA OF
SUPERFICIAL HUMAN NEOPLASMS[a]

Histology	Primary site	No. of patients	No. of courses of treatment	Responses CR(%)[b]	PR(%)[c]	NE(%)[d]
Squamous cell	Head and neck	9	12	1(8)	7(58)	4(33)
carcinoma	Lung	1	1	0	1	0
Adenocarcinoma	Ovary	2	2	0	1	1
	Breast	1	2	0	0	2
	Uterus	1	1	0	1	0
	Nose	1	1	0	0	1
Lymphoma	DHL[e]	2	2	0	0	2
	Mycosis fungoides	1	2	2	0	0
Melanoma		1	1	0	0	1
Medullary carcinoma	Thyroid	1	1	0	1	0
Neurofibrosarcoma		1	1	0	0	1
Total		21	26	3(12)	11(42)	12(46)

[a]From Marmor et al., 1979, with permission.
[b]CR = Complete clinical disappearance of tumore within the heated area.
[c]PR = Partial Response: 50% decrease in tumor volume within the heated area.
[d]NE = No Effect: <50% decrease in tumor volume, stasis, or growth of tumor within the heated area.
[a]DHL = Diffuse histiocytic lymphoma.

TABLE 7.5

OBJECTIVE TUMOR RESPONSES TO ULTRASOUND HYPERTHERMIA
ALONE, 43 to 50°C[a]

Histology	Evaluable patients	Complete response	Partial response	Overall response rate (%)
Melanoma	10	2	3	50
Sarcoma	7	1	4	71
Squamous cell carcinoma				
Head and neck	3	1	2	100
Lung	2	0	0	0
Adenocarcinoma	6	1	2	
Totals	28	5	11	

[a]E. Tilchen, P. Corry, B. Barlogie, and E. Armour. Manuscript submitted.

TABLE 7.6
EFFECT OF ULTRASOUND TREATMENT TEMPERATURE ON RESPONSE RATE AND DURATION

Institution	Temperature(°C)	Evaluable courses	Responses (complete and partial)	%	Median duration of response
Stanford[a]	43–44	23	9	39	6 weeks
M.D. Anderson[b]	43–44	15	8	53	29 days
Stanford	44.1–45	21	10	48	6 weeks
M.D. Anderson	45–47	7	3	43	45 days
M.D. Anderson	48–50	6	5[c]	83	250 days

[a]J.B. Marmor, D. Pounds, and G.M. Hahn, in press.
[b]E. Tilchen, P. Corry, B. Barlogie, and E. Armour, manuscript submitted.
[c]Several recent failures at this temperature, not included in this evaluation (P. Corry, personal communication).

missed. Particularly encouraging were the responses of tumors in heavily irradiated areas (Table 7.8).

Another study employing local heat is that of Storm *et al.* (1979). Radiofrequency heating employing an inductive method was used to heat designated lesions. Thirty tumors in thirty patients were treated. The study was unique in the sense that some tumors were heated to 50°C and even higher. Small tumors proved to be more difficult to heat than large tumors. Marked rises in temperature in tumors over that measured in skin, subcutaneous tissue, and tissue in the vicinity of the tumor were reported, with differences as high as 5 to 10°. This is contrary to the

TABLE 7.7
SIDE EFFECTS OF SUPERFICIAL LOCALIZED ULTRASOUND HYPERTHERMIA[a]

Side effect	Evaluable patients	Number with effect	Incidence (%)
Pain	52	12[b]	23
Superficial burn	52	10	19
Tumor ulceration	52	5	10
Miscellaneous:			
Vomiting	52	1	2
Laryngospasm	52	1	2

[a]J.B. Marmor, D. Pounds, and G.M. Hahn, unpublished.
[b]Tumor was located directly over bone in ten of these patients. Two had supraclavicular tumors and pain radiating down the arm, suggesting brachial plexus stimulation by the ultrasound.

TABLE 7.8
ULTRASOUND HEATING IN PREVIOUSLY IRRADIATED SITES[a]

Tumor and site[b]	Previous radiation dose[c] (rad)	Interval between radiation and heat (months)	No. of ultrasound treatments	Average temperature at tumor center (°C)	Tumor response[d]	Skin and subcutaneous radiation damage (prior to heat)	Skin effects of ultrasound
1. SCC—occipital node	5000(M)	16	14	43.5	PR	Moderate	0.5-cm burn[e]
2. AC—nose	8500(M + O)	7–15	3[f]	44.0	NE	Marked	None
3. SCC—scalp	4400(O)	5	5	44.5	PR	Minor	None
4. SCC—mandible	5000(M)	3	6	44.0	PR	Minor	None
5. AC—neck	5900(M)	1	14	43.5	CR	Marked	None
6. AC—sternum	6000(M)	16	4	44.0	PR	Marked	None
7. SCC—neck	5000(M)	32	7	45.0	NE	Marked	None
8. AC—abdomen	5000(M)	30	6	44.5	PR	Marked	None
9. SCC—neck	6200(M)	240	6[f]	43.0	NE	Marked	None
10. SCC—mastoid	8800(M + I)	29	11	43.5	CR	Marked	None
11. SCC—mandible	6000(M)	31	8	44.0	PR	Moderate	None
12. SCC—mastoid	9000(M)	19–38	25	44.0	PR	Marked	None
13. SCC—preauricular	11,000(I)	23–41	6	43.5	NE	Marked	0.5-cm burn[e]
14. SCC—maxilla	5500(M)	5	5	44.5	PR	Marked	None
15. SCC—mandible	5000(M)	24	6	44.5	NE	Marked	None
16. DHL—neck	4400(M)	14	6	44.0	NE	Marked	0.5-cm burn[e]
17. AC—supraclavicular	6900(M)	7–19	5	44.0	NE	Marked	None
18. SCC—neck	6000(M)	20	6	45.0	PR	Marked	None

[a]From Marmor and Hahn, 1978, with permission.

[b]SCC, squamous cell carcinoma; AC, adenocarcinoma; DHL, diffuse histiocytic lymphoma

[c]M. Megavoltage x rays; O, orthovoltage X rays; I, implant (^{192}Ir)

[d]CR, complete regression; PR, partial regression; NE, no effect.

[e]At site of thermocouple insertion; healed within one week.

[f]Treated with bleomycin along with heat.

findings of nearly all other investigators, who report only small (1 to 3°) differences between tumor and adjacent tissue. Marked tumor necrosis was seen in lesions heated to 50°C or higher during one session lasting 15–60 min. Visceral tumors after "effective" (i.e., presumably 50° or higher, although this is not specified) heating, however, remained intact with little change in size. These heated tumors produced no tumor breakdown products (e.g., serum creatinine, urate, or increased levels of urinary proteins). The authors postulated that the high temperature caused vascular necrosis and thrombosis, and therefore the usual means of tumor resorption were prevented from being active. In spite of the high tumor temperatures reached, no adverse normal tissue reactions were observed, except for some fibrosis in very obese patients. No attempts were made to quantify the rates of tumor responses nor the durations of the responses seen.

These results exemplify the type of tumor responses seen when heat alone is used as the treatment modality: about 50% of the cases respond at least partially; durations of responses are usually short, lasting on the average about six weeks. The lack of normal tissue damage is a clear indication that treatments at higher temperatures and/or longer durations of treatments would be feasible (except according to Storm's study) and these might result in longer remissions. However, the data also tend to point to a limit of the benefits of localized hyperthermia. Very likely tumor cells residing in areas of the tissue where the milieu reflects that of the normal tissue are not killed by the hyperthermic treatments, and these cells are responsible for tumor regrowth. Most of the data point to the advantage of combination therapy, since presumably such cells can be dealt with by either X irradiation or chemotherapy.

7.4.4. Discussion

Tumor responses following treatments employing hyperthermia are characterized by several features, which seem to be observed independently of the mode of heat induction, i.e., whole body, regional, or local. Reduction in tumor mass tends to be rapid (the exception to this appears to be in the case of Storm's work involving tumor temperatures in excess of 50°C). Relief from pain has been described as dramatic, occurring frequently after the first or second hyperthermic session. Although some histologies appear to be more likely to be affected by heat than others, considerable variation of responses is seen even within similar types of tumors. Complete disappearances of tumors are rare, ranging from less than 5% for whole-body hyperthermia to perhaps 10 to 20% for localized hyperthermia. Responses tend to be of short duration, rarely lasting more than a few months. It is possible to retreat tumors, and a measure of control of localized lesions can be maintained for considerable time. Normal tissue complications are minimal, even when tumors are treated in areas previously heavily irradiated.

Many of the observed tumor responses are related to known biological effects of heat on cells. For example, the rapid shrinking of heated tumor masses probably reflects the observed lysis of heated cells when they are maintained in unfavorable environments *in vitro* (low pH and poor nutrient supply). The range of tumor responses, as well as their short durations, can be explained on the basis of responses of cells in a range of tumor microenvironments. However, other aspects are more puzzling. The reduction of pain, unless it results from reduced pressure against nerves associated with rapid tumor shrinkage, obviously has no cellular analog. The almost total lack of normal tissue damage, as observed in most studies, is also difficult to comprehend. Particularly in previously irradiated volumes where vasculature may be compromised, I would have expected that considerable trouble would have been encountered. Clearly this was not the case.

The short durations of tumor responses clearly suggest that a non-negligible fraction of the tumor cells survived the hyperthermia. Two approaches immediately suggest themselves to deal with this situation. Longer treatment times or high temperatures might be appropriate. In view of the lack of normal tissue damage seen, higher temperatures or longer treatment times might well be tolerated. By analogy, radiation therapy did not reach its maximum effectiveness until radiation doses started to approach tissue tolerance limits; the same might well be true for hyperthermia. The other approach is to combine hyperthermia with either X irradiation or with chemotherapy, and let these modalities deal with the cells that have escaped killing by heat (or *vice versa*).

7.5. HUMAN CANCERS: HEAT PLUS IRRADIATION

7.5.1. Tumor Responses

There is by now a fairly large literature on the treatments of superficial lesions by radiation and by heat plus radiation. Some of these studies are essentially anecdotal, listing the effects of combined hyperthermia and radiation against surface tumors, but containing no controls for effects of hyperthermia alone or of radiation alone. Other studies attempt to answer the question of whether the addition of heat to radiation can be shown to modify, in a quantitative way, the response of the tumor over that seen with the single modality. The anecdotal studies go back to work by Stafford Warren, who in the 1930s treated several patients with a combination of heat and radiation therapy. Warren used a cabinet, not too different from the Pomp cabinet described in Chapter 6, to treat his patients. He raised the temperature to a maximum of 41.5°C, which he noted as the maximum safe temperature. It is interesting to point out that current wholebody treatments of 41.8°C also are characterized as reaching maximum temperatures. Thirty-two cases of "hopeless malignant disease" with widespread metastases were treated. The results obtained by Warren (1935) are shown in Table 7.9. Eighteen of these had received intensive irradiation (deep therapy and radium "packs") without results because of the appearance of widespread metastases. Fourteen cases had received no treatment, and these were too advanced to justify anything but palliative irradiation. He reported that in all cases but three heat treatment led to an immediate improvement in the general condition lasting variable periods of time (1–6 months), with patients gaining weight and strength, and tumors shrinking in mass and lessening in duration. Each of the treatments was associated with radiation therapy, but with small doses, typically of 500 rad, given in one session. Warren commented on the fact that these results were over and above what would have been expected from radiation therapy alone, and closed by saying that these results were sufficiently encouraging for further study.

Crile (1963) exposed a variety of near-surface tumors to the combination of heat and radiation therapy. Specifically, he thus treated cutaneous recurrences of breast cancer, malignant myoblastoma of the face, metastatic adenocarcinoma of the liver, osteogenic sarcoma, and metastatic carcinomas and sarcomas in bony sites. To quote from his paper,

"In the treatment of cutaneous recurrences of carcinoma of the breast, the chief value of the heat is in sensitizing the superficially heated tumors to radiation, so that after immersion of the skin in a bath at 44–46° for 1 hr, a single dose of 600 rads may suffice to destroy the tumor. In a conventional treatment, 1500 or more are required to accomplish the same biological result, and, in patients who have been irradiated before, such doses might cause further damage to underlying normal tissue such as breast or lung."

Clearly both Warren and Crile anticipated much of the work that is currently going on to establish the benefits of the combination of hyperthermia and X irradiation.

The more modern papers fall into three classes. The first consists of essentially anecdotal reports. Tumors are exposed to heat and radiation and the effects are noted. In the second group, investigators attempt to make a comparison usually between heat plus radiation and radiation alone, although in some studies a control using only heat is also included.

Marked improvement (marked shrinkage of tumor with very slow recurrence)

Hypernephroma (large subcutaneous masses and brain metastasis)	10 months	Clinical disappearance of tumor without other treatment than fever
Multiple myeloma	11 months[b]	Recalcification started
	7 months[b]	Recalcification started
Endothelioma of the bone marrow	23 months	Recalcification started
	12 months[b]	
Cancer of the rectum (with liver metastasis)	13 months	
	6 months	
Meduloblastoma (with spinal metastasis)	11 months	
	8 months	
	6 months[b]	

Moderate improvement (shrinkage of tumor with slow return)

Neurogenic sarcoma	8 months	
Osteogenic sarcoma	8 months	
	9 months	
Melanotic sarcoma	5 months	Massive cardiac invasion (no other treatment before or after fever treatment)
Cancer of the breast	2 months	Cerebral hemorrhage? (no other treatment before or after fever treatment)
	10 months[b]	

Slight improvement (marked shrinkage of tumor with rapid recurrence)

Embryoma of the ovary	5 months	
Embryoma of the testicle	5 months	
Carcinoma of the thyroid	4 months	
Carcinoma of the lung	4 months	
	4½ months	
	1½ months	
Lymphosarcoma	4 months	No other treatment

No improvement (slight shrinkage of tumor but rapid return of growth)

Cyst adenoma of the ovary	4 months	No follow-up treatment
	2 months	No follow-up treatment
Cancer of the breast	4 months	
	2 months	
	1 month	

No effect

Brain tumor—glioma	1 week
Hodgkin's disease	4 months
Died during fever treatment	
Cancer of the stomach (in extremis)	

[a]From Warren, 1935.
[b]Patient still living (as of 1935).

The final group, or to be specific, one study, is one in which a protocol was designed attempting specifically to optimize conditions for the combination of heat and radiation without regard to radiation-only or heat-only controls.

Brenner and Yerushalmi (1976) described results on six patients heated with 2.45 GHz microwaves and irradiated by a 250-kV X-ray machine. Some patients were also heated with a stream of hot air. Skin temperatures reached up to 46 to 47°C. Radiation doses ranged up to 3000 rad. The authors' impression was that heat plus radiation gave results far superior to those expected from radiation alone. Holt (1975) described results obtained with a combination of X irradiation and hyperthermia from a 434-MHz microwave unit. Very few details of the treatment are given; no temperature measurements were obtained. The results are very difficult to evaluate because of the lack of data presented and the seemingly exaggerated claims made. A very similar system was used by Hornbeck *et al.* (1977), and again the results are difficult to evaluate, largely because of the lack of details about temperature measurement. Much better described are the studies of U *et al.* (1980). Patients were treated with microwaves from either a 915-MHz or a 2.45-GHz system. Radiation was either cobalt, 250-kV X rays, or photons from a 4-MeV linear accelerator. Ionizing radiation was given in 200–600 rad fractions, two to five times per week, to a total of 1800–4200 rad. Hyperthermia was given at a 42 to 44°C intratumor temperature, two to three times per week up to a maximum of ten sessions over a 4-week period. The nineteen patients treated suffered from squamous cell carcinomas, adenocarcinomas, malignant melanomas, plasmacytomas, and undifferentiated carcinomas. The authors found that localized hyperthermia could be used effectively in combination with ionizing radiation with excellent "normal tissue tolerance," provided that local tissue temperature was carefully monitored, controlled, and maintained within the 42 to 44°C range. Tumor temperatures rose to higher values than those of normal tissues; in one example discussed, the tumor temperature was 43°C while adjacent normal tissue was 41°C. The repeated applications of hyperthermia at 42 to 43.5°C for 45 min per session immediately following X irradiation yielded what appeared to be a "favorable therapeutic result," and occasionally the result was dramatic.

The results of U *et al.* are very similar to those reported by Kim *et al.* (1978a). These latter investigators used an inductive radiofrequency technique at 27.12 MHz to induce hyperthermia. In a total of twenty-four patients, the mean tumor temperature rose to about 42°C, while "adjacent" normal tissue remained at an average temperature of 40.5°C (Figure 7.2). Shown in that figure is also the decay of temperature, both in normal and tumor tissue, following the termination of heating. It is somewhat

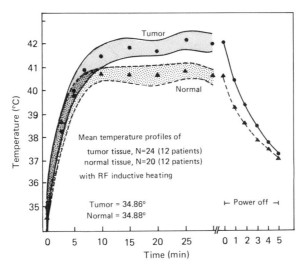

Figure 7.2. Average temperatures measured during RF (27 MHz) inductive heating of human tumors and "adjacent" normal tissue. Temperatures were measured with thermocouples during brief intervals (seconds) of power interruptions. The rapid rate of tumor temperature decay after the final power shut-off is puzzling, since it would indicate that blood flow in the tumor is greater, on average, than in the adjacent tissue. Data from Kim *et al.* (1978a), with permission.

difficult to reconcile the temperature decay with the usual claim that increased temperature in the tumor resulted from reduced blood flow rates. Had the blood flow indeed been low in the tumors, temperature decay should have been slower in the tumors than it was in normal tissue. In fact, the curves indicate that decay was more rapid, or at least as rapid in the tumor as in the adjacent nonmalignant volume. This is additionally puzzling, because after 30 min of heating, the increase in normal tissue blood flow resulting from homeostatic mechanisms would be expected to accentuate any preexisting differences between tumor and normal tissue blood flow rates.

A comparison was made by these authors of the responses of the lesions to radiotherapy alone and to radiotherapy plus heating. When radiotherapy alone was employed, 26% of the tumors regressed completely, while with the combination treatment 78% of the tumors showed a similar regression. While no specific scoring of normal tissue damage was done, the impression reported by Kim *et al.* was that the addition of hyperthermia to radiation when given in conventional dose fractionation, i.e., 200–300 rad per treatment, caused no increase in skin reaction from that caused by radiation therapy alone. This would suggest that the combined treatment gave a favorable "therapeutic gain factor." However, in patients treated more recently, in whom a high dose fractionation scheme was utilized, a concomitant enhanced skin reaction, although coupled with the rapid destruction of the tumor, was observed (Kim and Hahn, 1979). In the latter study the dose per fraction was approximately 500 rad.

Marmor and Hahn (1980) tested the combination of hyperthermia and radiation against radiation alone on matched nodules in individual patients. They found that the addition of hyperthermia (43°C, 15 min before radiation, 30 min after radiation) resulted in an objective improvement in treatment response in seven out of sixteen cases. In seven of the other cases there was no difference; this was in part because in some tumors radiation alone resulted in complete disappearance of the treated nodule without regrowth during the follow-up period; under such conditions the scoring system did not permit distinction between responses. In one case the heated nodule seemed to respond less well than those receiving no hyperthermia. Two patients showed enhanced skin reaction in the heated area; one of these was a severe wet desquamation.

Finally, Johnson et al. (1979) performed a study in which various fractionation schemes with and without heat were compared. The design of the study indicates that it was an attempt to determine a "rad equivalent" of the heating. Fractionation varied from 1 to 4 times, and total X-ray doses varied from 1000 to 3600 rad, with a dose per fraction of 100–700 rad. Tumor responses scored were: the rate of tumor regression and, when possible, duration of response. However, because of the advanced nature of the patients' disease, it was impossible to determine such a response. In addition skin response was scored, using a scoring system akin to that developed by Fowler et al. (1963). In comparing similar fractionation schemes with and without heat, in all cases both the tumor responses and the skin scores increased. There was too much scatter in the data to allow the authors to obtain a therapeutic gain factor, nor were they able to specify the radiation dose "saved" by the heat treatment.

Bicher (1980) and Arcangeli et al. (1980) have developed the only reported protocols of hyperthermia and X irradiation with the goal in mind to test the combination of the two treatments against potentially curable cancers, primarily those of the head and neck. Bicher's consists of the following: hyperthermia induced by microwaves at frequencies of 2.5 GHz or 915 or 300 MHz, depending upon the site of the tumor to be treated, is utilized initially as the exclusive modality. Patients are treated twice a week, with a 72-hr interval, at 45°C for 90 min. After four such treatments, the patients are given a week's rest. Then each hyperthermia treatment, now at 42°C for 2 hr, is preceded by a 400-rad fraction of X irradiation;

four such treatments are given, for a total of 1600 rad. Thus, a complete course of treatment consists of four treatments at 45°C without irradiation and four treatments at 42°C preceded by the 400-rad X-ray fractions. Only preliminary data were available up to the time of publication. A total of thirty-seven treatment fields had been exposed in twenty-three patients. Histologies included malignant melanomas, lymphomas, squamous cell carcinomas, adenocarcinomas, sarcomas, one glioma, one basal cell carcinoma, and a transitional cell carcinoma. Only marginal skin burns that healed completely were noted as adverse effects. Of the tumors treated, all in the head and neck region, there was a 67% total response and a 30% partial response rate. Only one patient showed no response at all. It should be emphasized that several of the patients were being retreated in previously irradiated areas. Obviously the protocol of Bicher *et al.* utilizes a radiation–hyperthermia combination in which unconventional X-ray fractionation is used, and a very low total dose. Yet, at least for the relatively short period of follow-up (6 months), the results so far must be termed exceedingly encouraging.

Somewhat in a similar vein is the ongoing study of Arcangeli *et al.* (1980). Strictly speaking, it is a comparison between a nonconventional X-ray fractionation scheme and a similar X-ray fractionation schedule to which hyperthermia has been added. Heating is accomplished by microwaves at 500 MHz. The basic plan of the program is to treat comparable lesions in the same patient with hyperthermia alone and with radiation combined with hyperthermia. A total of thirty-three neck nodes have been treated at the time of writing. Thirteen were treated with radiation alone and twenty with combined modalities. Irradiation followed a multiple daily fractionation schedule. It consisted of 200 + 150 + 150 rad per day, with a 4–5 hr interval between individual fractions. Patients were treated 5 days a week up to a total of 4000–7000 rads. While this is a relatively large dose range, all the lesions in each patient were irradiated with the same total dose, whether or not they received hyperthermia. Heat was applied on days 1, 3, and 5 of each week. Tumor core temperature was raised to at least 42°C and maintained for 40–50 min. The heat treatment was given immediately after the second irradiation of the day. The results of fifteen patients treated are shown. The multiple daily fractionation scheme plus hyperthermia resulted in a far superior response rate, 85%, when compared to multiple daily fractionation only, where the response rate was 46%. The complete response rate of an historical control, 30%, is probably not statistically different from that found for the multiple daily fractionation scheme.

The treatment was well-tolerated by almost all patients. No unusual skin reactions were seen, once microwave applicators had been developed that were able to fit an irregular surface. Again the preliminary results obtained here are very interesting.

7.5.2. Discussion

All the studies discussed in the previous section are uniform in one respect: they show that the addition of heat to X irradiation results in improved tumor responses when the comparison is made at similar X-ray dose levels and the two treatments are given in close temporal sequence.

Indeed, in view of all the cellular and animal data predicting such findings, a lack of enhanced tumor response in humans would have been remarkable. Less uniform are findings with regard to the ability of heat to improve therapeutic results, since at least some of the studies indicate that, under similar treatment conditions, skin reactions are also enhanced. There is a great danger that these latter results might be projected to imply that combinations of heat and irradiation do not lead to treatment advantages. There are many reasons why this is not likely to be the case. First of all, in all the investigations cited, the portal used for heating was similar to that used for the X-ray beam. Obviously, heating of normal tissue would therefore be expected to be associated with an exacerbated X-ray effect. I have already pointed out in Chapter 6 that in many cases it is quite feasible to use different geometries for heating than for X irradiation. If this is done, the radiation beam and the heated area overlap largely within the tumor volume, and augmentation of X-ray effects would only occur there. Whenever geometric isolation of this type is feasible, therapeutic gain relates only to the response of the normal tissue in and immediately adjacent to the tumor volume (and of course to the tumor itself).

Even in situations where the paths of heating and of X irradiation need to coincide, a favorable therapeutic situation may develop. Several of the studies show that many human tumors have a tendency to rise to higher temperatures than does surrounding normal tissue. Even small temperature differences can result in considerable differences in cell killing by X rays. This seems particularly true in the 41 to 44°C range. Thus, tumor and normal tissue physiology may provide some level of increased antitumor benefits of the X irradiation. In any case, skin effects can be bypassed by appropriate surface cooling, and few data exist on the possible adverse effects in other tissue. Obviously no definite conclusions can be drawn at this time regarding the conditions under which the close temporal association of heat and X irradiation is contraindicated; it is however clearly indicated whenever geometric isolation of the two treatments outside the tumor volume is possible and when measurements show a higher intratumor temperature than that measured in surrounding tissue.

While the close sequencing of the two treatments undoubtedly leads to a maximum antitumor effect, considerable merit lies in the suggestion that therapeutic advantages might be associated with spacing the two treatments by several hours or days in order to minimize interactions of heat and X rays. This would amount to using hyperthermia and X irradiation as independent modalities. The philosophy here would be to take advantage of the complementarity of the two modalities with respect to affecting different subpopulations of tumor cells, while the heat–time profile employed hopefully would not measurably increase normal tissue burden over that associated with X irradiation.

These considerations would suggest two different treatment strategies for X rays and hyperthermia: for those tumors where geometric separation of heat induction and X irradiation is possible, and for those where temperature rises two or three degrees above that of normal tissue, close temporal sequencing appears optimal. For other tumors, separation of the two treatments by several hours or even days may be the most prudent approach. A protocol such as the one of Bicher (1980) might be used for all tumors since it combines features of both strategies.

7.6. HUMAN CANCERS: HEAT PLUS DRUGS

Almost all the data in the literature on the combination of drugs and hyperthermia relate to either whole-body heating or to regional perfusion. Several of the studies on whole-body hyperthermia either contain or anticipate on arm in which anticancer drugs are administered either before or during hyperthermia. For example, Bull (1979) proposes the use of adriamycin or of a methyl-nitrosourea (MCCNU). Parks *et al.* (1979) suggest another nitrosourea, BCNU, while Larkin and Pettigrew (1980) have used multiple drug regimens. Use of chemotherapeutic agents is attractive, provided a good choice of agents is used. Care must be taken that drugs like actinomycin D, against which heat may protect, or adriamycin, be administered only in a time sequence that permits optimal drug action. Furthermore, it must be anticipated that heat, when it does augment drug activity, may do so not only against the tumor but also against critical normal tissue. *A priori*, one cannot in any way equate increased tumor cell killing with therapeutic benefits. The available data on patient responses to combined whole-body heating and systemic drug application are very fragmentary and do not allow one to decide whether or not the combination leads to superior responses than either of these modalities individually.

More data exist for this combination in regional treatments. Particularly noteworthy here are the results of Stehlin and his associates against melanoma (Stehlin, 1964; Stehlin *et al.*, 1975; 1979). This group started perfusions of the extremities in 1957, using melphalan at normal body temperatures, and in 1967 added hyperthermia induced by heating of the blood to the treatment. During treatment, muscle temperature is monitored continuously and blood temperature is raised or lowered to achieve an intramuscular reading of 40.0°C. Tourniquets are used to improve isolation of the treatment volume. The maximum time that the tourniquet is kept in place is 2.5 hr. In a comparison of 5-year survival rates of patients treated for stage IIIA melanomas with and without hyperthermia, Stehlin *et al.* (1979) found that the addition of the heat treatment improved the projected 5-year survival rate from 22 to 74%, a rather remarkable result, even though the controls were a group of patients analyzed retrospectively. Since melphalan was used for all patients, there is no way of knowing if heat by itself might not have yielded similar results. Such a possibility was suggested by Cavaliere *et al.* (1980), who compared hyperthermic perfusions against melanomas and osteogenic sarcomas with and without "antiblastic" agents, and found no difference in results.

There are no data in the literature that deal exclusively with the combination of chemotherapy and hyperthermia against localized lesions and tumors. For this reason I have to resort to quoting individual anecdotal reports in papers dealing primarily with other subjects. Barlogie *et al.* (1980), in a paper dealing primarily with synergism of the combination of hyperthermia and drug exposure *in vitro*, reported that,

> "We have since obtained clinical evidence of synergism between 43° ultrasound hyperthermia and DDP (cis-platinum) in one patient with a head and neck squamous cell carcinoma that had been refractory to hyperthermia and DDP alone. Interestingly, there was a 75% tumor regression with one treatment of DDP (25 mg/sq.m.) and one hour ultrasound hyperthermia at 43° administered concurrently on each of three subsequent days."

Synergism between hyperthermia and cis-DDP has also been noted by Arcangeli (1980). Patients treated with a combination of the two therapies responded even when individual therapy had failed.

Finally, at the Institut Gustave-Roussy, two individual responses to hyperthermia were noted. Patients had almost complete regression of heated tumors after only two to three sessions at 43°C, each of which lasting for about 1 hr. A reexamination of their charts showed that unknown to the physicians applying the hyperthermia, each patient had concurrently been on cyclophosphamide therapy, which until the application of hyperthermia had proven to be totally without response (J. M. Cosset, private communication).

It is extremely curious that no clinical studies have as yet been undertaken to carefully delineate the possible benefits of the combination of hyperthermia and drugs, at least against refractory isolated lesions during regular courses of chemotherapy. Clearly the drugs of most interest here would be cis-platinum and the nitrosoureas and other alkylating agents, as well as bleomycin. Heat should certainly have a role in palliative chemotherapy, particularly because of the many reports on its unusual and very rapid action in reducing pain.

7.7. CONCLUSION

Very likely the application of hyperthermia by itself, although resulting in a large number of regressions, has not cured a single patient of his tumor. Remissions, when induced, tend to be of short duration. The combination of hyperthermia and radiation therapy clearly offers considerable potential for improving the treatment of isolated lesions. Particularly encouraging are the findings that heavily irradiated volumes can be retreated with small doses of radiation, which, with the addition of hyperthermia, provide considerable benefit for the patient. The area of the combination of chemotherapy and heat for the treatment of localized lesions is essentially an unexplored field. It deserves much more attention than it has been getting in the past, and the current absence of adequate data is most surprising.

Anyone reading the literature that describes the historical evolution of cancer treatment by heat is surely struck by the frequently repeated cycle: initial excitement about the discovery of the "new" modality; then one or two reports of seemingly encouraging clinical results; finally silence and, presumably, abandonment of the technique. Coley, Westermark, Warren, and Crile, to name only a few, all more or less followed this pattern. Reasonably, the question must come to mind: are we now seeing a repeat of this process, albeit on a larger scale?

An answer to this question is perhaps contained in a short examination of the difficulties encountered by many of the early investigators and the range of their successes. The latter are perhaps most easily summarized; Warren (1935) pointed out clearly, "It should be emphasized that no results approaching cure have as yet been obtained with this procedure." "This procedure" involved treating patients with 41.5°C for up to 13 (!) hr using either local or regional heating. Obviously, during a period when the search for the cure of cancer was uppermost in many physicians' (and certainly the public's) mind, such a statement was enough to insure that few practitioners of hyperthermia would emerge.

Localized and regional hyperthermia were saddled with equipment problems. Apparatus for heat delivery was poor; as one reads some of the reports it is obvious that breakdown was the rule, rather than the exception. Heating was only possible for very superficial lesions. Obviously no definition of dose existed, but even time–temperature relationships were frequently not appreciated. Temperature measurement in any human tumor was very difficult. These problems were superimposed on those still with us: lack of knowledge about normal tissue tolerance and of optimum fractionation intervals. Thus any type of cost–benefit analysis surely suggested to the investigators concerned that the probability was low of developing hyperthermia as a routine clinical tool. Furthermore, neither surgery nor radiotherapy was anywhere near its limit in terms of improving treatment, and additionally, hope for finding the "magic bullet" was widely held.

Today the situation is certainly different. Both radiotherapy and cancer surgery are mature disciplines; chemotherapy, although still developing, has hardly produced the hoped-for miracle cure. On the other hand, information about the response of cells and tissue to heat is being acquired rapidly, and the technology of heating and of temperature measurements is advancing at a rapid rate. For these reasons potential benefits from hyperthermia are much more highly appreciated, while the costs in terms of money as well as hours of needed research for developing adequate techniques appear reasonable. Finally, the success of the preliminary preclinical studies has not been an isolated event, but a repeatable and verifiable result. Thus, it seems unlikely that hyperthermia will undergo another cycle of early enthusiasm followed by later disappointment.

7.8. SUMMARY

The rationale for the use of hyperthermia against human cancers is based in part on the many anecdotal reports of "spontaneous" remissions observed in patients who had episodes of high fevers. Reviews of these and other reports have shown that a high percentage of all reported spontaneous remissions were associated with such episodes.

Preclinical studies of heat against spontaneous tumors first involved dogs and cats. The evolution of cancers in such animals was affected materially by multiple sessions of moderate, localized hyperthermia (42 to 45°C; 45–60 min). Complete regressions were sometimes seen, but these were rare; however, many tumors regressed partially. Overall response rates were in excess of 50%. Normal tissue damage, except for minor local burns, was not seen.

Whole-body heating of humans suffering from advanced cancers of a variety of histologies has at times brief or temporary beneficial effects. Results presumably depend critically on the heat sensitivity of the tumor cells, since normal tissue tolerance limits exposures to temperatures below 42°C. Although several techniques have been used to induce whole-body heating, it is not clear that any one of them yields superior results. Heating rates are lowest when techniques are used that depend upon heat conduction into the body from an outside source, and perhaps are most rapid when extracorporeally heated blood is recirculated. Observed response rates range from 10 to 50%; complete tumor regressions are very rare and responses tend to be of short durations, rarely exceeding 6–12 months, and frequently are of much shorter duration.

Regional heating of tumors has been employed primarily for the treatment of tumors located in extremities. Histologies are primarily melanomas and osteogenic and soft-tissue sarcomas. The technique used is perfusion of extracorporeally heated blood. Amputation has usually followed the heat treatment, though new studies are under way that test the need for amputation. Five-year survival rates of 50% and better have been reported in patients with melanomas; the results of course depend strongly upon the stage of the disease at the time treatment commenced. The observation that patients with local metastases or local recurrences respond quite well to hyperthermic perfusions is encouraging. Complications with currently used methods are not a problem.

Localized heat can also cause regressions of tumors so treated. Several studies have shown that six sessions of hyperthermia, each lasting 45 min and at tumor temperatures of 44 to 45°C, result in complete or partial regressions of about 50% of the tumors treated. Squamous cell carcinomas, lymphomas, and mycosis fungoidis respond well, though responses are not limited to those histologies. Normal tissue damage is minimal, even in patients whose tumors are heated in areas irradiated previously to maximum tissue tolerance. Durations of responses tend to be short, a few weeks usually, but retreatment of tumors is found to be quite feasible.

The addition of heating to fractionated regimens of radiotherapy results in improved rates of tumor response (at similar X-ray dose levels). Increased normal tissue damage (to skin) has been reported in some studies, suggesting that therapeutic gain does not necessarily match the improved tumor response. In all the reported studies, the geometries of the heated and irradiated volumes are more or less similar, and X rays and heat are given in close temporal sequence. Considerable cellular and mouse data suggest that such schedules may not be optimal.

A treatment protocol involving an intense initial series of treatments at 45°C without X irradiation followed by a limited amount of X rays sequenced with 42°C hyperthermia has yielded some highly encouraging preliminary results.

The use of heat in augmenting tumor responses to chemotherapy has found surprisingly few advocates, in spite of much positive cellular and animal data, as well as the existence of one long-term study in humans. That work, involving the perfusion of limbs with blood to which an alkylating agent was added, suggests that the addition of hyperthermia to the perfusion increases the 5-year survival rate of stage IIIA melanoma from 22% (drug perfusion only) to 74% (perfusion of the drug in heated blood). While improvement for the treatment of other histologies was not as dramatic, nevertheless addition of hyperthermia to the perfusion of the drug led to significant improvements in tumor response rates.

References

Alexandrov, V.Y., 1977, *Cells, Molecules and Temperature—Conformational Flexibility of Macromolecules and Ecological Adaptation,* Springer-Verlag, Berlin, Heidelberg, and New York.

Allison, A.C., and Paton, G.R., 1975, Chromosome damage in human diploid cells following activation of lysosomal enzymes, *Nature* 207:1170–1173.

Alper, T., 1974, The role of membrane damage in irradiated cells, *Br. J. Radiol.* 47:240.

Anderson, R.L., Minton, K.W., Li, G.C., and Hahn, G.M., 1981, Temperature-induced homeoviscous adaptation of Chinese hamster ovary cells, *Biochim. Biophys. Acta* 641:334–348.

Arcangeli, G., Barni, E., Cividalli, A., Mauro, F., Morelli, D., Nervi, C., Spano, M., and Tabocchini, A., 1980, Effectiveness of mocrowave hyperthermia combined with ionizing radiation: Clinical results on neck node metastases, *Int. J Radiat. Oncol. Biol. Phys.* 6:143–148.

Arcangeli, G., Cividalli, A., Lovisolo, G., Mauro, F., Creton, G., Nervi, C., and Pavin, G., 1979, Effectiveness of local hyperthermia in association with radiotherapy or chemotherapy: Comparison of multimodality treatments on multiple neck node metastases, in: *Proceedings of the First Meeting of the European Group on Hyperthermia in Radiation Oncology* (G. Arcangeli and F. Mauro, eds.), pp.257–265.

Ashburner M., and Bonner, J.S., 1978, The induction of gene activity in *Drosophila* by heat shock, *Cell* 17:241–254.

Ashby, B.S., 1966, pH studies in human malignant tumors, *Lancet,* 2:312–315.

Atkinson, E.R., 1977, Hyperthermia dose definition, *J. Bioengineering* 1:487–492.

Aurell, E., and Tengroth, B., 1973, Lenticular anoretinal changes secondary to microwave exposure, *Acta Ophthalmol.* 51:764–771.

Bacher, J.E., and Kauzmann, W., 1952, The kinetics of hydrolysis of ribonucleic acid, *J. Am. Chem. Soc.* 74:3779–3786.

Barlogie, B., Corry, P.M., and Drewinko, B., 1980, *In vitro* thermochemotherapy of human colon cancer cells with cis-dichlorodiammineplatinum (II) and mitomycin C, *Cancer Res.* 40:1165–1168.

Bass, H., Moore, J.L., and Coakely, W.T., 1978, Lethality in mammalian cells due to hyperthermia under oxic and hypoxic conditions, *Int. J Radiat. Biol.* 33:57–67.

Belli, J.A., and Bonte, F.J., 1963, Influence of temperature on the radiation response of mammalian cells in tissue culture, *Radiat. Res.* 18:272–276.

Ben-Hur, E., and Elkind, M.M., 1974, Thermally enhanced radioresponse of cultured Chinese hamster cells: Damage and repair of single-stranded DNA and a DNA complex, *Radiat. Res.* 59:484–495.

Ben-Hur, E., and Riklis, E., 1978, Enhancement of thermal killing by polyamines: II. Uptake and metabolism of exogenous polyamines in hyperthermic Chinese hamster cells, *Int. J. Cancer* **22:**607–610.

Ben-Hur, E., and Riklis, E., 1979, Enhancement of thermal killing by polyamines: III. Synergism between spermine and γ-radiation in hyperthermic Chinese hamster cells, *Radiat. Res.* **78:**321–328.

Ben-Hur, E., Bronk, V.B., Elkind, M.M., 1972, Thermally enhanced radiosensitivity of cultured Chinese hamster cells, *Nature [New Biol.]* **238:**209–211.

Ben-Hur, E., Elkind, M.M., and Bronk, B.V., 1974, Thermally enhanced radioresponse of cultured Chinese hamster cells: Inhibition of repair of sublethal damage and enhancement of lethal damage, *Radiat. Res.* **58:**38–51.

Ben-Hur, E., Prager, A., and Riklis, E., 1978, Enhancement of thermal killing by polyamines: I. Survival of Chinese hamster cells, *Int. J. Cancer* **22:**602–606.

Bertazzoni, U., Stefanni, M., Noy, G., Giulotto, E., Nuzzo, F., Flaschi, A., and Spadari, S., 1976, Variation of DNA polymerase-α and -β during prolonged stimulation of human lymphocytes, *Proc. Natl. Acad. Sci. USA* **73:**785–789.

Bichel, P., and Overgaard, J., 1977, Hyperthermia effect on exponential and plateau ascites tumor cells *in vitro* dependent on environmental pH, *Radiat. Res.* **70:**449–454.

Bicher, H.I., 1980, The physiological effects of hyperthermia, *Radiology* **137:**511–513.

Bicher, H.I., Hetzel, F.W., Sandhu, T.S., Frinak, S., Vaupel, P., O'Hara, M.D., O'Brien, T., 1980, Effects of hyperthermia on normal and tumor microenvironment, *Radiology* **137:**523–530.

Bieri, V., and Wallach, D., 1975, Variation of lipid–protein interactions in erythrocyte ghosts as a function of temperature and pH in physiological and non-physiological ranges: A study using paramagnetic quenching of protein fluorescence by nitroxide lipid analogues, *Biochim. Biophys. Acta* **406:**415–423.

Bishop, F.W., Horton, C.B., and Warren, S.L., 1932, A clinical study of artifical hyperthermia induced by high frequency currents, *Am. J. Med. Sci.* **184:**515–533.

Blair, R.M., and Levin, W., 1978, Clinical experience on the induction and maintenance of whole body hyperthermia, in: *Cancer Therapy by Hyperthermia and Radiation*, proceedings of the Second International Symposium, Essen, Germany, June 2–4, 1977 (C. Streffer, D. van Beuningen, F. Dietzel, E. Röttinger, J.E. Robinson, E. Scherer, S. Seeber, and K.R. Trott, eds.), Urban and Schwarzenberg, Baltimore and Munich, p. 318.

Blair, O.C., Winward, R.T., and Roti Roti, J.L., 1979, The effect of hyperthermia on the protein content of HeLa cell nuclei: A flow cytometric analysis, *Radiat. Res.* **78:**474–484.

Bleehan, N.M., Honess, D.J., and Morgan, J.E., 1977, Interaction of hyperthermia and the hypoxic cell sensitizer RO-07-0582 on the EMT6 mouse tumor, *Br. J. Cancer* **35:**299–306.

Bleiberg, I., and Sohar, E., 1975, The effect of heat treatment on the damage and recovery of the protein synthesis mechanism of human kidney cell-line, *Virchows Arch. [Zellpathol.]* **17:**269–278.

Bollum, F.U., 1975, Mammalian DNA polymerases, *Prog. Nucleic Acid Res. Mol. Biol.* **15:**109–144.

Bootsma, D., 1965, Changes induced in the first post-rradiation generation cycle of human cells studied by double labeling, *Exp. Cell Res.* **38:**429–431.

Bowen T., Connor, W., Nasoui, R., Pifes, D., and Shozles, R., 1975, *Measurement of the Temperature Dependence of the Velocity of Ultrasound in Soft Tissue*, Ultrasonics Symposium Proceedings IEEE Cat. No. 75:CW0 994–995.

Bowler, K., Duncan, C.J., Gladwell, R.T., and Davison, T.F., 1973, Cellular heat injury, *Comp. Biochem. Physiol.* **45A**:441–450.

Braun, J., and Hahn, G.M., 1975, Enhanced cell killing by bleomycin and 43° hyperthermia and the inhibition of recovery from potentially lethal damage, *Cancer Res.* **35**:2921–2927.

Brenner, H.J., and Yerushalmi, A., 1976, Combined local hyperthermia and x-irradiation in the treatment of metasatic tumors, *Br. J. Cancer* **33**:91–95.

Brock, T.D., 1978, *Thermophilic Microorganisms and Life at High Temperatures*, Springer-Verlag, New York, Heidelberg, and Berlin.

Bronk, B.V., Wilkins, R.J., and Regan, J.C., 1973, Thermal enhancement of DNA damage by an alkylating agent in human cells, *Biochem. Biophys, Res. Commun.* **52**:1064–1070.

Brown, J.M., 1979, Evidence for acutely hypoxic cells in mouse tumors and a possible mechanism of reoxygenation, *Br. J. Radiol.* **52**:650–656.

Brown, L.A., and Crozier, W.J., 1927, Rate of killing of cladocerans at higher temperatures, *J. Gen. Physiol.* **11**:25–36.

Bull, J.M., 1979, Summary of the informal discussion of animal models and clinical studies, *Cancer Res.* **39**:2262–2263.

Bull, J.M., Lees, D., Schuette, W., Whang-Pang, J., Smith, R., Bynum, G., Atkinson, E.R., Gottdiener, J.S., Gralnick, H.R., Shawker, T.H., and DeVita, V.T., Jr., 1979, Whole body hyperthermia: A phase I trial of a potential adjuvant to chemotherapy, *Ann. Intern. Med.* **90**:317–323.

Busch, W., 1866, Über den Einfluss welche heftigere Erysipeln zuweilig auf organisierte Neubildungen ausüben, *Vrh. Naturhist. Preuss Rhein. Westphal* **23**:28–30.

Capon, A., 1970, Utilisation d'une méthode à thermodiffusion pour l'évaluation du débit sanguin dans les tumeurs cérébrales, *Acta Clin. Belg.* **25**:174–178.

Cavaliere, R., Moricca, G., and Caputo, A., 1975, Regional hyperthermia by perfusion, in: *Proceedings of the International Symposium on Cancer Therapy by Hyperthermia and Radiation* (M. Wizenberg and J.E. Robinson, eds.), American College of Radiology Press, Baltimore, pp. 251–265.

Cavaliere, R., Ciocatto, E.C., Giovanella, B.C., Heidelberger, C., Johnson, R.O., Moricca, G., and Rossi-Fanelli, A., 1967, Selective heat sensitivity of cancer cells (biochemical and clinical studies), *Cancer* **20**:1351–1381.

Cavaliere, R., Moricca, G., DiFilippo, F., Caputo, A., Monticelli, G., and Santori, F.S., 1980, Heat transfer problems during local perfusion in cancer treatment, *Ann. NY Acad. Sci.* **338**:311–327.

Ceri, H., and Wright, J.A., February, 1977, Temperature sensitive hamster cell lines with altered membrane properties, *Exp. Cell Res.* **104**:388–398.

Cetas, T.C., 1975, Biological effects of electromagnetic waves, in: *Proceedings of the 1975 USNC/URSI Symposium* (C. Johnson and M. Shore, eds.), Bureau of Radiological Health, Rockville, Md., NEW Publ. (FDA) 77-8011, Vol. II, p. 239.

Cetas, T.C., Connor, W.G., and Manning, M.R., 1980, Monitoring of tissue temperature during hyperthermia therapy, *Ann. NY Acad. Sci.* **335**:281–297.

Chen, M.M., Cain, C.A., Lam, K.L., and Mullin, J., 1977, The viscometric thermometer: A non-perturbing instrument for measuring temperature in tissues under electromagnetic radiation, *J. Bioeng.* **1**:547–554.

Chen, T.T., and Heidelberger, C., 1969, Quantitative studies on the malignant transformation of mouse prostate cells by carcinogenic hydrocarbons *in vitro*, *Int. J. Cancer* **4**:166 178.

Christensen, D.A., 1979, Thermal dosimetry and temperature measurements, *Cancer Res.* **39**:2325–2327.

Clark, E.P., and Lett, J.T., 1978, Possible mechanisms for hyperthermic inactivation of the rejoining of x-ray induced DNA strand breaks, in: *Cancer Therapy by Hyperthermia and Radiation*, proceedings of the Second International Symposium, Essen, Germany, June 2–4, 1977 (C. Streffer, D. van Beuningen, F. Dietzel, E. Röttinger, J.E. Robinson, E. Scherer, S. Seeber, and K.R. Trott, eds.), Urban and Schwarzenberg, Baltimore and Munich, pp. 144–145.

Clark, E.P., Hahn, G.M., and Little, J.B., 1981, Hyperthermic modulation of X-ray-induced oncogenic transformation in C3H 10T1/2 cells, *Radiat. Res.* **88**:619–622.

Cleary, S.F., 1970, Considerations in the evaluation of the biological effects of exposure to microwave radiation, *Am. Ind. Hyg. Assoc. J.* **31**:52–59.

Cohen, S.S., and Barnes, H.D., 1954, Studies on unbalanced growth in *Escherichia coli, Proc. Natl. Acad. Sci USA* **40**:885–892.

Coley, W.B., 1893, The treatment of malignant tumors by repeated inoculations of erysipelas, with a report of ten original cases, *Am. J. Med. Sci.* **105**:488–511.

Coley, W.B., 1894, Treatment of inoperable malignant tumors with the toxins of erysipelas and the *Bacillus prodigiosus, Am. J. Med. Sci.* **108**:50–66.

Coley, W.B., 1911, A report of recent cases of inoperable sarcoma successfully treated with mixed toxins of erysipelas and *Bacillus prodigiosus, Surg. Gynecol. Obstet.* **13**:174–190.

Coley-Nauts, H., Swift, W., and Coley B., 1946, The treatment of malignant tumors by bacterial toxins as developed by the late William B. Coley, M.D.: Reviewed in light of modern research, *Cancer Res.* **6**:205–216.

Connor, W.G., Gerner, E.W., Miller, R.C., and Boone, M.L.M., 1977, Prospects for hyperthermia in human cancer therapy: Part II, *Radiology* **123**:497–503.

Cooper, K.E., Veale, W.L., Kasting, N., and Pittman, Q.J., 1979, Ontogeny of fever, *Fed. Proc.* **38**:35–38.

Corry, P.M., Robinson, S., and Getz, S., 1977, Hyperthermic effects on DNA repair mechanisms, *Radiology* **123**:475–482.

Corry, P.M., Spanos, W., Tilchen, E., and Barlogie, B., 1980b, Combined ultrasound–radiation therapy of human superficial tumors, *Radiat. Res.* **83**:464.

Corry, P.M., Barlogie, B., Spanos, W., Armour, E., Barkley, H., and Gonzales, M., 1980a, Approaches to clinical application of combinations of nonionizing and ionizing radiation, in: *Radiation Biology in Cancer Research* (R.E. Meyn and H.R. Withers, eds.), Raven Press, New York, pp. 637–645.

Cossins, A.R., and Prosser, C.L., 1978, Evolutionary adaptation of membranes to temperature, *Proc. Natl. Acad. Sci. USA* **75**:2040–2043.

Cress, A.E., and Gerner, E.W., 1980, Cholesterol levels inversely reflect the thermal sensitivity of mammalian cells in culture, *Nature* **283**:677–679.

Crile, G., Jr., 1963, The effects of heat and radiation on cancers implanted in the feet of mice, *Cancer Res.* **23**:372–380.

Cronquist, S., Ingvar, D., and Lassen, N., 1966, Quantitative measures of regional cerebral blood flow related to neuroradiological findings, *Acta Radiol. [Diagn.] (Stockh.)* **5**:760–766.

Cullen, J., Phillips, M.C., and Shipley, G.G., 1971, The effects of temperature on the composition and physical properties of the lipids of *Pseudomonas fluorescens, Biochem. J.* **125**:733–742.

Czerski, P., and Siekierznski, M., 1975, An analysis of occupational exposure to microwave radiation, in: *Fundamental and Applied Aspects of Nonionizing Radiation* (S.M. Michelson, M.W. Miller, R. Magin, and E.R. Carstensen, eds.), Plenum Press, New York, pp. 367–377.

Damir, Y., Gulyayev, G., Kalantarov, K., Akselrod, A., Yevdokimou, Y., Tsipis, A., and Zhanabayeu, K., 1972, Clinical investigation of microcirculation using radioactive xenon (preliminary report), *Vestn. Akad. Med. Nauk SSSR* **8**:26–30.

DeKruyff, B., Van Dijck, P.W.M., Goldback, R.W., Demel, R.A., and Van Deenan, L.L.M., 1973, Influence of fatty acid and sterol composition on the lipid phase transition and activity of membrane-bound enzymes in Acholeplasma laidlawii, *Biochim. Biophys, Acta* **330**:269–273.

Dewey, W.C., and Sapareto, S.A., 1978, Radiosensitization by hyperthermia occurs through an increase in chromosomal aberrations, in: *Cancer Therapy by Hyperthermia and Radiation,* proceedings of the Second International Symposium, Essen, Germany, June 2–4, 1977, (C. Streffer, D. van Beuningen, F. Dietzel, E. Röttinger, J.E. Robinson, E. Scherer, S. Seeber, and K.R. Trott, eds.) Urban and Schwarzenberg, Munich, Baltimore, pp. 149–151.

Dewey, W.C., and Miller, H.H., 1970, Effect of temperature (37°C) on x–ray-induced cell lethality and chromosomal aberrations, *Int. J. Radiat. Biol.* 18:91–93.

Dewey, W.C., Westra, A., Miller, H.H., and Magasawa, H., 1971, Heat-induced lethality and chromosomal damage in synchronized Chinese hamster cells treated with 5-bromodeoxyuridine, *Int. J. Radiat. Biol.* 20:505–520.

Dewey, W.C., Sapareto, S.A., and Betten, D.A., 1978, Hyperthermic radiosensitization of synchronous Chinese hamster cells: Relationship between lethality and chromosomal aberrations, *Radiat. Res.* **76**:48–59.

Dewey, W.C., Freeman, M.L., Raaphorst, G.P., Clark, E.P., Wong, R.S., Highfield, D.P., Spiro, J.S., Tomasovic, S.P., Denman, D.L., and Coss, R.A., 1980, Cell biology of hyperthermia and radiation, in: *Radiation Biology in Cancer Research* (R.E. Meyn and H.R. Withers, eds.), Raven Press, New York, pp. 589–623.

Dickson, J.A., 1977, The effects of hyperthermia in animal tumor systems, in: *Selective Heat Sensitivity of Cancer Cells* (A. Rossi-Fanelli and R. Cavaliere, eds.), Springer-Verlag, New York and Berlin, pp. 43–100.

Dickson, J.A., and Calderwood, S.K., 1980, Temperature range and selective sensitivity of tumors to hyperthermia: A critical review, in: *Thermal Characteristics of Tumors: Applications in Detection and Treatment* (R.K. Jain and P.M. Gullino, eds.), *Ann. NY Acad. Sci.* **335**:180–207.

Dickson, J.A., and Ellis, H.A., 1976, The influence of tumor volume and the degree of heating on the response of the solid Yoshida sarcoma to hyperthermia (40–42 degrees), *Cancer Res.* **36**:1188–1195.

Dickson, J.A., and Oswald, B.E., 1976, The sensitivity of a malignant cell line to hyperthermia (42 degrees) at low intracellular pH, *Br. J. Cancer* **34**:262–271.

Dickson, J.A., and Suzangar, M., 1974, *In vitro–in vivo* studies on the susceptibility of the solid Yoshida sarcoma to drugs and hyperthermia (42 degrees C), *Cancer Res.* **34**:1263–1274.

Dickson, J.A., and Suzangar, M., 1976, A predictive *in vitro* assay for the sensitivity of human solid tumors to hyperthermia (42°C) and its value in patient management, *Clin. Oncol.* **2**:141–155.

Dietzel, F., 1975, *Tumor und Temperatur,* Urban and Schwarzenberg, Munich and Berlin.

Dikomey, E., 1978, Repair of DNA strand breaks in Chinese hamster ovary cells at 37 degrees or at 42 degrees C, in: *Cancer Therapy by Hyperthermia and Radiation,* proceedings of the Second International Symposium, Essen, Germany, June 2–4, 1977 (C.

Streffer, D. van Beuningen, F. Dietzel, E. Röttinger, J.E. Robinson, E. Scherer, S. Seeber, and K.R. Trott, eds.), Urban and Schwarzenberg, Munich and Baltimore, pp. 146–49.

Di Mayorca, G., Greenblatt, M., Trauthen, T., Soller, A., and Giordano, R., 1973, Malignant transformation of BHK_{21} clone 13 cells *in vitro* by nitrosamines—a conditional state, *Proc. Natl. Acad. Sci. USA* **70:**46–49.

Djordjevic, O., Kostic, L., Brkic, G., and Astaldai, G., 1978, Effects of hyperthermia and drug in cultured mammalian cells, *Biomedicine* **28:**323–327.

Donaldson, S.S., Gordon, L.F., and Hahn, G.M., 1978, Protective effect of hyperthermia against the cytotoxicity of actinomycin D on Chinese hamster cells, *Cancer Treat. Rep.* **62:**1489–1495.

Doss, J.D., 1974, Use of RF fields to produce hyperthermia in animal tumors, in: Proceedings of the International Symposium on Cancer Therapy by Hyperthermia and Radiation (M. Wizenberg and J.E. Robinson, eds.), American College of Radiology Press, Baltimore, Md., pp. 226–228.

Douglass, M.A., Parks, L.C., and Bebin, J., 1981, Sudden myelopathy secondary to therapeutic total body hyperthermia after spinal cord irradiation, *N. Engl. J. Med.* **304:**583–585.

Durand, R.E., 1978, Potentiation of radiation lethality by hyperthermia in a tumor model: Effects of sequence, degree and duration of heating, *Int. J. Radiat. Oncol. Biol. Phys.* **4:**401–406.

Eddy, H.A., 1980, Alterations in tumor microvasculature during hyperthermia, *Radiology* **137:**515–521.

Eden, M., Haines, B., and Kahler, H., 1955, The pH of rat tumors measured in vivo, *J. Natl. Cancer Inst.* **16:**541–556.

Edwards, M.S., 1967, Congenital defects in guinea pigs following induced hyperthermia during gestation, *Arch: Pathol.* **84:**42–48.

Elkind, M.M., and Sutton, H., 1959, X-ray damage and recovery in mammalian cells in culture, *Nature* **184:**1293–1295.

Elkind, M.M., Sutton, H., and Moses, W.B., 1967, Sublethal and lethal radiation damage, *Nature* **214:**1088–1092.

Elkind, M.M., Kano, E., and Sutton-Gilbert, H., 1969, Cell killing by actinomycin D in relation to the growth cycle of Chinese hamster cells, *J. Cell. Biol.* **42:**366–377.

Esser, A.F., and Souza, K.A., 1974, Correlation between thermal death and membrane fluidity in *Bacillus stearothermophilus*, *Proc. Natl. Acad. Sci. USA* **71:**4111–4115.

Euler, J., Priesching, A., Wenzel, J., Sauermann, G., Klockler, K., and Kretschmer, G., 1974a, Hyperthermia peritoneal perfusion in ascites tumors in rats, *Wien. Klin. Wochenschr.* **86:**220–225.

Euler, J., Sauermann, G., Priesching, A., and Klockler, K., 1974b, Effect of temperature, pH and thio-tepa on tumor take rates and thymidine incorporation in ascites tumor cells, *Wien. Klin, Wochenschr.* **86:**211–220.

Euler-Rolle, J., Prieschling, A., Vormittag, E., Tschakaloff, C., and Polterauer, P., 1978, Prevention of cardiac complications during whole body hyperthermia by beta receptor blockage, in: *Cancer Therapy by Hyperthermia and Radiation*, proceedings of the Second International Symposium, Essen,Germany, June 2–4, 1977 (C. Streffer, D. van Beuningen, F. Dietzel, E. Röttinger, J.E. Robinson, E. Scherer, S. Seeber, and K.R. Trott, ets.), Urban and Schwarzenberg, Baltimore and Munich, p. 302.

Fabricius, H.A., Neumann, H., Stahn, R., Engelhardt, R., and Lohr, G.W., 1978, Changes in clinical and immunological laboratory parameters of healthy adults after exposure to a one-hour 40° whole-body hyperthermia, *Klin, Wochenschr.* **56:**1049–1056.

Fajardo, L.F., Egbert, B., Marmor, J., and Hahn, G.M., 1980, Effects of hyperthermia in a malignant tumor, *Cancer* **45**:613–623.

Faria, S.L., and Hahn, G.M., 1982, Differences between heat and radiation damages in RIF tumors, *J. Natl. Cancer Inst. Monograph* (in press).

Fehleisen, R., 1883, *Die Atiologie des Erysipels*, T. Fischer Verlag, Berlin.

Field, S.B., 1978, The response of normal tissue to hyperthermia alone or in combination with x-rays, in: *Cancer Therapy By Hyperthermia and Radiation*, proceedings of the Second International Symposium, Essen, Germany, June 2–4, 1977 (C. Streffer, D. van Beuningen, F. Dietzel, E. Rottinger, J.E., Robinson, E. Scherer, S. Seeber, and K.R. Trott, eds.), Urban and Schwarzenberg, Baltimore and Munich, pp. 37–48.

Field, S.B., Hume, S., Law, M.P., Morris, C., and Meyers, R., 1976, Some effects of combined hyperthermia and ionizing radiation on normal tissues, in: *Proceedings of the International Symposium on Radiobiology Research Needed for the Improvement of Radiotherapy*, I.A.E.C., Vienna.

Fisher, G.A., Li, G.C., and Hahn, G.M., 1982, Modification of the thermal response by D_2O: Cell survival and the temperature shift. *Radiat. Res.*, (in press).

Fowler, G.A., and Nauts, H.C., 1964, *Effects of Acute Concurrent Infection on Cancer in Man*, New York Cancer Research Institute, New York.

Fowler, J., Morgan, R., Sylvester, J., Bewley, D., and Turner, B., 1963, Experiments with fractionated X-ray treatment of the skin of pigs: I. Fractionation up to 28 days, *Br. J. Radiol.* **36**:188–196.

Frazier, O.H., 1979, Discussion on Parks, I., Minaberry, D., Smith, D., and Neely, W. article, "Treatment of far advanced bronchogenic carcinoma for extracorporeally induced systemic hyperthermia," *J. Thorac, Cardiovasc. Surg.* **78**:892.

Freeman, M.L., Dewey, W.C., and Hopwood, L.E., 1977, Effect of pH on hyperthermic cell survival, *J. Natl. Cancer Inst.* **58**:1837–1839.

Friedgood, H.B., 1928, On the thermal death point of sarcoma and normal mononuclear cells, *Arch. Exp. Zellforsch.* **7**:243–248.

Fuhr, J.E., 1974, Effect of hyperthermia on protein biosynthesis in L5178Y murine leukemic lymphoblasts, *J. Cell. Physiol.* **84**:365–371.

George, K.C., Hirst, D.G., and McNally, N.J., 1977, Effect of hyperthermia on cytotoxicity of the radiosensitizer RO-07-0582 in a solid mouse tumor, *Br. J. Cancer* **35**:372–275.

Gerner, E.W., and Leith, J.T., 1977, Interaction of hyperthermia with radiation of different linear energy transfer, *Int. J. Radiat. Biol.* **31**:238–288.

Gerner, E.W., and Russell, D.H., 1977, The relationship between polyamine accumulation and DNA replication in synchronized Chinese hamster ovary cells after heat shock, *Cancer Res.* **37**:482–489.

Gerner, E.W., Connor, W.G., Boone, M.L.M., Doss, J.D., Mayer, E.G., and Miller, R.G., 1975, The potential of localized heating as an adjunct to radiation therapy, *Radiology* **116**:433–439.

Gerner, E.W., Leith, J.T., and Boone, M.L.M., 1976, Mammalian cell survival response following irradiation with 4 MeV x-rays or accelerated helium ions combined with hyperthermia, *Radiology* **119**:715–720.

Gerner, E.W., Boone, R., Connor, W.G., Hicks, J.A., Boone, M.L.M., 1976b, A transient thermotolerant survival response produced by single thermal doses in HeLa cells, *Cancer Res.* **36**:1035–1040.

Gerner, E.W., Holmes, P.W., and McCullough, J.A., 1979, Influence of growth state on several thermal responses of EMT6/Az tumor cells *in vitro*, *Cancer Res.* **39**:981–986.

Gerner, E.W., Cress, A., Stickney, D., Holmes, D., and Culver, P., 1980, Factors regulating membrane permeability alter thermal resistance, *Ann. NY Acad. Sci.* **335**:215–233.

Gerweck, L.E., 1977, Modification of cell lethality at elevated temperatures: The pH effect. *Radiat. Res.* **70**:224–235.

Gerweck, L.E., 1978, Influence of microenvironmental conditions on sensitivity to hyperthermia or radiation for cancer therapy, in: *Proceedings of the Symposium on Clinical Prospects of Hypoxic Cell Sensitizers and Hyperthermia* (W. Caldwell and R. Durand, eds.), University of Wisconsin, Madison.

Gerweck, L.E., and Dewey, W.C., 1975, Variation in response to heat during the mammalian cell cycle, *Proceedings of the International Symposium, on Cancer Therapy By Hyperthermia and Radiation*, (M. Wizenberg and J.E. Robinson, eds.), American College of Radiology Press, Baltimore, Md., pp. 16–26.

Gerweck, L.E., Gillette, E.L., and Dewey, W.C., 1975, Effect of heat and radiation on synchronous Chinese hamster cells: Killing and repair, *Radiat. Res.* **64**:611–623.

Gerweck, L.E., Nygaard, T.G., and Burlett, M., 1979, Response of cells to hyperthermia under acute and chronic hypoxic conditions, *Cancer Res.* **39**:966–972.

Gillette, E.L., 1979, Large animal studies of hyperthermia and irradiation, *Cancer Res.* **39**:2242–2244.

Gillette, G.L., and Ensley, B.A., 1979, Effect of heating order on radiation response of mouse tumor and skin, *Int. J. Radiat. Oncol. Biol. Phys.* **5**:209–213.

Gilman, M.Z., and Thilly, W.G., 1977, Cytotoxicity and mutagenicity of hyperthermia for diploid human lymphoblasts, *J. Thermal Biol.* **2**:95–99.

Ginoza, W., 1958, Kinetics of heat inactivation of ribonucleic acid of tobacco mosaic virus, *UCLA Medical Project Reports* **1958**:1–16.

Ginoza, W., and Giold, W.R., 1961, On the inactivation of transforming DNA by temperatures below the melting point, *Proc. Natl. Acad. Sci. USA* **47**:633–639.

Giovanella, B.C., and Mondovi, B., 1977, Introduction, in: *Selective Heat Sensitivity of Cancer Cells*, (A. Rossi-Fanelli, R. Cavaliere, B. Mondavi, and G. Moricca, eds.), Springer-Verlag, Berlin, Heidelberg, and New York, pp. 1–7.

Giovanella, B.C., Lohman, W.A., and Heidelberger, C., 1970, Effects of elevated temperatures and drugs on the viability of L1210 leukemia cells, *Cancer Res.* **30**:1623–1631.

Giovanella, B.C., Morgan, A.C., Stehlin, J.A., and Williams, L.J., 1973, Selective lethal effect of supranormal temperatures on mouse sarcoma cells, *Cancer Res.* **33**:2568–2578.

Giovanella, B.C., Stehlin, J.S., and Morgan, A.C., 1976, Selective lethal effects of supranormal temperatures on human neoplastic cells, *Cancer Res.* **36**:3944–3950.

Giovanella, B.C., Stehlin, J.S., Shepard, R.C., and Williams, L.J., 1979, Hyperthermic treatment of human tumors heterotransplanted into nude mice, *Cancer Res.* **39**:2236–2241.

Giovanella, B.C., Stehlin, J.S., Williams, L.J., Lee, S.S., and Shepard, R.C., 1978, Heterotransplantation of human cancers into nude mice: A model system for human cancer chemotherapy, *Cancer* **42**:2269–2281.

Goetze, O., and Schmidt, K.H., 1931, Örtliche homogene Überwärmung gesunder und kranker Gliedmassen, *Deutsche Z. Chir.* **234**:623–670.

Goffinet, D.R., Choi, K.Y, and Brown, J.M., 1977, The combined effects of hyperthermia and ionizing radiation on the adult mouse spinal cord, *Radiat. Res.* **73**:238–244.

Goss, P., and Parsons, P.G., 1977, The effect of hyperthermia and melphalan on survival of human fibroblast strains and melanoma cell lines, *Cancer Res.* **37**:152–156.

Greer,S., and Zamenhof, S., 1962, Studies of depurination of DNA by heat, *J. Mol. Biol.* **4**:123–141.

Gullino, P.M., Grantham, F.H., Smith, S.H., and Haggerty, A.C., 1965, Modifications of the acid-base status of the internal millieu of tumors, *J. Natl. Cancer Inst.*, **34**:857–869.

Gwozda, B., Dyduch, A., Grzybek, H., and Panz, B., 1978, Structural changes in brain mitochondria of mice subjected to hyperthermia, *Exp. Pathol. (Jeng)* **15:**124-126.

Hagler, A.N., and Lewis, M.J., 1974, Effect of glucose on thermal injury of yeast that may define the maximum temperature of growth, *J. Gen. Microbiol.* **80:**101-109.

Hahn, E.W., Alfieri, A.A., and Kim, J.H., 1974, Increased cures using fractionated exposures of x-irradiation and hyperthermia on the local treatment of the Ridgeway osteogenic sarcoma in mice, *Radiology* **113:**199-202.

Hahn, E.W., Alfieri, A.A., and Kim, J.H., 1979, The significance of local tumor hyperthermia/radiation on the production of disseminated disease, *Int. J. Radiat. Oncol. Biol. Phys.* **5:**819-823.

Hahn, E.W., Feingold, S.M., and Kim, J.H., 1980, Single dose radiation and hyperthermia and growth of the rat tail, *Int. J. Radiat. Oncol. Biol. Phys.* **6:**457-481.

Hahn, E.W., Canada, T.R., Alfieri, A.A., and McDonald, J.C., 1976, The interaction of hyperthermia with fast neutrons or x-rays on local tumor response, *Radiat. Res.* **68:**39-56.

Hahn, G.M., 1974, Metabolic aspects of the role of hyperthermia in mammalian cell inactivation and their possible relevance to cancer treatment, *Cancer Res.* **34:**3117-3123.

Hahn, G.M., 1976, Recovery of cells from induced, potentially lethal damage, *Cancer Treat. Rep.* **60:**1791-1798.

Hahn, G.M., 1978, Interactions of drugs and hyperthermia *in vitro* and *in vivo,* in: *Cancer Therapy by Hyperthermia and Radiation,* proceedings of the Second International Symposium, Essen, Germany, June 2-4, 1977 (C. Streffer, D. van Beuningen, F. Dietzel, E . Röttinger, J.E., Robinson, E. Scherer, S. Seeber, and K.R. Trott, eds.), Urban and Schwarzenberg, Baltimore and Munich, pp. 72-79.

Hahn, G.M., 1979, Potential for therapy of drugs and hyperthermia, *Cancer Res.* **39:**2264-2268.

Hahn, G.M., 1980, Comparison of the malignant potential of 10T ½ cells and transformants with their survival responses to hyperthermia and to amphotericin B, *Cancer Res.* **40:**3763-3767.

Hahn, G.M. and Li, G.C., 1982, The interactions of hyperthermia and drugs: Treatments and probes, *J. Natl. Cancer Inst. Monograph* (in press).

Hahn, G.M., Li, G.C., and Shiu, E.C., 1977, Interaction of amphotericin B and 43° hyperthermia. *Cancer Res.* **37:**761-764.

Hahn, G.M., and Little, J.B., 1972, Plateau-phase cultures of mammalian cells: An *in vitro* model for human cancer, *Curr. Top. Radiat. Res. Quarterly* **8:**39-83.

Hahn, G.M., and Pounds, D., 1976, Heat treatment of solid tumors: Why and how, *Appl. Radiol.* **6:**131-144.

Hahn, G.M., and Strande, D.P., 1976, Cytotoxic effects of hyperthermia and adriamycin on Chinese hamster cells, *J. Natl. Cancer Inst.* **57:**1063-1067.

Hahn, G.M., Bagshaw, M.A., Evans, R.C., and Gordon, L.F., 1973, Repair of potentially lethal lesions in x-irradiated, density-inhibited Chinese hamster cells: Metabolic effects and hypoxia, *Radiat. Res.* **55:**280-290.

Hahn, G.M., Braun, J., and Har-Kedar, I., 1975, Thermochemotherapy: Synergism between hyperthermia (42-43°C) and adriamycin (or bleomycin) in mammalian cell inactivation, *Proc. Natl. Acad. Sci. USA* **72:**937-940.

Hahn, G.M., Marmor, J.B., and Fajardo, L.J., 1978a, Kinetics of EMT-6 cellular survival after curative doses of hyperthermia, *Bull. Cancer (Paris)* **65:**473-474.

Hahn, G.M., Steinberg, D., and Fisher, G., 1978b, Protection by deuterium oxide against hyperthermic inactivation of Chinese hamster cells, *Radiat. Res.* **74:**476-477.

Hahn, G.M., Kernahan, P., Martinez, A., Pounds, D., Prionas, S., Anderson, T., and

Justice, G., 1980, Some heat transfer problems associated with heating by ultrasound, microwaves or radiofrequency, *NY Acad. Sci.* **335**:327–346.

Hahn, G.M., Marmor, J.B., Pounds, D.W., 1981, Induction of hyperthermia by ultrasound, *Bull. Cancer* **68**:249–254.

Hall, E.J., 1978, *Radiobiology for the Radiologist,* 2nd ed., Harper and Row, New York, pp. 52–53.

Hanawalt, P.C., Cooper, P.K., Ganesan, A.K., and Smith, C.A., 1979, DNA repair in bacteria and mammalian cells, *Annu. Rev. Biochem.* **48**:783–836.

Harisiadis, L., Hall, E.J., Kraljevic, U., and Borek, C., 1975, Hyperthermia: Biological studies at the cellular level, *Radiology* **117**:447–452.

Harisiadis, L., Sung, D.I., Lessaris, N., and Hall, E., 1978, Hyperthermia and low dose-rate irradiation, *Radiology* **129**:195–198.

Harisiadis, L., Miller, R.C., Harisiadis, S., and Hall, E.J., 1980, Oncogenic transformation and hyperthermia, *Br. J. Radiol.* **55**:479–482.

Harris, J.W., and Meneses, J.J., 1978, Effects of hyperthermia on the production and activity of primary and secondary cytolytic T-lymphocytes *in vitro, Cancer Res.* **38**:1120–1126.

Harris, M., 1966, Criteria of viability in heat-treated cells, *Exp. Cell. Res.* **44**:658–661.

Harris, M., 1967, Temperature-resistant variants in clonal populations of pig kidney cells, *Exp. Cell Res.* **46**:301–314.

Harris, M., 1969, Growth and survival of mammalian cells under continuous thermal stress, *Exp. Cell Res.* **56**:382–386.

Harris, M., 1980, Stable heat resistant variants in populations of Chinese hamster cells, *J. Natl. Cancer Inst.* **64**:1495–1501.

Haveman, J., 1981, The capacity of lysosomes of cultured mammalian cells to accumulate acridine orange is destroyed by hyperthermia, *Cell Tissue Res.* **213**:343–350.

Haveman, J., and Hahn, G.M., 1981, The role of energy in hyperthermia-induced mammalian cell inactivation: A study of the effects of glucose starvation and an uncoupler of oxidative phosphorylation, *J. Cell Physiol.* **107**:237–241.

Hazel, J.R., and Prosser, C.L., 1974, Molecular mechanisms of temperature compensation in poikilotherms, *Physiol. Rev.* **54**:620–677.

Heine, U., Severak, L., Kondratick, J., and Bonar, R.A., 1971, The behavior of HeLa-S$_3$ cells under the influence of supranormal temperatures, *J. Ultrastruct. Res.* **34**:375–396.

Henderson, M.A., and Pettigrew, R.T., 1971, Induction of controlled hyperthermia in treatment of cancer, *Lancet* **1**:1275–1278.

Henle, K.J., and Dethlefsen, L.A., 1978, Heat fractionation and thermotolerance: A review, *Cancer Res.* **38**:1843–1851.

Henle, K.J., and Leeper, D.B., 1976, Interaction of hyperthermia and radiation in CHO cells: Recovery kinetics, *Radiat. Res.* **66**:505–518.

Henle, K.J., and Leeper, D.B., 1979, Effects of hyperthermia (45°) on macromolecular synthesis in Chinese hamster ovary cells, *Cancer Res.* **39**:2665–2674.

Henle, K.J. and Roti Roti, J.L., 1980, Time temperature conversions in biological applications of hyperthermia, *Radiat. Res.* **82**:1387–1394.

Henle, K.J., Karamuz, J.E., and Leeper, D.B., 1978, Induction of thermotolerance in Chinese hamster ovary cells by high (45°) or low (40°) hyperthermia, *Cancer Res.* **38**:570–574.

Henle, K.J., Bitner, A.F., and Dethlefsen, L.A., 1979, Induction of thermotolerance by multiple fractions in Chinese hamster ovary cells, *Cancer Res.* **39**:2486–2491.

Henriques, F.C., Jr., 1947, Studies of thermal injury, *Arch. Pathol.* **43**:489–502.

Hermans, J., Jr., and Scheraga, H.A., 1959, The thermally induced configurational change of ribonuclease in water and deuterium, *Biochim. Biophys. Acta* **36**:534–535.

Hill, S.A., and Denekamp, J., 1979, Response of six mouse tumours to combined heat and X rays—implications for therapy, *Br. J. Radiol.* **52**:209–218.

Hofer, K.G., Hofer, M.G., and Ieracitano, J., 1977, Radiosensitization of hypoxic tumor cells by simultaneous administration of hyperthermia and nitroimidazoles, *Radiat. Res.* **70**:362–377.

Holt, J.A.G., 1975, The use of V.H.F. radiowaves in cancer therapy, *Australas. Radiol.* **19**:223–241.

Holt, J.A.G., 1977, Increase in X ray sensitivity of cancer after exposure to 434 MHz electromagnetic radiation, *J. Bioeng.* **1**:479–485.

Hornbeck, N.B., Shupe, R.E., Shidnia, H., Joe, B.T., Sayoc, E., and Marshall, C., 1977, Preliminary clinical results of combined 433 megahertz microwave therapy and radiation therapy on patients with advanced cancer, *Cancer* **40**:2854–2863.

Horvath, J., 1944, Ultraschallwirkung beim menschlichen Sarkom, *Strahlentherapie* **75**:119–1125.

Huang, L., Lorch, S.K., Smith, G.G., and Haug, A., 1974, Control of membrane lipid fluidity in *Acholeplasma laidlawii, FEBS Lett.* **43**:1–5.

Hubbell, W.L., and McConnell, H., 1971, Molecular motion in spin-labeled phospholipids and membranes, *J. Chem. Soc. [Perkin I]* **93**:314–326.

Hughes, W.L., Nussbaum, G.H., Connolly, R., Emani, B., and Reilly, P., 1979, Tissue perfusion rate determined from the decay of oxygen-15 activity after photon activation *in situ, Science* **204**:1215–1217.

Hume, S.P., and Field, S.B., 1977, Acid phosphatase activity following hyperthermia of mouse spleen and its implication in heat potentiation of X ray damage, *Radiat. Res.* **72**:145–153.

Hume, S.P., Rogers, M.A., and Field, S.B., 1978, Heat-induced thermal resistance and its relationship to lysosomal response, *Int. J. Radiat. Biol.* **34**:503–511.

Huth, E., 1957, Die Rolle der Bakteriellen Infektion bei Spontanremission maligner Tumoren und Leukosen, *Korpereigene Abwehr und Bosartige Geschwülste*, (H. Lampert and O. Selawry, eds.), K.F. Haug Verlag, Ulm, pp. 23–37.

Huth, E., 1977, Experimentelle Grundlagen der Immumtherapie maligner Tumoren mit mikrobiellen Substanzen, *Fortschr. Med.* **95**:1359–1364.

Jain, M., Gleeson, J., Upreti, A., and Upreti, G., 1978, Intrinsic perturbing ability of alkanols in lipid bilayers, *Biochim. Biophys. Acta* **509**:1–8.

Janki, R.M., Aithal, H.N., Tussanof, E.R., and Ball, A.S.S., 1975, Biogenesis of mitochondrial membranes in yeast *Saccharomyces cerevisiae, Biochim. Biophys. Acta* **3**:375–446.

Johnson, C.C., and Guy A.W., 1972, Non-ionizing electromagnetic wave effects in biological materials and systems, *Proc. IEEE* **60(6)**:692–718.

Johnson, C.C., and Shore, M.L., 1975, Biological Effects of Electromagnetic Waves, Selected papers of the USNC/URSI Annual Meeting, Boulder, C., Oct. 20–23, U.S. Dept. of Health, Education, and Welfare, Rockville, Md.

Johnson, H.A., and Pavelec, M., 1973, Thermal enhancement of thio-TEPA cytotoxicity, *J. Natl. Cancer Inst.* **50**:903–908.

Johnson, R.J., Sandhu, T.S., Hetzel, F.W., Song, S.Y., Bicher, H.J., Surseck, S.R., and Kowal, H.S., 1979, A pilot study to investigate skin and tumor thermal enhancement ratios of 41.5–42.0°C hyperthermia with radiation, *Int. J. Radiat. Oncol. Biol. Phys.* **5**:947–953.

Johnson, S.A., Greenleaf, J.F., Samayoa, W.A., Duck, F.A., and Sidstand, J., 1975, Reconstruction of three dimensional velocity fields and other parameters by acoustic ray tracing, *Ultrasonics Symposium Proceedings IEEE* Cat. No. 75: CWO 994–995.

Joines, W.T., Jirtle, R.J., Rafal, M.D., and Schaefer, D.J., 1980, Microwave power absorption differences between normal and malignant tissue, *Int. J. Radiat, Oncol. Biol. Phys.* **6**:681–687.

Joshi, D.S., and Jung, H., 1979, Thermotolerance and sensitization induced in CHO cells by fractionated hyperthermic treatments at 38°–45°C, *Eur. J. Cancer* **15**:345–350.

Joshi, D.S., Deys, B.F., Kipp, J.B.A., Barendsen, G.W., and Kralendonk, J., 1977, Comparison of three mammalian cell lines with respect to their sensitivities to hyperthermia, gamma-rays and UV radiation, *Int. J. Radiat. Biol.* **31**:485–492.

Joshi, D.S., Barendsen, G.W., and van der Schueren, E., 1978, Thermal enhancement of the effectiveness of gamma radiation for induction of reproductive death in cultured mammalian cells, *Int. J. Radiat. Biol.* **34**:233–243.

Kal, H.B., and Hahn, G.M., 1976, Kinetic responses of murine sarcoma cells to radiation and hyperthermia *in vivo* and *in vitro*, *Cancer Res.* **36**:1923–1929.

Kal, H.B., Hatfield, M., and Hahn, G.M., 1975, Cell cycle progression of murine sarcoma cells after x-irradiation or heat shock, *Radiology* **117**:215–217

Kapitulnik, J., Tshershedsky, M., and Yechezkel, B., 1979, Fluidity of the rat liver microsomal membrane: Increase at birth, *Science* **206**:843–844.

Kapp, D.S., and Hahn, G.M., 1979, Thermosensitization by sulfhydryl compounds of exponentially growing Chinese hamster cells, *Cancer Res.* **39**:4630–4635.

Kase, K., and Hahn, G.M., 1975, Differential heat response of normal and transformed human cells in tissue culture, *Nature* **255**:228–230.

Kase, K., and Hahn, G.M., 1976, Comparison of some responses to hyperthermia by normal human diploid cells and neoplastic cells from the same origin, *Eur. J. Cancer* **12**:481–491.

Kaufman, E.R., and Davidson, R.L., 1976, Novel phenotypes arising from selection for resistance to 5-bromodeoxyuridine, *J. Cell Biol.* **70**:199a.

Kelley, P., and Schlesinger, M., 1978, the effect of amino acid analogues and heat shock on gene expression in chicken embryo fibroblasts, *Cell* **15**:1277–1286.

Kiefer, J., Kraft-Weyrather, W., and Hlawica, M., 1976, Cellular radiation effects and hyperthermia influence of exposure temperature on survival of diploid yeast irradiated under oxygenated and hypoxic conditions, *Int. J. Radiat. Biol.* **30**:293–300.

Kim, J.H., and Hahn, E.W., 1979, Clinical biological studies of localized hyperthermia, *Cancer Res.* **39**:2258–2261.

Kim J.H., Kim, S.H., and Hahn, E.W., 1974, Thermal enhancement of radiosensitivity using cultured normal and neoplastic cells, *Am. J. Roentgenol. Radium Ther. Nucl. Med.* **121**:860–864.

Kim, J.H., Hahn, E.W., and Tokita, M., 1978a, Combination hyperthermia and radiation therapy for cutaneous malignant melanoma, *Cancer* **41**:2143–2148.

Kim, J.H., Kim, S.H., Hahn, E.W., and Song, C.W., 1978b, 5-thio-D-glucose selectivity potentiates hyperthermic killing of hypoxic tumor cells, *Science* **200**:206–207.

Kim, S.H., Kim, J.H., and Hahn, E.W., 1975a, The radiosensitization of hypoxic tumor cells by hyperthermia, *Radiology* **114**:727–728.

Kim, S.H., Kim, J.H., and Hahn, E.W., 1975b, Enhanced killing of hypoxic tumor cells by hyperthermia, *Br. J. Radiol.* **48**:872–874.

Kim, S.H., Kim, J.H., and Hahn, E.W., 1976, The enhanced killing of irradiated HeLa cells in synchronous culture by hyperthermia, *Radiat. Res.* **66**:337–345.

Kim, S.H., Kim, J. H., and Hahn, E.W., 1978, Selective potentiation of hyperthermia killing of hypoxic cells by 5-thio-D-glucose, *Cancer Res.* **38**:2935–2938.

Kluger, M.J., Tarr, R.S., and Heath, J.E., 1973, Posterior hypothalamic lesions and disturbances in behavioral thermoregulation by the lizard *Disposaurus dorsalis, Physiol. Zool.* **101**:219–229.

Koch, C., and Painter, R., 1975, The effects of extreme hypoxia on the repair of DNA single-strand breaks in mammalian cells, *Radiat. Res.* **64**:256–269.

Kramer, P., Guy, A.W., Emery, A.F., and Harris, C., 1976, Acute microwave irradiation and cataract formation in rabbits and monkeys, *J. Microwave Power* **11**:135–136.

Kreshover, S.J., and Clough, O.W., 1953, Prenatal influences on tooth development: Artificially induced fever in rats, *J. Dent. Res.* **32**:565–577.

Kumar, A., Bandman, E., and Melvin, W., 1976, Ribosome metabolism in temperature-sensitive mutant of BHK cells, *Nature* **259**:692–694.

Kurokawa, T., Hattori, T., and Furne, H., 1972, Clinical experiences with the streptococcal anticancer preparation OK-432, *Cancer Chemother. Rep.* **56**:211–220.

Kutchai, H., Barenholz, Y., Ross, T., and Wermer, D., 1976, Developmental changes in plasma membrane fluidity in chick embryo heart, *Biochim. Biophys. Acta* **436**:101–112.

Kwock, L., Lin, P-S., Hefter, K., and Wallach, D.F.H., 1978, Impairment of Na^+-dependent amino acid transport in a cultured human T-cell line by hyperthermia and irradiation, *Cancer Res.* **38**:83–87.

Landry, J., and Marceau, N., 1978, Rate-limiting events in hyperthermic cell killing, *Radiat. Res.* **75**:573–585.

Landry, J., and Marceau, N., 1979, Cell growth recovery after treatments at various supraoptimal temperatures, *Cancer Res.* **39**:1218–1223.

Langridge, J., 1968, Thermal responses of mutant enzymes and temperature limits to growth, *Mol. Gen. Genet.* **103**:116–126.

Larkin, J.M., 1979, A clinical investigation of total-body hyperthermia as cancer therapy, *Cancer Res.* **39**:2252–2254.

Larkin, J.M., Edwards, W.S., and Smith, D.E., 1976, Total body hyperthermia and preliminary results in human neoplasms, *Surg. Forum* **27**:121–123.

Larkin, J.M., Edwards, W.J., Smith, D.E., and Clark, P.J., 1977, Systemic thermotherapy: Description of a method and physiologic tolerance in clinical subjects, *Cancer* **40**:3155–3159.

Law, H.T., and Pettigrew, R.T., 1980, Heat transfer in whole body hyperthermia, *Ann. NY Acad. Sci.* **335**:298–310.

Law, M.P., Ahier, R.G., and Field, S.B., 1978, The response of the mouse ear to heat applied alone or combined with x-rays, *Br. J. Radiol.* **51**:132–138.

Law, M.P., Ahier, R.G., and Field, S.B., 1979, The effect of prior heat treatment on the thermal enhancement of radiation damage in the mouse ear, *Br. J. Radiol.* **52**:315–321.

Lea, D.E., 1947, *Actions of Radiations on Living Cells*, 1st ed., Cambridge University Press, London, pp. 261–276.

Lecyk, M., 1966, The effect of hyperthermia applied in the given stages of pregnancy on the number and form of vertebrae in the offspring of white mice, *Experientia* **22**:254–255.

Lehmann, J.F., and Krusen, F.H., 1955, Biophysical effects of ultrasonic energy on carcinoma and their possible significance, *Arch. Phys. Med. Rehabil.* **36**(7): 452–459.

Lele, P.P., 1979, A strategy for localized chemotherapy of tumors using ultrasonic hyperthermia, *Ultrasound Med. Biol.* **5**:95–97.

LeVeen, H.H., Wapnick, S., Piccone, V., Falk, G., and Ahmed, N., 1976, Tumor eradication by radiofrequency therapy, *JAMA* **235**:2198–2200.

Levine, E.M., and Robbins, E.B., 1970, Differential temperature sensitivity of normal and cancer cells in culture, *J. Cell Physiol.* **76**:373–379.

Li, D.S., Want, C.Q., Qiu, S.L., and Shao, L.F., 1982, Intraluminal microwave hyperthermia in the combined treatment of esophageal cancer: A preliminary report on 103 cases, in: *Third International Symposium on Cancer Therapy by Hyperthermia, Drugs and Radiation,* Ft. Collins, Co., June 1980, *J. Natl. Cancer Inst. Monograph* (in press).

Li, G.C., and Hahn, G.M., 1978, Ethanol-induced tolerance to heat and to adriamycin, *Nature* 274:699–701.

Li, G.C., and Hahn, G.M., 1980a, A proposed operational model of thermotolerance based on effects of nutrients and the initial treatment temperature, *Cancer Res.* 40:4501–4508.

Li, G.C., and Hahn, G.M., 1980b, Adaptation to different growth temperatures modifies some mammalian cell survival responses, *Exp. Cell Res.* 128:475–485.

Li, G.C., and Kal, H.B., 1977, Effect of hyperthermia on the radiation response of two mammalian cell lines, *Eur. J. Cancer* 13:65–69.

Li, G.C., Evans, R.G., and Hahn, G.M., 1976, Modification and inhibition of repair of potentially lethal X-ray damage by hyperthermia, *Radiat. Res.* 67:491–501.

Li, G.C., Hahn, G.M., and Shiu, E.C., 1977a, Cytoxicity of commonly used solvents at elevated temperatures, *J. Cell Physiol.,* 93:331–334.

Li, G.C., Hahn, G.M., and Tolmach, L.J., 1977b, Cellular inactivation by ultrasound, *Nature* 267:163–165.

Li, G.C., Shiu, E.C., and Hahn, G.M., 1978, Interaction of 43°C hyperthermia and polyene antibiotics: Amphotericin B, lagosin and filipin, in: *Cancer Therapy by Hyperthermia and Radiation,* Proceedings of the Second International Symposium, Essen, Germany, June 2–4, 1977 (C. Streffer, D. van Beuningen, F. Dietzel, E. Röttinger, J.E. Robinson, E. Scherer, S. Seeber, and K.R. Trott, eds.) Urban and Schwarzenberg, Baltimore and Munich, pp. 283–287.

Li, G.C., Shiu, E.C., and Hahn, G.M., 1980a, Recovery of cells from heat-induced potentially lethal damage: Effects of pH and nutrient environment, *Int. J. Radiat. Oncol. Biol. Phys.* 6:577–582.

Li, G.C., Shiu, E.C., Hahn, G.M., 1980b, Similarities in cellular inactivation by hyperthermia or by ethanol, *Radiation Res.* 82:257–268.

Li, G.C., Petersen, N.S., and Mitchell, H.K., 1982a, Induced thermal tolerance and heat shock protein synthesis in Chinese hamster ovary cells. *Int. J. Radiat. Oncol. Biol. Phys.* 8:63–67.

Li, G.C., Fisher, G.A., Hahn, G.M., 1982b, Induction of thermotolerance and evidence for a well-defined thermotropic cooperative process, *Radiation Res.* 89:361–368.

Liebeskind, D., Bases, R., Mendez, F., Elquin, F., and Koenigsberg, M., 1979, Sister chromatic exchanges in human lymphocytes after exposure to diagnostic ultrasound, *Science* 205:1273–1275.

Lin, P.A., Butterfield, C.E., and Wallach, D.F.H., 1977, Hyperthermia treatment (43°) rapidly impedes attachment of fibroblasts to culture substrates, *Cell Biol. Int. Reports* 1:51–55.

Lin, P.S., Wallach, D.F.H., and Tsai, S., 1973, Temperature-induced variations in the surface topology of cultured lymphocytes are revealed by scanning electron microscopy, *Proc. Natl. Acad. Sci. USA* 70:2492–2496.

Lindahl, T., and Nyberg, B., 1972, Rate of depurination of native deoxyribonucleic acid, *Biochemistry* 11:3610–3618.

Loshek, D.D., Orr, J.S., and Solomonidis, E., 1977a, Interaction of hyperthermia and radiation: The survival surface, *Br. J. Radiol.* 50:893–901.

Loshek, D.D., Orr, J.S. and Solomonidis, E., 1977b, Interaction of hyperthermia and radiation: Temperature coefficient of interaction, *Br. J. Radiol.* 50:902–907.

Lücke-Huhle, C., 1978, Hyperthermic response of tetraploid Chinese hamster cells with respect to growth phase and cell-to-cell contact, in: *Cancer Therapy by Hyperthermia and Radiation,* proceedings of the Second International Symposium, Essen, Germany, June 2–4, 1977 (C. Streffer, D. van Beuningen, F. Dietzel, E. Röttinger, J.E. Robinson, E. Scherer, S. Seeber, and K.R. Trott, eds.) Urban and Schwarzenberg, Baltimore and Munich, pp. 261–263.

Lücke-Huhle, C., and Dertinger, H., 1977, Kinetic response of an *in vitro* "Tumor Model" (V99 spheroids) to 42°C hyperthermia, *Eur. J. Cancer* **13**:23–28.

Mäntylä, M.J., Kuikka, J., and Rekonen, A., 1976, Regional blood flow in human tumors with special reference to the effect of radiotherapy, *Br. J. Radiol.* **49**:335–338.

Marmor, J.B., 1979, Interactions of hyperthermia and chemotherapy in animals, *Cancer Res.* **39**:2269–2276.

Marmor, J.B., and Hahn, G.M., 1978, Ultrasound heating in previously irradiated sites, *Int. J. Radiat. Oncol. Biol. Phys.* **4**:1029–1032.

Marmor, J.B., and Hahn, G.M., 1980, Combined radiation and hyperthermia in superficial human tumors. *Cancer* **46**:1986–1991.

Marmor, J.B., Hahn, N., and Hahn, G.M., 1977, Tumor cure and cell survival after localized radiofrequency heating, *Cancer Res.* **37**:879–883.

Marmor, J.B., Pounds, D., Hahn, N., and Hahn, G.M., 1978, Treating spontaneous tumors in dogs and cats by ultrasound-induced hyperthermia, *Int. J. Radiat. Oncol. Biol. Phys.* **4**:967–973.

Marmor, J.B., Pounds, D., Postic, T., and Hahn, G.M., 1979, Treatment of superficial human neoplasms by local hyperthermia induced by ultrasound, *Cancer* **43**:196–205.

Marmor, J.B., Pounds, D., and Hahn, G.M., 1982, Clinical studies with ultrasound-induced hyperthermia, *J. Natl. Cancer Inst. Monograph* (in press).

Martinez, A., Fajardo, L.F., Kernahan, P., Prionas, S., Hahn, G.M., 1980, The effects of radio frequency heating on normal fat and muscular tissues: A histologically based tissue injury grading system. Presented at the Third International Symposium: Cancer Therapy by Hyperthermia, Drugs and Radiation, held in Fort Collins, Co., June 22–26.

Martinez, A., Faria, S.L., Flores, S., and Hahn, G.M., 1982, The effects of heat on wound healing in mice, *J. Natl. Cancer Inst.* (in press).

Maurer, H.R., and Wenzel, M., 1977, Temperature dependence of the proliferation of mouse bone marrow cells cultured in H_2O and D_2O media, *Virchows Arch. B* **26**:187–193.

McAllister, L., and Finkelstein, D., 1980, Heat shock proteins and thermal resistance in yeast, *Biochem. Biophys. Res. Commun.* **93**:819–824.

McCormick, W., and Penman, S., 1969, Regulation of protein synthesis in HeLa cells: Translation at elevated temperatures, *J. Mol. Biol.* **39**:315–333.

Mendecki, J., Friendenthal, E., and Botstein, C., 1977, Microwave applicators for localized hyperthermia treatment of malignant tumors, *J. Bioeng.* **1**:511–518.

Meyer, K.A., Kammerling, E.M., Amtman, L., Koller, M., and Hoffman, S.J., 1948, pH studies of malignant tissues in human beings, *Cancer Res.,* **8**:513–518.

Meyn, R.E., Corry, P.M., Fletcher, S.E., and Demetriades, M., 1980, Thermal enhancement of DNA damage in mammalian cells treated with cis-diaminedichloroplatinum (II), *Cancer Res.* **40**:1136–1139.

Mikkelsen, R., and Wallach, D., 1977, Temperature sensitivity of the erythrocyte membrane potential as determined by cyanine dye fluorescence, *Cell Biol. Int. Rep.* **1**:51–55.

Miller, J.B., and Koshland, D.E., Jr., 1977, Membrane fluidity and chemotaxis: Effects of temperature and membrane lipid construction on the swimming behavior of *Salmonella typhimurium* and *Escherichia coli, J. Mol. Biol.* **111:**183–201.

Miller, R.C., Connor, W.G., Heusinkveld, R.S., and Boone, M.L.M., 1977. Prospects for hyperthermia in human cancer therapy, *Radiology* **123:**489–495.

Miller, P., Smith, D.W., and Shepard, T.H., 1978, Maternal hyperthermia as a possible cause of anencephaly, *Lancet* **1:**519–520.

Minton, K., Stevenson, M.A., Kendig, J., and Hahn, G.M., 1980, Pressure inhibits thermal killing of Chinese hamster ovary fibroblasts, *Nature* **285:**482–483.

Mitchell, H.K., and Lipps, L.S., 1978, Heat shock and phenocopy induction in *Drosophila, Cell* **15:**907–918.

Mitchell, H.K., Moller, G., Petersen, N.S., and Lipps-Sarmiento, L., 1979, Specific protection from phenocopy induction by heat shock, *Dev. Genet.* **1:**181–192.

Mittler, S., 1979, Hyperthermia and radiation induced genetic aberrations in *Drosophila melanogaster, Mutat. Res.* **59:**123–128.

Myakoshi, J., Ikebuchi, R., Furukawa, M., Yamagata, K., Sugahara, T., and Kano, E., 1979, Combined effects of x-irradiation and hyperthermia (42 and 44°C) on Chinese hamster V-79 cells *in vitro, Radiat. Res.* **79:**77–88.

Mondovi, B., Strom, B., Rotilio, G., Agro, A.F., Cavaliere, R., and Rossi-Fanelli, A., 1969a, The biochemical mechanisms of selective heat sensitivity of cancer cells: I. Studies on cellular respiration, *Eur. J. Cancer* **5:**129–136.

Mondovi, B., Agro, A.F., Rotilio, G., Strom, R., Moricca, G., and Rossi-Fanelli, A., 1969b, The biochemical mechanisms of selective heat sensitivity of cancer cells: II. Nucleic acid and protein synthesis, *Eur. J. Cancer* **5:**137–146.

Mondovi, B., Santoro, A.S., Strom, R., Faiola, R., and Rossi-Fanelli, A., 1972, Increased immunogenicity of Ehrlich ascites cells after heat treatment, *Cancer* **30:**885–888.

Moressi, W., 1964, Mortality patterns of mouse sarcoma 180 cells resulting from direct heating and chronic microwave radiation, *Exp. Cell Res.* **33:**240–253.

Morgan, J., Honess, D., and Bleehen, N., 1979, The interaction of thermal tolerance with drug cytotoxicity *in vitro, Br. J. Cancer* **39:**422–428.

Moricca, G., Cavaliere, R., and Caputo, A., 1977, Hyperthermic treatment of tumors: Experimental and clinical applications, *Cancer Res.* **59:**112–152.

Moritz, A., and Henriques, F.C., 1947, Studies of thermal injury: II. The relative importance of time and surface temperature in the causation of cutaneous burns, *Am. J. Pathol.* **23:**695–720.

Muckle, D., and Dickson, J., 1973, Hyperthermia (42°C) as an adjuvant to radiotherapy and chemotherapy in the treatment of the allogenic VX-2 carcinoma in the rabbit, *Br. J. Cancer* **27:**307–315.

Myers, P.C., Sadowsky, N.L., and Barrett, A.H., 1979, Microwave thermography: Principles, methods and clinical applications, *J. Microwave Power* **17:**105–114.

Naeslund, J., and Swenson, K.E., 1953, Investigations of the pH of malignant tumors in mice and humans after the administration of glucose. *Acta Obstet. Gynecol. Scand.,* **32:**359–367.

Nagle, W., Moss, A., and Baker, M., 1982, Increased lethality from 42°C hyperthermia for hypoxic Chinese hamster cells heated under conditions of energy deprivation, *J. Natl. Cancer Inst. Monograph* (in press).

Nauts, H.C., 1975, Pyrogen therapy of cancer: A historical overview and current activities, in: *Proceedings of the International Symposium on Cancer Therapy by Hyperthermia and Radiation* (M. Wizenberg and J.E. Robinson, eds.), American College of Radiology Press, Baltimore, Md., pp. 239–250.

Nielsen, O., and Overgaard, J., 1979, Effect of extracellular pH on thermotolerance and recovery of hyperthermic damage *in vitro*, *Cancer Res.* **39**:2772–2778.

Nilsson, S., 1975, Skin temperature over an artificial heat source implanted in man, *Phys. Med. Biol.* **20**:366–383.

Nyström, C., Forssman, L., and Roos, B., 1969, Myometrial blood flow studies in carcinoma of the corpus uteri, *Acta Radio.. [Ther.] (Stockh.)* **8**:193–198.

Okamoto, H., Minami, M., Shoin, S., Koshimura, S., and Shimizu, R., 1966, Experimental anti-cancer studies: Part XXXI. On the streptococcal preparation having potent anti-cancer activity, *Jpn. J. Exp. Med.* **36**:175–186.

Okumura, Y., and Reinhold, H., 1978, Heat sensitivity of rat skin, *Eur. J. Cancer* **14**:1161–1166.

Oleson, J., and Paulson, O., 1971, The effect of intra-arterial papaverine on the regional cerebral blood flow in patients with stroke or intracranial tumor, *Stroke* **2**:148–159.

Ormerod, M., and Stevens, U., 1971, The rejoining of x-ray induced strand breaks in the DNA of murine lymphoma cells (L5178Y), *Biochim. Biophys. Acta* **232**:72–82.

Osieka, R., and Maginiera, L.L., 1978, The effect of hyperthermia on human colon cancer xenografts in nude mice, in: *Cancer Therapy by Hyperthermia and Radiation,* proceedings of the Second International Symposium, Essen, Germany, June 2–4, 1977 (C. Streffer, D. van Beuningen, F. Dietzel, E. Röttinger, J.E. Robinson, E. Scherer, S. Seeber, and K.R. Trott, eds.) Urban and Schwarzenberg, Baltimore and Munich, pp. 287–290.

Osieka, R., Madreiter, H., and Schmidt C., 1976, The effect of hyperthermia on DNA repair, *Z. Krebsforsch.* **88**:1–10.

Overgaard, J., 1975, Effect of hyperthermia on the cytochrome C oxidase activity in tumour cells, *IRCS Med. Sci. Biochem. Cancer* **3**:225.

Overgaard, J., 1976, Ultrastructure of a murine mammary carcinoma exposed to hyperthermia *in vivo, Cancer Res.* **36**:983–995.

Overgaard, J., 1977, Effect of hyperthermia on malignant cells *in vivo:* A review and hypothesis, *Cancer* **39**:2637–2646.

Overgaard, J., 1978, The effect of local hyperthermia alone and in combination with radiation on solid tumors, in: *Cancer Therapy by Hyperthermia and Radiation,* Proceedings of the Second International Symposium, Essen, Germany, June 2–4, 1977 (C. Streffer, D. van Beuningen, F. Dietzel, E. Röttinger, J.E. Robinson, E. Scherer, S. Seeber and K.R. Trott, eds.), Urban and Schwarzenberg, Baltimore and Munich, pp. 49–61.

Overgaard, J., and Overgaard, K., 1975, The effect of environment acidity on the hyperthermic treatment of tumor cells, *IRCS Med. Sci. Biochem. Cancer. Cell Membrane Biol.* **3**:386.

Overgaard, J., and Suit, H., 1979, Time–temperature relationship in hyperthermic treatment of malignant and normal tissue *in vivo, Cancer Res.* **39**:3248–3253.

Overgaard, K., 1934, Über Wärmtherapie bösartiger Tumoren, *Acta Radiol. [Ther.] (Stockh.)* **15**:89–99.

Overgaard, K., 1935, Combined diathermy and roentgenotherapy of Wood sarcoma: Preliminary report, *Ugeskr. Laeger* **97**:333–337.

Overgaard, K., and Overgaard, J., 1972, Investigations on the possibility of a thermic tumour therapy: II. Action of combined heat–roentgen treatment on a transplanted mouse mammary carcinoma, *Eur. J. Cancer* **8**:573–575.

Overgaard, K., and Overgaard, J., 1974, Radiation sensitizing effect of heat, *Acta Radiol. [Ther.] (Stockh.)* **13**:501–511.

Overgaard, K., and Overgaard, J., 1977, Hyperthermic tumour-cell devitalization *in vivo, Acta Radiol. [Ther.] (Stockh.)* **16**:1–16.

Paliwal, B.R., Cardozo, C., Safari, F., Hanson, S., and Caldwell, W., 1980, Heating patterns produced by 434 MHz Erbotherm UHF 69, *Radiology* **135**:511–512.

Palzer, R., and Heidelberger, C., 1973, Influence of drugs and synchrony on the hyperthermic killing of HeLa cells, *Cancer Res.* **33**:422–427.

Parks, L.C., Minaberry, D., Smith, D.P., and Neely, W., 1979, Treatment of far-advanced bronchogenic carcinoma by extracorporeally induced systemic hyperthermia, *J. Thorac. Cardiovasc. Surg.* **78**:883–892.

Pedersen, P.L., 1978, Tumor mitochondria and the bioenergetics of cancer cells, in: *Progress in Experimental Tumor Research*, Karger Publishing Co., Basel, Switzerland, pp. 190–275.

Pettigrew, R.T., 1975, Cancer therapy by whole body heating, in: *Proceedings of the International Symposium on Cancer Therapy by Hyperthermia and Radiation*, (M. Wizenberg and J.E. Robinson, eds.), American College of Radiology Press, Baltimore, pp. 282–288.

Phillips, R.A., and Tolmach, L.S., 1966, Repair of potentially lethal damage in x-irradiated HeLa cells, *Radiat. Res.* **29**:413–432.

Pincus, G., and Fischer, A., 1931, The growth and death of tissue cultures exposed to supranormal temperatures, *J. Exp. Med.* **54**:323–332.

Pomp, H., 1978, Clinical applications of hyperthermia in gynecological malignant tumors, in: *Cancer Therapy by Hyperthermia and Radiation*, proceedings of the Second International Symposium, Essen, Germany, June 2–4, 1977 (C. Streffer, D. van Beuningen, F. Dietzel, E. Röttinger, J.E. Robinson, E. Scherer, S. Seeber, and K.R. Trott, eds.), Urban and Schwarzenberg, Baltimore and Munich, pp. 326–327.

Power, J., and Harris, J., 1977, Response of extremely hypoxic cells to hyperthermia: Survival and oxygen enhancement ratios for exponential and plateau-phase cultures, *Radiology* **123**:767–770.

Raaphorst, G., Romano, S., Mitchell, J., Bedford, J., and Dewey, W.C., 1979, Intrinsic differences in heat and/or x-ray sensitivity of seven mammalian cell lines cultured and treated under identical conditions, *Cancer Res.* **39**:396–401.

Reeves, O., 1972, Mechanism of acquired resistance to acute heat shock in cultured mammalian cells, *J. Cell Physiol.* **79**:157–159.

Reinhold, H., Blachiewicz, B., and Berg-Blok, A., 1978, Decrease in tumor microcirculation during hyperthermia, in: *Cancer Therapy by Hyperthermia and Radiation*, proceedings of the Second International Symposium, Essen, Germany, June 2–4, 1977 (C. Streffer, D. van Beuningen, F. Dietzel, E. Röttinger, J.E. Robinson, E. Scherer, S. Seeber, and K.R. Trott, eds.), Urban and Schwarzenberg, Baltimore and Munich, pp. 231–232.

Reznikoff, C., Brankow, D., and Heidelberger, C., 1973, Establishment and characterization of a cloned line of C3H mouse embryo cells sensitive to post confluence inhibition of division, *Cancer Res.* **33**:3231–3238.

Robinson, J.E., 1975, Hyperthermia and the oxygen enhancement ratio, in: *Proceedings of the International Symposium on Cancer Therapy by Hyperthermia and Radiation* (M. Wizenberg and J.E. Robinson, eds.), American College of Radiology Press, Baltimore, pp. 66–74.

Robinson, J.E., and Wizenberg, M.J., 1974, Thermal sensitivity and the effect of elevated temperatures on the radiation sensitivity of Chinese hamster cells, *Acta Radiol. [Ther.] (Stockh.)* **13**:241–249.

Robinson, J.E., Wizenberg, M.J., and McCready, W., 1974a, Radiation and hyperthermal response of normal tissue *in situ*, *Radiology* **133**:195–198.

Robinson, J.E., Wizenberg, M.J., McCready, W., and Scheltema, J., 1974b, Combined hyperthermia and radiation suggest an alternative to heavy particle therapy for reduced oxygen enhancement ratios, *Nature* **251**:521–522.

Robinson, J.E., Harrison, G., MaCready, W., and Samaras, G., 1978, Good thermal dosimetry is essential to good hyperthermia research, *Br. J. Radiol.* **51**:532–534.

Rockwell, S., and Kallman, R., 1973, Cellular radiosensitivity and tumor radiation response in the EMT6 tumor cell system, *Radiat. Res.* **53**:281–294.

Rockwell, S., and Rockwell, C., 1976, Surface morphology of EMT6 tumor cells: Scanning electron microscope observations of irradiated and unirradiated cells in exponential growth and plateau phase. *Radiat. Res.* **67**:564.

Roti Roti, J., and Winward, R., 1978, The effects of hyperthermia on the protein-to-DNA ratio of isolated HeLa cell chromatin, *Radiat. Res.* **74**:159–169.

Roti Roti, J., Henle, K., and Winward, R., 1979, The kinetics of increase in chromatin protein content in heated cells: A possible role in cell killing, *Radiat. Res.* **78**:522–531.

Rowell, L.B., 1974, Circulation to skeletal muscles, in: *Physiology and Biophysics* (T.C. Ruch and H.D. Patton, eds.), W.L. Saunders, Philadelphia, London and Toronto, pp. 200–213.

Rozell, T.C., Johnson, C.C., Durney, C.H., Lords, J.L., and Olsen, R.T., 1974, Nonperturbing temperature sensor for measurements in electromagnetic fields, *J. Microwave Power* **9**:241–249.

Sachs, T.C., and Tanney, C.S., 1977, A two-beam acoustic system for tissue analysis, *Phys. Med. Biol.* **22**:327–340.

Sapareto, S., Hopwood, L., Dewey, W., Raju, M., and Gray, J., 1978, Effects of hyperthermia on survival and progression of Chinese hamster ovary cells, *Cancer Res.* **38**:393–400.

Sapareto, S., Raaphorst, G., and Dewey, W.C., 1979, Cell killing and the sequencing of hyperthermia and radiation, *Int. J. Radiat. Oncol. Biol. Phys.* **5**:343–347.

Schechter, M., Stowe, S., and Moroson, H., 1978, Effects of hyperthermia on primary and metastatic tumor growth and host immune response in rats, *Cancer Res.* **38**:498–502.

Schrek, R., 1966, Sensitivity of normal and leukemic lymphocytes and leukemic myeloblasts to heat, *J. Natl. Cancer Inst.* **37**:649–654.

Schulman, N., and Hall, E., 1974, Hyperthermia: Its effect on proliferative and plateau phase cell cultures, *Radiology* **113**:207–209.

Schwan, H., and Piersol, G., 1954, The absorption of electromagnetic energy in body tissues: Part I, *Am. J. Phys. Med.* **33**:371–404.

Schwan, H., and Piersol, G., 1955, The absorption of electromagnetic energy in body tissues: Part II, *Am. J. Phys. Med.* **34**:425–448.

Selawry, O., Goldstein, M., and McCormick, T., 1957, Hyperthermia in tissue-culture cells of malignant origin, *Cancer Res.* **17**:785–791.

Selawry, O., Carlson, J., and Moore, G., 1958, Tumor response to ionizing rays at elevated temperatures, *Am. J. Roentgenol. Radium Ther. Nucl. Med.* **80**:833–839.

Shinitzky, M., and Barenholz, Y., 1978, Fluidity parameters of lipid regions determined by fluorescence polarization, *Biochim. Biophys. Acta* **515**:367–394.

Simard, R., and Bernhard, W., 1967, A heat-sensitive cellular function located in the nucleolus, *J. Cell Biol.* **34**:61–76.

Simard, R., Amalric, F., and Zolta, J., 1969, Effet de la Température Supraoptimale sur les Ribonucléoproteines et la RNA Nucléolaire, *Exp. Cell Res.* **55**:359–369.

Simchen, G., 1978, Cell cycle mutants, *Annu. Rev. Genet.* **12**:161–191.

Smith, L., and McKinley, T., Jr., 1967, Influence of temperature on the x-ray sensitivity of mouse bone marrow cells *in vitro, Radiat. Res.* **32**:441–451.

Smith, S.W., Clarren, S.K., Harvey, M.A.S., 1978, Hyperthermia as a possible teratogenic agent, *J. Pediatr.* **92**:878–883.

Song, C.W., 1978, Effect of hyperthermia on vascular functions of normal tissues and experimental tumors, *J. Natl. Cancer Inst.* **60**:711–713.

Song, C.W., Clement, S.S., and Levitt, S.H., 1977, Cytotoxic and radiosensitizing effects of 5-thio-D-glucose on hypoxic cells, *Radiology* **123**:201–205.

Song, C.W., Kang, M., Rhee, J., and Levitt, S., 1980, Vascular damage and delayed cell death in tumours after hyperthermia, *Br. J. Cancer* **41**:309–312.

Spencer, T., and Lehninger, A., 1976, L-lactate transport in Ehrlich ascites-tumor cells, *Biochem. J.* **154**:405–414.

Stehlin, J.S. Sr., 1964, Perfusion for melanoma of the extremities: 6½ years experience with 221 cases, *Proc. Natl. Cancer Conf.* **5**:525–581.

Stehlin, J.S., Jr., Giovanella, B., deIpolyi, P., Muenz, L., and Anderson, R., 1975, Results of hyperthermic perfusion for melanoma of the extremities, *Surg. Gynecol. Obstet.* **140**:339–348.

Stehlin, J.S., Jr., Giovanella, B.C., deIpolyi, P.D., and Anderson, R.F., 1979, Eleven years experience with hyperthermic perfusion for melanoma of the extremities, *World J. Surg.* **3**:305–307.

Stevenson, M.A., Minton, K.W., and Hahn, G.M., 1981, Survival and concanavalin-A induced capping in CHO fibroblasts after exposure to hyperthermia, ethanol, and x-irradiation, *Radiat, Res.* **86**:467–479.

Stitt, J.T., 1979, Fever versus hyperthermia, *Fed. Proc.* **38**:39–43.

Stone, H., 1978, Enhancement of local tumour control by misonidazole and hyperthermia, *Br. J. Cancer* **37**(Supp. III):178–183.

Storm, F., Harrison, W., Elliott, R., and Morton, D., 1979, Normal tissue and solid tumor effects of hyperthermia in animal models and clinical trials, *Cancer Res.* **39**:2245–2251.

Strom, R., Santoro, S., Crifo, C., Bozzi, A., Mondovi, B., and Rossi-Fanelli, A., 1973, The biochemical mechanism of selective heat sensitivity of cancer cells: IV. Inhibition of RNA synthesis, *Eur. J. Cancer* **9**:103–112.

Strom, R., Crifo, C., Bozzi, A. and Rossi-Fanelli, A., 1975, Inhibition by elevated temperatures of ribosomal RNA maturation in Ehrlich ascites cells, *Cancer Biochem. Biophys.* **1**:57–62.

Strom, R., Crifo, C., Rossi-Fanelli, A., and Mondovi, B., 1977, Biochemical aspects of heat sensitivity of tumor cells, in: *Selective Heat Sensitivity of Cancer Cells* (A. Rossi-Fanelli, R. Cavaliere, B. Mondovi, and G. Morricca, eds.) Springer-Verlag, Berlin, Heidelberg, and New York, pp. 7–35.

Suit, H.D., 1975, Hyperthermia in the treatment of tumors, in: *Proceedings of the Internation Symposium on Cancer Therapy by Hyperthermia and Radiation* (M. Wizenberg and J.E. Robinson, eds.), American College of Radiology Press, Baltimore , pp. 105–106.

Suit, H.D., and Blitzer, P.H., 1980, Thermally induced resistance to hyperthermic damage, *Ann. NY Acad. Sci.* **335**:379–382.

Suit, H.D., and Shwayder, M., 1974, Hyperthermia: Potential as an anti-tumor agent, *Cancer* **34**:122–129.

Suit, H.D., Sedlacek, R., and Wiggins, S., 1977, Immunogenicity of tumor cells inactivated by heat, *Cancer Res.* **37**:3836–3837.

Suit, H.D., Sedlacek, R., Fagundes, L., Goitein, M., and Rothman, K.J. 1978, Time distributions of recurrences of immunogenic and nonimmunogenic tumors following local irradiation, *Radiat. Res.* **73**:251–266.

Suryanarayan, C.R., 1966, Certain interesting observations during and after hydrohyperthermic chemotherapy in advanced malignancies (preliminary survey), *Indian J. Cancer* **3:**176–181.

Sutherland, R., and Durand, R., 1976, Radiation response of multicell spheroids: An *in vitro* tumor model, *Top. Rad. Res.* **11:**87–139.

Suzuki, K., 1967, Application of heat to cancer chemotherapy: Experimental studies, *Nagoya J. Med. Sci.* **30:**1–21.

Swan, H., 1974, *Thermoregulation and Bioenergetics,* Elsevier Publishing Co., Amsterdam, pp. 330–331.

Szmigielski, S., and Janiak, M., 1978, Reaction of cell-mediated immunity to local hyperthermia of tumors and its potentiation by immunostimulation: A review, in: *Cancer Therapy by Hyperthermia and Radiation* (C. Streffer, D. van Beuningen, F. Dietzel, E. Röttinger, J.E. Robinson, E. Scherer, S. Seeber, K.R. Trott, eds.), Urban and Schwarzenberg, Baltimore and Munich, pp. 80–89.

Tansey, M., and Brock, T., 1972, The upper temperature limit for eukaryotic organisms, *Proc. Natl. Acad. Sci. USA* **69:**2426–2428.

Taylor, L.S., 1978, Devices for microwave hyperthermia, in: *Cancer Therapy by Hyperthermia and Radiation,* proceedings of the Second International Symposium, Essen, Germany, June 2–4, 1977 (C. Streffer, D. van Beuningen, F. Dietzel, E. Röttinger, J.E. Robinson, E. Scherer, S. Seeber, and K.R. Trott, eds.), Urban and Schwarzenberg, Baltimore and Munich, pp. 115–118.

Terasima, T., and Tolmach, L.J., 1963a, Variations in several responses of HeLa cells to x-irradiation during the division cycle, *Biophys. J.* **3:**11–33.

Terasima, T., and Tolmach, L.J., 1963b, X-ray sensitivity and DNA synthesis in synchronously dividing populations of HeLa cells, *Science* **140:**490–492.

Terzaghi, M., and Little, J., 1976, Oncogenic transformation *in vitro* by x-rays: Influence of repair processes, in: *Biology of Radiation Carcinogenesis* (J.M. Yuhas, R.W. Tennant, and J.D. Regan, eds.), Raven Press, New York, pp. 327–334.

Tomasovic, S., Turner, G., Dewey, W.C., 1978, Effect of hyperthermia on non-histone proteins isolated with DNA, *Radiat. Res.* **73:**535–552.

Touloukian, R., Rickert, R., Lane, R., and Spencer, R., 1971, The microvascular circulation of lymphangiomas: A study of Xe[133] clearance and pathology, *Pediatrics* **48:**36–40.

Twentyman, P., Morgan, J., and Donaldson, J., 1978, Enhancement by hyperthermia of the effect of BCNU against the EMT6 mouse tumor, *Cancer Treat. Rep.* **62:**439–443.

U.R., Noell, K.T., Woodward, K.T., Worde, B.T., Fishburn, R.I. and Miller L.S., 1980, Microwave-induced local hyperthermia in combination with radiotherapy of human malignant tumors, *Cancer* **45:**638–646.

Van Den Thillart, G., and Modderkolk, J., 1978, The effect of acclimation temperature on the activation energies of state III respiration and on the unsaturation of membrane lipids of goldfish mitochondria, *Biochim. Biophys. Acta* **510:**38–51.

Verma, S., and Wallach, D., 1976, Multiple thermotropic state transitions in erythrocyte membranes: A laser–raman study of the CH-stretching and acoustical regions, *Biochim. Biophys. Acta* **436:**307–318.

Vig, B., 1979, Hyperthermic enhancement of chromosome damage and lack of effect on sister-chromatid exchanges induced by bleomycin in Chinese hamster cells *in vitro*, *Mutat. Res.* **61:**309–317.

Von Ardenne, M., 1971, The cancer multi-step therapy concept, *Panminerva Med.* **13:**509–519.

Von Ardenne, M., 1975, Prinzipien und Konzept 1974 der "Krebs-Mehrschritt-Therapie", *Radiobiol. Radiother.* **16**:99–119.

Von Ardenne, M., 1978, On a new physical principle for selective local hyperthermia of tumor tissues, in: *Cancer Therapy by Hyperthermia and Radiation,* proceedings of the Second International Symposium, Essen, Germany, June 2–4, 1977 (C. Streffer, D. van Beuningen, F. Dietzel, E. Röttinger, J.E. Robinson, E. Scherer, S. Seeber, and K.R. Trott, eds.), Urban and Schwarzenberg, Baltimore and Munich, pp. 96–104.

Von Ardenne, M., and Reitnauer, P., 1970, Erythembildung als Folge der Zellschädigungskettenreaktion mit Aufgiftung lysosomaler Enzyme beim niedrigen Haut-pH Erythemvermeidung bei Krebs-mehrschritt-therapie ohne immunologische Attacke, *Arch. Geschwulstforsch.* **30**:319–330.

Von Ardenne, M., and Reitnauer, P., 1976, Verstärkung der mit Glukoseinfusion erzielbaren Tumorübersäuerung *in vivo* durch NAD, *Arch. Geschwulstforsch.* **46**:197–203.

Von Ardenne, M., Chaplain, R., and Reitnauer, P., 1969, Selektive Krebszellenschädigung durch eine Attackenkombination mit Übersäuerung Hyperthermie, Vitamin A, Dimethylsulfoxid und weiteren die Freisetzung lysomaler Enzyme fördernden Agenzien, *Arch. Geschuwulstforsch.* **33**:331–344.

Walker, A., McCallum, H., Wheldon. T., Nias, A., and Abdelaal, A., 1978, Promotion of metastasis of C3H mouse mammary carcinoma by local hyperthermia, *Br. J. Cancer* **38**:561–563.

Wallach, D., 1977, Basic mechanisms in tumor thermotherapy, *J. Molecular Med.* **2**:381–403.

Wallach, D., Bieri, V., Verma, S.P., and Schmidt-Ullrich, R.R., 1975, Modes of lipid–protein interactions in biomembranes, *Ann. NY Acad. Sci.* **264**:142–160.

Wallach, D., Verma, S.P. and Fookson, S., 1979, Application of laser, raman. and infrared spectroscopy to the analysis of membrane structure: Review, *Biochim. Biophys. Acta* **559**:153–208.

Wang, C.Q., 1982, A specially designed intralumenal microwave antenna for the hyperthermic treatmenal of esophageal cancer, *J. Natl. Canc. Inst. Monograph* (in press).

Warocquier, R., and Scherrer, K., 1969, RNA metabolism in mammalian cells at elevated temperatures, *Eur. J. Biochem.* **10**:362–370.

Warren, S.L., 1935, Preliminary study of the effect of artificial fever upon hopeless tumor cases, *Am. J. Roentgenol.* **33**:75–87.

Watson, K., Houghton, R.L., Bertoli, E., and Griffiths, D.E., 1975, Membrane-lipid unsaturation and mitochondrial function in *Saccharomyces cerevisiae*, *Biochem. J.* **146**:409–416.

Weichselbaum, R., Little, J., and Nove, J., 1977, Response of human osteosarcoma *in vitro* to irradiation as evidence for unusual cellular repair activity, *Int. J. Radiat. Biol.* **31**:295–299.

Weniger, P., Wawra, E., and Dolejs, I., 1979, The action of hyperthermia on DNA repair, *Radiat, Environ. Biophys.* **16**:135–141.

Wenzel, M., and Stohr, W., 1970, Schutzeffeke von D_2O gegen die Hyperthermieschädigung von Ascites-tumorzellen, *Hoppe Seylers Z. Physiol. Chem.* **351**:737–740.

Westermark, N., 1927, The effect of heat on rat tumors, *Skand. Arch. Physiol.* **52**:257–322.

Westra, A., 1971, The influence of radiation on the capacity of *in vitro* cultured mammalian cells to proliferate, published in Academic Doctoral Thesis, University of Amsterdam, Holland.

Westra, A., and Dewey, W.C., 1971, Heat shock during the cell cycle of Chinese hamster cells *in vitro*, *Int. J. Radiat. Biol.* **19**:467–477.

Wickersheim, K.A., and Alves, R.B., 1979, Recent advances in optical temperature measurement, *Industrial Research/Development*, December, **1979**:82–89.

Withers, H.R., and Romsdahl, M.M., 1977, Post-operative radiotherapy for adenocarcinoma of the rectum and rectosigmoid, *Int. J. Radiat. Oncol. Biol. Phys.* **2**:1069–1074.

Wood, T., 1956, Lethal effects of high and low temperatures on unicellular organisms, *Adv. Biol. Med. Phys.* **4**:119–165.

Woodhall, B., Pickerell, K., Georgiade, N., Mahaley, M., and Dukes, W., 1960, Effect of hyperthermia on cancer chemotherapy: Application to external cancer of head and face structures, *Ann. Surg.* **151**:750–759.

Yatvin, M., 1977, The influence of membrane lipid composition and procaine on hyperthermic death of mice cells, *Int. J. Radiat. Biol.* **32**:513–523.

Yatvin, M., Clifton, K., and Dennis, W., 1979, Hyperthermia and local anesthetics: Potentiation of survival of tumor-bearing mice, *Science* **205**:195–196.

Yerushalmi, A., 1975, Cure of a solid tumor by simultaneous administration of microwaves and x-ray irradiation, *Radiat. Res.* **64**:602–610.

Yerushalmi, A., 1976, Treatment of a solid tumor by local simultaneous hyperthermia and ionizing radiation: Dependence on temperature and dose, *Eur. J. Cancer* **12**:807–813.

Yerushalmi, A., 1978, Simulation of resistance against local tumor growth of hosts: Pretreated by combined local hyperthermia and x-irradiation, *Bull. Cancer* **65**:475–478.

Yerushalmi, A., and Hazan, G., 1979, Control of Lewis lung carcinoma by combined treatment with local hyperthermia and cyclophosphamide: Preliminary results, *Isr. J. Med. Sci.* **15**:462–463.

Zaret, M.M., 1964, An experimental study of the cataractogenic effects of microwave radiation, *Rome Air Development Center Report* (RADC-TDR) **1964**:273–275.

Index